MIXED MESSAGES

Mixed Messages

NORMS AND SOCIAL CONTROL AROUND TEEN SEX
AND PREGNANCY

Stefanie Mollborn

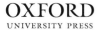

OXFORD
UNIVERSITY PRESS

OXFORD
UNIVERSITY PRESS

Oxford University Press is a department of the University of Oxford. It furthers
the University's objective of excellence in research, scholarship, and education
by publishing worldwide. Oxford is a registered trade mark of Oxford University
Press in the UK and certain other countries.

Published in the United States of America by Oxford University Press
198 Madison Avenue, New York, NY 10016, United States of America.

© Oxford University Press 2017

CIP data is on file at the Library of Congress
ISBN 978-0-19-063327-1 (hbk.); 978-0-19-063328-8 (pbk.)

9 8 7 6 5 4 3 2 1

Paperback printed by WebCom, Inc., Canada
Hardback printed by Bridgeport National Bindery, Inc., United States of America

For my family

Contents

Preface

WHEN I WAS 15, I spent a year as an exchange student in Sweden. Coming from a highly religious, lower-income rural community in Ohio, I was startled by two facts, one more obvious than the other. First, the teenagers I met in Sweden experienced very different social rules than what I was accustomed to. Second, when fellow American exchange students and I were asked to describe what life was like in the United States, our answers were sometimes so disparate that they sounded like we were describing different worlds.

At a meeting of exchange students, I found some of my U.S. compatriots blowing up large white balloons and laughing hysterically. They laughed even harder when I asked them what was so funny about balloons. The balloons were actually condoms that were being distributed freely to teenagers. My friends, most of whom were 18 years old, found this free availability so unbelievable as to be hilarious. Having gone through my school's sex education curriculum, I had heard the word "condom" but had never seen one and did not understand how they worked. In Sweden, it seemed that condoms and other contraceptives were treated matter-of-factly and teen sex wasn't seen as a major social issue. Sociologist Amy Schalet calls a similar dynamic in the Netherlands the "normalization" of teen sex, in contrast to the "dramatization" that happens in the United States (Schalet, Amy T. 2011. *Not under My Roof: Parents, Teens, and the Culture of Sex*. Chicago: University of Chicago).

In my small school at home, my first classmate to get pregnant was about 12 years old. She left school shortly before childbirth, never to return. As the years went by, more classmates became mothers, most vanishing quietly from school. I never knew who the fathers were. In the rural Swedish town where I was sent, I never heard about teens having children, even though high school students talked regularly about having sleepovers at girlfriends' and boyfriends' houses. Everyone, including parents, seemed to treat this situation in a matter-of-fact way. Sexual content was included in movies shown on public television, and advertisements for contraceptives were posted in public places. Even though my U.S. and Swedish communities were demographically fairly similar, their norms about teen sexuality were worlds apart.

There were also big differences between my experiences at home and those of other U.S. exchange students I met. As I was accustomed to from home, the American teens didn't really talk about their sexual experiences, but dating was another thing. Most exchange students I knew were taught a rule for their behavior that they called "the four Ds": no drinking, drugs, driving, or dating (in other words, no serious romantic relationships). I had coincidentally not been warned off dating by my local U.S. sponsors, which led to many conversations with other exchange students about that part of the rule. Those from more privileged communities didn't worry much about the ban on romantic relationships, saying that they were in high school, so why would they have a serious relationship anyway? To me this attitude seemed foreign. My parents had dated throughout high school, and many of my friends' parents were also high school sweethearts. Meeting a future spouse in high school was normatively appropriate for teenagers in my town, so proscribing romantic relationships for a whole year was a serious rule indeed.

Social norms can be hard to recognize unless you violate them or end up in a climate with different ones. My experience as an exchange student was formative in this way, leading me to realize how different normative climates can be from country to country, but also within the United States. How do these differences arise, and do they matter for understanding how the people in a country or community behave?

My journey to answer these questions has been supported by many people. Thanks to my teachers in the Washington Court House public schools for encouraging my interests in social science and writing. I thank the Harvard University Department of Sociology, particularly Mary Waters, William Julius Wilson, and my wonderful thesis advisor Peter Marsden, for making the sociology curriculum so fascinating that even my timid, disorganized undergraduate self couldn't help but be drawn in. My Stanford University dissertation committee members Karen Cook, Nancy Tuma, Michael Rosenfeld, and Dan McFarland—but most of all my adviser Cecilia Ridgeway—taught me, among many other things, not to be scared of theory and that social norms really are important to understand. Friends and fellow graduate students Cynthia Brandt, Chris Bourg, Kjersten Bunker Whittington, Shelley Correll, Julie Dubrouillet, Sean Everton, Gabriel Ignatow, Yan Li, Tony Lee, Heili Pals, Irena Stepanikova, Justine Tinkler, and Jennifer van Stelle were a huge support and gave me academic confidence.

The entire research process for this book has taken place since I became a faculty member at the University of Colorado Boulder. Financial support for the teen parent interviews came from a University of Colorado/IGP Seed Grant Program Innovative Grant (with research collaborator Janet Jacobs). The college student interview work was supported by a Scholar Grant from the Center to Advance Research and Teaching in the Social Sciences at the University of Colorado Boulder. Other research and administrative support came from the NIH/NICHD-funded CU Population Center (P2C HD066613).

At the Institute of Behavioral Science, I'm deeply indebted to the world-class mentoring team that supported the writing of this book, even though it wasn't a typical project for the demographers I work with there. Jane Menken and Richard Jessor encouraged me to take the time I needed and follow my preferred, theoretically focused but riskier, approach. Together with leaders like Richard Rogers, Jason Boardman, Lori Hunter, Fred Pampel, and more recently Myron Gutmann, they have created an interdisciplinary intellectual community that has pushed me and many others to do our best work. Colleagues such as Tania Barham, Fernando Riosmena, and Elisabeth Root have encouraged me to look outside my sociological training for ideas and debates. Lindy Schultz provided impeccable and prompt bibliographic support. Steve Graham, Rajshree Shrestha, Joel Colvin, Cheryl Graham, and Judith McCabe have been sources of all kinds of help, from grant and administrative questions to moral support on tough days.

I'm equally grateful for the unstinting support of my colleagues and my wonderful graduate and undergraduate students in the Department of Sociology. The junior faculty reading group (whose members are almost all no longer junior) provided crucial intellectual support and feedback at different stages of this project— my thanks go out to wonderful friends and colleagues Jennifer Bair, Jill Harrison, Ryan Masters, Sanyu Mojola, Hillary Potter, Isaac Reed, Christina Sue, and Amy Wilkins. Thanks to the department's many book writers for unlocking the mysteries of the process for me. The support of the department's many and wonderful senior mentors, especially Janet Jacobs and Sara Steen, was very important. In particular, as chairs during data collection and initial writing, Michael Radelet, Richard Rogers, and Joyce Nielsen helped make this work possible.

Many people read drafts and provided invaluable feedback. Thanks to generous colleagues and friends Tracy Deyell, Paula Fomby, Laurie James-Hawkins, Elizabeth Lawrence, Yan Li, Christie Sennott, Christina Sue, Justine Tinkler, and Amy Wilkins for reading and editing chapters. Four wonderful people—Janet Jacobs, Richard Jessor, Sanyu Mojola, and Fredrik Mollborn—read and provided crucial feedback on the entire book. Members of the University of Colorado Boulder and University of Georgia Departments of Sociology and the Lund University School of Social Work in Sweden, as well as undergraduates in several different classes and audiences at conference presentations, provided feedback on early versions of this work.

Anonymous reviewers of the book manuscript gave me crucial, insightful feedback, and I thank them for making this work better. Oxford University Press editor James Cook has supported my vision for this work and provided valuable input for improving it. The teen parent and college student interview participants, as well as staff at the two teen parent interview sites, gave time and energy to this project. I hope I have told interviewees' stories and analyzed their experiences faithfully.

Without my research collaborators, this project would not have been possible. I particularly thank Janet Jacobs, who collaborated on the teen parent interview project, coauthored articles, and provided crucial mentoring and feedback. Leith Lombas, Nicole Moore, and Devon Thacker were the tireless, first-rate student members of that research team. Amy Wilkins facilitated some of the peer interviews for the college student project, and Danielle Denardo, Laurie James-Hawkins, Katherine McCune, Christie Sennott, and Aleeza Zabriskie Tribbia, together with the undergraduate peer interviewers, made a fabulous research team. Christie Sennott and I published two articles together from this project, one of which (Mollborn, Stefanie and Christie Sennott. 2015. "Bundles of Norms about Teen Sex and Pregnancy." *Qualitative Health Research* 25(9):1283–1299. DOI: 10.1177/1049732314557086) is included in this book in partial, revised form with permission from Sage Publications.

Finally, I thank my family. The Swedish side of the family put up with my odd book-writing habits and general air of distraction during our sabbatical and our subsequent annual visits, and they helped make those trips happen. The U.S. side provided every possible kind of logistical support. Justin Bailey and Kate Leslie cheered me on, and little Owen provided much-needed distraction from work. My parents Susan and Timothy Bailey read the manuscript on top of all their other invaluable help. My husband Fredrik Mollborn read the book with a Swede's eye, questioning my assumptions and always having faith in the project and in me. And my sons Benjamin and Simon, who give meaning to every day, grew up together with this book. Becoming the mother of a teenager one month from now is giving me an entirely new perspective on the subject matter, and writing this book has changed the way I will parent my teens.

Stefanie Mollborn
May 2016
Boulder, Colorado

MIXED MESSAGES

1

NORMS AND SOCIAL CONTROL AROUND TEEN SEXUALITY

MANY PEOPLE WORRY about the messages teenagers hear about sex and sexuality in the United States. Ratings systems regulate the sexual content young people are exposed to in the media, and interest groups struggle for control over the sex education curricula students receive in schools. Parents wonder how to talk to their teens about sex, and news outlets report that cliques of teenagers are convincing each other to get pregnant.[1] I argue that most of the social influences on teens' sexual behaviors go beyond mere messages. Instead, they are *norms*—social rules about how to behave that result in negative sanctions when violated. Norms are important for understanding teen sexuality because they shape sexual behaviors and because the negative sanctioning of violators affects teens' lives. Struggles over norms and enforcement around teen sexuality are also a major cultural battleground. What are the norms about teen sexuality in different areas of the United States, and how do they matter? Talking to young people is the key to answering this question.[2] Listening to their stories, like Claudia's, Julie's, and Fernando's below, reveals a fascinating and complicated world of communication and silence, rules and inconsistencies, control and evasion, hidden behaviors and threatened reputations.

Claudia grew up in a fairly wealthy, predominantly White Western university town she describes as very liberal.[3] She says she and her high school classmates took comprehensive sex education and "were really well educated" about sex and contraception. Although Claudia and some of her friends didn't have sex during high school, many teenagers did, and their peers didn't consider it a big deal. Claudia said most of her friends were on birth control pills. Parents' biggest focus wasn't on preventing teens from having sex, she said, because "it's not something you can control—it's frustrating if you try to." Instead, parents tried "to help your teen out as far as being healthy and safe." This meant encouraging them to prevent teen pregnancy through consistent contraception. If one of Claudia's friends had gotten pregnant, friends and family would have recommended abortion as "the easiest, cleanest, most discreet thing."

Claudia's community sounds like the kind of sex-positive, liberal place that some Americans love and others hate. But it's more complicated than that. As in most other communities, it seems that adults often tolerated teen sex because they felt they had no other choice, but they didn't encourage it. And like nearly everywhere else, this tolerance evaporated when it came to teens having babies. Claudia says people didn't bring teen parenthood up much, but they were "really turned off by it. I think it's something that people are really scared of, especially in our community." She says that in her community, as in others in this book, pregnancy is only supposed to happen once you are married, have graduated from college, and have a job. Doing things "in the right time frame" is very important. Claudia says her parents, like many other community members, "are really not okay" with teen parenthood. "I don't think I ever heard it being spoken about in a positive light. It was always like, 'Wow, what is she going to do? How is she going to support a baby? How is she going to get her own education and take care of a family?'" Nobody talked about the babies' fathers.

Less than an hour's drive away in the same metropolitan area, Julie grew up in another solidly middle-class, mostly White suburb that she describes as very conservative. Like Claudia, Julie is White and has middle-class parents who are well off enough to help with some, but not all, of her college expenses. But when it comes to norms about teen sex and pregnancy, Julie and Claudia might as well have come from different worlds. Julie's community was highly religious, with conservative Christian groups and a large Latter-day Saints (Mormon) population. Teens received abstinence-only sex education that Julie says focused on "scaring" them. The main norms communicated to teens were not to have sex, not to have an abortion (although this was controversial), and not to become a parent. Julie says her community and family were "*so* negative" about teen parenthood. Although Julie thinks religion shaped many people's perceptions of teen mothers, it went beyond religious groups: "I think the fact that people were getting pregnant so young was viewed negatively by the whole community."

Even though *norms* about teen sex and related behaviors were very different for Julie, the sexual activity and contraceptive *behaviors* she described among teens sounded like those in Claudia's community. Julie says, "Everybody was doing it. I mean, even people that were quote unquote 'religious,' they were still having sex." Julie's impression was that many teens had multiple sexual partners during high school, and like her, most consistently used contraception to avoid pregnancy (even though their parents didn't often know they were sexually active or using birth control). But there was no "easy, clean" way out of pregnancy through abortion for girls in this community—Julie tells us that a girl who got an abortion was ostracized throughout her senior year when others in the school found out.

Fernando lives halfway between Julie and Claudia in a large Western city, but his financial situation and opportunities for future success are worlds away. He and the people around him didn't have much money when he was growing up, and he spent some time in jail. Fernando became a father at age 17. Even though Fernando is from a high-risk demographic group for teen parenthood and comes from an area where it's fairly common, he grew up hearing lots of negative messages about teen parents. Fernando's older brother lectured him sternly about avoiding negative consequences of sex, saying, "You've got to put your mind first and think, wear condoms, use protection. Don't let all the emotions make you forget." When his brother found out about Fernando's girlfriend's unintended pregnancy, he was upset: "Are you stupid or what? You can't afford that." Fernando's friends were all shocked about the pregnancy. He stopped spending time with them, and ultimately he and his girlfriend switched high schools before he dropped out to start working. Fernando says that after his son was born, "I really isolated myself from everybody," perhaps in response to their negative reactions. Even though one might have expected Fernando's friends and family to be more encouraging of teen pregnancy than people like Julie and Claudia who come from wealthier families and communities, in fact he faced considerable stigma and a lack of support.

In this book, I rely on the stories of young people like Claudia, Julie, and Fernando, as well as those of others from a wide range of communities and backgrounds, to answer three main questions: *What norms about teen sexuality are being communicated to U.S. teens by their families, friends, schools, and communities? How are these norms conveyed and enforced? And what strategies do teens use to negotiate the normative pressures they experience?* You may not have been surprised to read that teen sexuality norms in Claudia's liberal, secular community are different from those in Julie's conservative, highly religious community. It may be more unexpected that the norms against teen pregnancy aren't very different in Fernando's low-income urban community than they are in Claudia's or Julie's towns. Researchers don't know much about the content of all these norms, nor about how norm enforcers and teens are responding to the norms they're exposed to. This book fills a gap in knowledge by focusing on how and why teen sexuality norms are different in different places and how those differences matter. In-depth studies have painted detailed pictures of particular communities and groups, but it's important to understand the diversity of teen sexuality norms throughout the United States. Particularly little is known about the sexuality norms communicated to boys and to middle-class White teens, who are a focus of this book together with girls and less advantaged teens.[4] Other studies of teen sexuality tend to focus on teens' narrative constructions or on a specific social context, like parents, schools, or friends.[5] Following the lead of the interviewees, who described their own social worlds, I look in depth at each of these contexts and at the communities teens live in. Finally, little is known about how people try to enforce social norms around teen sexuality, how well that enforcement works, and how teens respond to attempts to control their behaviors.

Past research has looked in depth at cultural messages around teen sexuality in specific places or particular populations, but for this book I took a different approach. I sought out young people from a wide variety of communities that provide a fairly broad cross-section of the United States. But instead of trying to capture young people's experiences in numbers, as survey researchers do, I asked them to describe those experiences in their own words. This open-ended approach to exploring social norms can help us understand them better. In this book, I develop theoretical tools for understanding teenagers' complex normative environments and assessing which social control strategies are effective and which aren't. These tools can help us understand how the very different norms in Claudia's and Julie's communities can result in similar sexual behaviors, but still have different implications for both young women's futures.

A message becomes a social norm when people are willing to enforce it by sanctioning those who don't behave appropriately.[6] This kind of enforcement, or social control,[7] is an important part of teen sexuality norms—people try to influence teens to behave in the right way and sanction them through socially excluding or withholding resources from them if they behave in the wrong way, such as by having a baby. But teens can make their own decisions and push back against control.[8] Teens may seek sex in order to experience pleasure, to feel more adult, or to gain approval from romantic partners or friends who encourage it. To analyze current cultural struggles over teen sexuality in the United States, it's important to consider both people's attempts to control teens' sexual behaviors and teens' responses to those attempts. A perspective focused on norms encompasses all sides of the issue. Using a norms perspective, the battles over sex education playing out in state legislatures and school boards make sense. The winners will control the sexuality messages teens hear in schools and will be able to exclude alternative norms about appropriate sexual behaviors. But similar struggles are also happening outside official institutions in communities across the United States. Parents and other adults are communicating norms about sex, contraception, abortion, and pregnancy to teens, working to control teens' opportunities to be sexual, and threatening sanctions if teens break the rules. But teens are also learning norms from peers and collaborating with friends to weigh the social costs and benefits of sexual behavior. Because sexual behaviors are private, teens ultimately have leeway to make their own behavioral decisions and try to keep them secret. Norms and social control can help us make sense of the complicated and conflict-filled arena of teen sexuality.

Besides being a flashpoint for cultural conflict, teen sexuality is important for understanding human lives. The *life course perspective* on understanding human development emphasizes that reaching sexual maturity and learning how to engage in intimate relationships with others are important aspects of the transition to adulthood. But there is a lot of variation in how those things happen. Some young people start having sex early, while others wait. Some have sex in risky ways—leaving themselves vulnerable to sexually transmitted infections (STIs), unintended pregnancy, or damaging intimate relationships—and some don't. Risky sex is one of many unhealthy behaviors, like drug use, binge drinking, and delinquency, that can cause problems for teens' futures. Sometimes teens have sex as part of a larger pattern of risky behaviors, and sometimes it happens in a safer way. Investigating the many ways in which young people adapt to becoming sexual is important for understanding the rest of their lives. Although other factors besides norms and social control also shape teens' behaviors, the conceptual tools developed in this book can help improve that understanding.

I argue that teens hear mixed messages about sexuality from the people and institutions around them, who all work hard to try to control teens' behavior and bring it in line with their norms. But this control has unintended consequences. It doesn't stop most teens from having sex before finishing high school. Instead, it often strengthens the negative consequences of sex and pregnancy in a multitude of ways.

NORMS AND SOCIAL CONTROL

The research in this book contributes to two areas of knowledge: norms and social control, and contemporary U.S. teens' sexual behaviors. A lot is known about how social norms and their enforcement work in the abstract, thanks to the mostly experimental research coming from fields like psychology, sociology, and economics.[9] These studies tend to focus on single norms that are manipulated in a laboratory setting. This approach is ideal for isolating the effects of a particular norm but can tell us less about how norms and social control work in everyday life and what surrounding phenomena they may shape or be influenced by. A lab-based approach yields less information about how norms work together, how to conceptualize conflict or change in norms, and how to understand people's negotiation strategies in response to social control.[10] Limited scholarly attention to these issues has led some researchers studying culture to disregard norms as part of an outdated "motivational paradigm."[11] In this book, I study norms qualitatively from the perspectives of teenagers in complex real-world settings to consider both how norms shape behavior and how they operate in ways that have not previously been considered.[12]

This "grounded" approach to studying social norms can only focus on one real-life example at a time. I chose teen sexual behavior because it is normatively contested and because young people's behaviors don't always match what the norms prescribe. These inconsistencies are useful when investigating the effectiveness and ineffectiveness of norms and social control. Teen sexual behavior is also an interesting issue to study because *actual* sexual behaviors and young people's *public portrayals* of their behaviors don't necessarily match, which creates interesting strategic options for teens when negotiating social pressures. Finally, the stakes are high. There are risky negative consequences that can have serious implications for the lives of young people and their sexual partners and families, and these problems are more widespread in the United States than in many other places. Researchers often point to norms as a possible way to improve teens' sexual health, but we don't know enough about these norms to figure out yet if a norm-based approach to policy is promising. The research in this book can help answer this question.

Using young people's descriptions of their real-world experiences, I demonstrate the importance of social norms for understanding teen sexuality. Norms have long been recognized as an important way in which society can shape people's behavior, but because they are a group-level phenomenon, they are hard for social scientists to measure.[13] Social norms are widespread, they are more visible when they are contested or violated, and people learn norms from monitoring others' reactions. Norms are also difficult to study because looking at people's behavior doesn't necessarily tell you much about the norm in play: The ways people behave don't always follow the social rules. Teen sexual behavior is a good example. Despite strong norms discouraging these behaviors, a majority of high school seniors have had sex, many don't use condoms or other contraception, and about one in seven teen girls becomes a mother. Sexuality is also a particularly interesting case for studying norms because the struggle for control over reproduction is a major way that power plays out in societies.[14]

This book focuses not only on norms, but also on the social control exerted over people and institutions to encourage them to conform to norms or to punish norm violators. I also explore people's responses to social control, which sometimes work in sync with it and sometimes conflict. When a person has internalized a social norm, she believes in its rightness and voluntarily follows the rule. Teenagers in the "virginity pledge" movement are an example. They have pledged to abstain from sex until marriage because they personally feel they aren't ready or because they agree with religious teachings that premarital sex is a sin.[15] But when people don't personally agree with a norm, they can choose either to conform anyway in order to avoid social sanctions or to break the rule, follow their hearts, and potentially face negative sanctions such as social exclusion or the withholding of socioeconomic opportunities. I show that social control affects which decision a person in this situation will make. Someone who doesn't expect to see the people he is interacting with ever again might break the rule, while someone who has no possibility of leaving the situation or joining other social groups might choose to conform.[16] As this suggests, people who have more options for interacting with groups that have different norms may feel less bound to follow a particular group's social rules if they don't agree with them. Moreover, people belong to different reference groups (such as family, classmates, friends, or community members) that may hold different norms. For example, some teens' parents and religious communities discourage sexual activity, while their close friends accept it. In this kind of situation in which there are heterogeneous norms, social control is weaker and teens are more able to do what they want.[17]

This study of teen sexuality shows that norms and social control are not just influenced by the different groups in a person's social environment but also shape those groups. A group's social rules—for example, rules about religious practices or substance use—can be part of its identity, helping distinguish it from other groups and build cohesion among its members.[18] And holding different norms about a particular behavior, such as teen sex, can heighten social divides between different groups. Researcher Julie Bettie showed how different norms about sexuality and romantic relationships solidified social boundaries between different racial and socioeconomic groups of girls in a U.S. high school. But even more important than the actual norms in those groups was the perception of the norms the groups held. People assumed that the lower-income Latina groups were more sexually active and welcomed teen pregnancy, even when this was not true.[19] Teachers often made inaccurate assumptions about the girls' sexual behavior from the racial and socioeconomic makeup of their friendship groups and the presumed norms within those groups, and treated the girls differently as a result. A Latina girl would often be assumed to be sexually active, welcoming of teen motherhood, and not interested in school. This differential treatment led to disparate opportunities for girls' future educations. In my book, like in Bettie's study, people's perceptions of norms are rooted in race-, class-, and gender-based social inequalities, and these perceptions also perpetuate the inequalities. I find that the norms held by the dominant group in an unequal social system tend to become the rules that people are ultimately held to. Even if a girl finds a friendship group that accepts her sexual activity, teachers, other adults, and many peers will still hold her to the dominant norm that opposes that behavior.

This book complicates our understanding of norms by showing that they occur not in isolation, but in what I call "norm sets."[20] There is not one single norm about teen sex—instead, multiple norms regulate related behaviors. For example, many teens experience a norm against teen sex and another encouraging contraception if teens violate the first norm. If a teen gets pregnant, competing norms sometimes encourage abortion to protect the teen's future and sometimes discourage abortion on religious or ethical grounds. This complexity arising from sets of norms isn't often studied because experimental research generally seeks to isolate a single norm and document its effects. I argue that not just norms prescribing behaviors, but also norms prescribing public portrayals of behaviors and emotion norms regulating how people should feel about their behaviors, are part of a norm set. Metanorms, or norms about how to enforce norms, are often included in norm sets as well.[21] I find that people who don't enforce a norm correctly may themselves face social sanctions. The friends or parents of a pregnant teenager are expected by their community to sanction the girl in certain ways, and if they don't, they may be socially excluded.[22]

Although research on norms about teen sexuality hasn't studied norm sets or metanorms much, there is some quantitative evidence, including my own work, that documents a norm against teen pregnancy. On average, both adults and teens in the United States perceive that there is a social norm against teen pregnancy and believe teen pregnancy is embarrassing and a bad idea.[23] There are racial and class differences in this norm, with more advantaged racial and socioeconomic groups tending to have stronger norms against teen pregnancy.[24] I have shown that people who have a stronger norm against teen pregnancy are less willing to provide support to a hypothetical teen parent in their family, suggesting that young people who violate the norm against teen childbearing are negatively sanctioned.[25]

Gender is more complicated than race or class in terms of its relationship to sexuality norms, I find in past research as well as in this book. Perhaps surprisingly, my earlier quantitative research found that boys and girls perceive similar norms against teen pregnancy. But different reference groups affect this perception: The average teen pregnancy norms experienced by schoolmates matter more for boys' perceptions, while friends' norms matter more for girls.[26] I have found that the relationship between teen pregnancy norms and sexual behavior also differs by gender. Girls' own embarrassment at the prospect of a teen pregnancy reduces their sexual activity and raises their likelihood of using contraception, but for boys, their own embarrassment isn't very important for understanding their behavior unless they are also in a school or peer environment that discourages teen pregnancy. When their own perception is reinforced by their social context, boys are less likely to have sex and more likely to use contraception.[27]

This book digs deeper into these dynamics through interviews with both girls and boys. Including both genders is fairly rare, as are in-depth interviews with teen boys about sexuality. I find that male and female teens and those who influence them are the most concerned about pregnancy as a negative consequence of teen sex. Pregnancy is a serious worry for girls more than for boys, and religious strictures around sex are usually targeted more strongly to women than men. This book shows that even when both genders perceive similar sexuality norms, girls are held more strictly to those norms, facing greater sanctions if they break the rules. Sexuality appears to be central to other people's perceptions of girls, especially if they are racial minorities or have lower socioeconomic status (SES), but this is less true for boys.[28]

A final important factor in understanding teen sexuality norms in the United States is religion. Most Americans are religious, and religious teachings underlie many communities' norms, particularly in the area of sexuality.[29] In past quantitative research I have found that teen girls who believe that a religious text is the literal word of God (an indicator of fundamentalist religious beliefs) are more embarrassed by the prospect of a teen pregnancy, which reduces their likelihood of having sex, but the same is not true for boys.[30] Having more students with fundamentalist beliefs in a school is not correlated with a stronger school-level norm against teen pregnancy or a greater consensus about the norm, but it is correlated with a higher rate of teen pregnancies in the school.[31] This may sound counterintuitive, but other research has also found that counties and states with more conservative religious beliefs have higher teen birth rates.[32] This may be because many teens in these settings still have sex but use contraception less consistently.[33]

The different norms about teen sexuality that Claudia, Fernando, and Julie described arise from two different explanations for *why* a particular norm set is appropriate, which I call the *practical rationale* and the *moral rationale*.[34] Claudia's secular, liberal community and Fernando's urban community support a practical rationale. Teen sexual behavior is explicitly linked to academic achievement and future socioeconomic success. Avoiding outcomes that jeopardize that future is the most important goal, so consistent contraception and avoidance of teen parenthood are the main focuses of the practical rationale. Teen sex and abortion of teen pregnancies are tacitly tolerated, even if many people don't approve. Julie's conservative, highly religious community is a stark contrast. The moral rationale adopted there focuses on the right thing to do based on religious principles. Sinful behavior is strongly discouraged, so even if many teens engage in this behavior, they work hard to hide it. The moral rationale focuses mostly on discouraging teen sex, pregnancy, and abortion for moral reasons. Contraception isn't discussed much, even though it can prevent pregnancy and abortion among sexually active teenagers. This book shows that a seemingly inconsistent set of norms makes sense once the underlying rationale explaining it is taken into account. The practical and moral rationales can coexist to some extent. In Julie's community, ongoing controversies over teen abortion (which is strongly discouraged by the moral rationale but encouraged in case of pregnancy by the practical rationale) suggest that both rationales are at least somewhat in play—but usually only one rationale is the dominant, publicly articulated message underlying norms about teen sexuality in a community.

In terms of religion and in many other ways, the social norms people experience have complicated and sometimes unexpected links to their behaviors. Documenting how social control and people's responses to this control work in the realm of teen sexuality norms is important for understanding these complexities. In this book, I find that the importance of religion in a community is the main influence on the content of teen sexuality *norms*, but not teens' actual behaviors, in that community. Religion determines whether the moral rationale or the practical rationale is used to justify why norms prescribe certain kinds of behavior. Despite different norms, though, differences in teens' actual sexual *behaviors* are mostly shaped not by religion, but by the community's social class, which influences how teens view their future prospects. The implications of norms and behaviors for teenagers' lives vary for different groups of teens because of differences in social control. Girls and racially and socioeconomically disadvantaged teens are held to stricter standards, given less leeway to make forgivable "mistakes," and sanctioned more severely if they violate norms.

The processes around norms and social control articulated in this book show how complex norms are and how much conflict and negotiation happens around them. Understanding this helps illuminate what makes norms effective in real-world settings. Even though they are heavily dependent on adults for resources and peers for social interaction, teenagers have many options for negotiating normative pressures. Teenagers and the people and institutions seeking to control them can comply with or deviate from norms and metanorms, communicate or evade communication, choose from among conflicting norms, say one thing and do another, or work to justify their choices to others. The many strategies available to social actors complicate the links between norms and both behaviors and social sanctions. Conflict, change, and social inequalities are important for understanding the success and failure of different strategies. This perspective on norms reflects real life and incorporates ideas from recent decades of sociological thinking.

Can the normative processes described for the case of teen sexuality help us understand norms and social control around *other* types of behavior? I argue that they can, but a grounded approach to understanding other cases of norms will be important for expanding on this book's ideas. Most obvious are their implications for sexual behaviors at other ages and for other groups such as sexual minorities; for example, this book's ideas about norms and social control can help us understand sexuality among college students. But the book's implications extend beyond sexuality. Closely related sets of behaviors, such as parenting practices or types of substance use, are likely regulated by sets of norms that may be internally inconsistent but likely have coherent underlying rationales. Private behaviors that are distinct from people's public portrayals, like marijuana use or tax evasion, probably open up considerable strategic options for social actors and those who seek to control them. And many of the normative processes detailed in this book, like the role of social inequalities for norm enforcement, the importance of multiple reference groups, and the conflicts within and between social actors who are working to control behaviors, may be applicable for many types of social norms.

TEEN SEXUALITY, THEN AND NOW

To understand teen sexuality norms, it is important to remember that illicit teen sex is not new. Historical records suggest that "shotgun weddings," in which a man is forced to marry his already pregnant girlfriend, have been common as far back as the United States has existed. Historians estimate that around the time of the American Revolutionary War, about one third of first births were conceived premaritally.[35] As cars became common and teenagers' freedoms increased in the first half of the twentieth century, so did opportunities for sexual contact.[36] Before the advent of hormonal contraception in the 1960s, young people from all walks of life were generally expected to marry if their sexual activity resulted in a pregnancy. Historians believe that teen sexual activity was fairly widespread,[37] so there were a lot of teen births. The teen birth rate was high from the 1940s through the early 1970s, a time when women were also marrying at younger ages.[38] At the peak of the teen birth rate in the mid-1950s, almost 1 in 10 girls between the ages of 15 to 19 gave birth *every year*. Today, the teen birth rate is less than one third as high as it was then and less than half as high as the most recent peak in the mid-1990s.[39]

Today's teens are coming of age in a rapidly changing world in which sexual behaviors are in flux while norm changes lag behind. Compared to their parents and grandparents, many face bleaker economic prospects, and education beyond high school is more important for making a living wage. These educational pressures, combined with greatly increased technology use, are changing teens' leisure time and social interactions. As the typical ages for getting married and having children continue to rise into the late 20s and more young people enroll in college, many teens now anticipate having an extended period of "emerging adulthood"—an "age of independence" from their parents' and home communities' social control, before settling into adult roles.[40] This experience depends a lot on social class and race, but for more privileged teens it means that high school is no longer the time to find a mate and get ready to start full-time work.[41] With public attitudes shifting toward acceptance of gay and lesbian relationships, today's teens are sometimes less constrained by heteronormative sexuality than their parents were.[42] For some teens, "hooking up" is an available alternative to dating or long-term relationships, and a hookup's ambivalent meaning (it can be anything from a kiss to sexual intercourse) gives them some flexibility to keep their casual sexual activities private.[43] Newer contraceptive options, such as hormone shots and today's intrauterine devices (IUDs), provide more reliable protection from pregnancy and greater convenience, but their expense may mean getting parents' permission or not being able to use them.[44] The combination of these social trends means that many teens are under increasing pressure to do everything they can to ensure a bright future and to avoid serious relationships in high school, instead waiting many years to marry. At the same time, expectations of their sexual behavior are strict and their sexual options are broadening, incentivizing them to keep their sexual behavior secret. This is a recipe for complex norms, social control, and negotiation strategies.

The hard facts about teen sexual behavior are overshadowed by the cultural disputes surrounding them. Even though teen parenthood rates have been falling sharply, Americans are more likely to guess that teen parenthood is increasing than that it's staying the same or decreasing.[45] This disjoint between perception and reality suggests an outsized cultural concern about teen parents. Why does it strike many people as surprising that teen parenthood is so much less common now than in the past? Sociologist Frank Furstenberg, Jr. writes that it's because most teen births now occur outside of marriage.[46] Through the mid-1960s, less than 20 percent of births to teens were to an unmarried mother, but now that figure is nearly 90 percent.[47] This decoupling of teen motherhood from marriage has given rise to the perception that teen pregnancy is a *social problem*, even though in reality it's much less common than it once was. In a 2004 U.S. opinion poll, 79 percent of adults called teen pregnancy an "important" or "very serious" problem for the United States.[48] Although the teen pregnancy rate fell by nearly half from 1990 to 2008 and the teen abortion rate fell even more in roughly the same period, both are still relatively high compared to other countries.[49] About 5 percent of girls aged 15 to 19 get pregnant each year, and about one third of U.S. teen pregnancies end in abortion.[50]

In 2011, just under half of all high school students had ever had penile–vaginal intercourse (called "sex" here), a statistic that is no different than a decade before but a bit lower than in the early 1990s.[51] Although only one third of high school freshmen had had sex, nearly two thirds of seniors had.[52] Other estimates have found that nearly three quarters of teens have sex by age 19.[53] Riskier types of sex, like having many partners and not using protection, are common among U.S. youth. About a third of sexually experienced high school students have had four or more sexual partners during their lifetimes. When high school students last had sex, 40 percent did not use a condom and 13 percent did not use any contraceptive at all. Use of more effective pregnancy prevention methods such as hormonal methods (including birth control pills) and intrauterine devices was low, at less than one quarter of sexually active students.

Negative experiences with sex are also common. Among high school students, 12 percent of girls and 5 percent of boys have ever been forced to have sexual intercourse.[54] Just a third of young women describe their first teen sex as "really wanted," and most young people wish they had waited longer to have sex.[55] STIs are also common among teens. Tests from 2004 found that almost one quarter of all teen girls, and nearly two out of five sexually experienced girls, had an STI.[56]

This paints a fairly bleak picture of sex and its associated physical and emotional risks among U.S. teenagers. How does the United States compare to other developed countries?[57] The age at which U.S. teens start to have sex is quite similar to that of many other places, but the similarities end there. American teenagers' contraceptive use lags considerably behind many other developed countries, even though it has improved in recent years. The consequences of this difference are what one might expect. The prevalence of teen pregnancy, abortion, and childbearing is higher than in other developed countries. U.S. youth also tend to have higher rates of HIV and, to the extent statistics are available for comparison, other STIs as well.[58] But these statistics hide a lot of variation within the United States. The teen birth rate is 3.4 times higher in New Mexico than in New Hampshire, which has the lowest teen birth rate.[59] But even New Hampshire's teen birth rate is about double that of Sweden or Germany and about triple that of the Netherlands or Japan.

Sex education is another way in which the United States is different from many other developed countries. It has greater diversity in curricula and less reliance on comprehensive sex education—which teaches about contraceptives and how to use them, as well as about abstinence and negative consequences of sex.[60] In 2014, 76 percent of U.S. high schools taught that abstinence from sex is the most effective way to prevent pregnancy and sexually transmitted infections. Most high schools also taught about the risks associated with having multiple sexual partners and how to resist peer pressure to be sexually active. These topics fit within either an "abstinence-only" or "abstinence-plus"/comprehensive sex education curriculum. In contrast, just 35 percent of schools taught students how to use a condom correctly, which would often be taught in a comprehensive/"abstinence-plus" sex education curriculum. "Abstinence-only" curricula do not teach this information to students. This suggests, and interviewees confirmed, that there is a lot of variation among U.S. schools in the way sex education is taught.

In opinion polls, Americans seem conflicted about what they think the best sex education policies would be. Among parents of minor children, 91 percent agreed that high school sex education programs should be telling teens not to have sex until after high school (and 79 percent thought the message should be to wait altogether with sex until it is with the person they want to marry).[61] This suggests a preference for abstinence-focused sex education. But another poll of U.S. adults has found a fairly even split between preferences for reducing teen pregnancy "by emphasizing morality and abstinence" versus "by emphasizing sex education and birth control."[62] And almost two thirds of adults agree that "making birth control available to teenagers would reduce the number of pregnancies among teenagers."[63] To me, these polling data suggest that adults aren't sure about the best approach to educating teens about sex and pregnancy. But they do seem to agree that our current sex education curricula aren't the answer: Only 15 percent consider school sex education programs to be very effective at reducing teen pregnancy.[64] It may not be surprising that sex education is a major site of conflict among parents, teachers, schools, and communities.[65]

This book focuses on heterosexual teen sex, both because of its emphasis on teen pregnancy and because interviewees were almost totally silent about other types of sex and about the experiences of sexual minorities—such as gay, lesbian, bisexual, and transgender students—in high school. As later chapters suggest, such a silence may indicate a deep disapproval of non-heterosexual teen sexuality. Indeed, at the time the interviewees were in high school, only about half of Americans thought that gay and lesbian *adult* sexual relations should even be legal.[66] Recent years have seen considerable weakening of these norms against non-heterosexual sex and marriage,[67] so new explorations of these changing norms are needed. This book's silence on the topic should be read as a lack of data rather than a statement on its importance.

In the United States, like elsewhere, teen sexual behaviors are linked to social inequalities. Disadvantaged groups in our social structure experience conditions—like poverty, lower school quality, and less attractive career prospects—that shape their sexual behaviors.[68] Sexual minority youth, who experience stigma and discrimination, have compromised sexual health.[69] In terms of race, teen births are twice as common among Latina and Black girls as among White girls, with Native Americans in the middle and Asian Americans with by far the lowest rates.[70] Black high school students are more likely to have had sex than Whites; Latino boys are more likely than White boys to have had sex, but Latina girls are slightly less likely than White girls to have done so.[71] For both boys and girls, White teens are more likely to have used some method of contraception than Latino and Black teens. Besides race, social class is an important factor. Not only are the majority of teen mothers' families living in or near poverty, but the majority of children living in poverty have a mother who was a teen at their own or an older sibling's birth.[72] The socioeconomic backgrounds not just of teens themselves, but also of their neighborhoods and communities, are related to their likelihood of experiencing a teen pregnancy.[73] These social inequalities in teen sexual behaviors may further drive the sense that these behaviors are a "problem" because the racially and socioeconomically disadvantaged teens who are often viewed by U.S. society as "problems" are the ones experiencing these behaviors the most.

Researchers have long recognized that what happens during the teen years has implications for the rest of a person's life course. Social inequalities in the age norms that regulate sexuality during adolescence can therefore have reverberating effects later in life, both for teen parents who violate those norms and for all the teenagers who are regulated by them. This book emphasizes that not only teenagers' sexual behaviors, but also the norms, sanctions, and other social control surrounding them, matter for human lives.

THE STUDY

Claudia, Julie, and Fernando are three of the 133 young people who participated in in-depth interviews to talk about their teenage years and the messages they heard about teen sexuality. Interviews allow researchers access to people's accounts, self-presentations, descriptions of social contexts and interactions, and discussions of emotions, all of which are important for this book.[74] As sociologist Allison Pugh writes, interviews "can tap into the interactive edge where embodied culture and external pressures to feel or think a certain way collide."[75] The 57 interviewees who appear most often in this book, including Julie and Claudia, were college students at a large public Western university who came from a wide variety of communities across the United States. Along with typical students, our research team targeted those from communities with a lower social class and those from rural areas, resulting in a geographically dispersed and diverse cross-section of U.S. communities.[76] Targeting a large university campus made it feasible to reach a broad set of communities in a way that other sampling strategies could not have. Another 76 interviewees who appear less frequently, including Fernando, were teen mothers and fathers from a clinic and school in a large metropolitan area in the mountain West. These interviewees came from disadvantaged communities and can tell us what it's like to violate social norms around teen pregnancy and parenthood.[77]

The college student interviews are the main data source for this book because they better represent a cross-section of the United States. Teen parents very frequently come from strikingly disadvantaged contexts and the teen parent study was conducted in an urban area, so those interviews mostly tell us about one particular type of community. Teen parents from advantaged communities are very rare and could not be discussed in this study. The college student interviewees represented a variety of high school sexual experiences, from those who were never sexually active in high school, to those who were and used contraception consistently, to those who used birth control inconsistently, to people who experienced teen pregnancies. Their retrospective accounts of their high school years provide a clearer sense of the normative contexts they were embedded in during high school than if my research team had interviewed them during high school, because the contrast between their college and high school settings brought the high school norms into sharper focus.

College student interviews happened in two phases. The first 43 were peer interviews completed by trained undergraduate interviewers. These interviews tended to follow a consistent set of questions. Interviewees were willing to speak in a less politically correct way and disclose more sensitive information, such as past abortions, than when they spoke with non-peer researchers. The last 14 interviews were conducted by a small research team including me. We ranged more widely in our questions, some of which followed up on theoretical ideas that emerged from the first set of interviews.

The college student interviewees were three years out of high school on average (Table 1.1), and their ages ranged from 18 to 24. Although more than half of interviewees came from the Western state in which the university was located, there was regional variation. Interviewees attended high school in 14 different states representing all regions of the United States. Most interviewees went to high school somewhere in the Western region, which is a large and diverse geographic area with all of the normative community models described in Chapter 6 well represented. Interviewees identified the communities in which they attended high school as ranging politically from very conservative to very liberal, with similar variation in community-level SES and religious composition. Because communities loomed so large for understanding the norms teens experienced, I use their community characteristics to describe them when introducing interview quotes. Sixty percent of interviewees had sex during high school, and a third of those didn't use contraception consistently. Two disclosed teen abortions, but none were teen parents, which is not surprising given that most teen parents don't end up attending four-year colleges.[78] See the Appendix for a description of the teen parent interviewees and more information about the college student interviewees.

TABLE I.I

Characteristics of the 57 college student interviewees

Characteristic	Mean or % of interviewees
Age	20.8 years
Years in college	3.1 years
Female	63%
Race/ethnicity	
Hispanic/Latino	2%
Asian	4%
White	94%
U.S. region of high school	
Mountain West	74%
Pacific West	7%
South	9%
Midwest	6%
Northeast	4%
Parent has college degree	57%
Community SES	
(% of those mentioned, N = 44)	
Higher	53%
Mixed	31%
Lower	18%
Community religious composition	
(% of those mentioned, N = 47)	
Conservative/"very" Christian	26%
Evangelical Christian	19%
Catholic	34%
Mainline Protestant	6%
Mormon/LDS	15%
Sexual orientation in college	
Sexual minority	8%
Heterosexual	92%
Sexual experience in high school	
No heterosexual intercourse	40%
Had sex, always used contraception	40%
Had sex, didn't always use contraception	20%
Reported aborted teen pregnancy	4%
Teen parent	0%

Both phases of interviews targeted interviewees' experiences during high school, drawing some comparisons to their college experiences. Asking interviewees to look back on their high school years, when they were still close enough to remember them well, was helpful because they were now in a new setting and could therefore see their high school normative contexts more clearly (norms can be hard to identify when you're in the midst of them). Among other topics, our research team asked about the norms interviewees perceived about teen sex, contraception, pregnancy, abortion, and parenthood in their social contexts (such as families, schools, etc.) during high school, how the norms were communicated and enforced, how norms shaped their own and other teens' behaviors, and how they responded to attempts at social control. Questions started out fairly open-ended so teens could define their own communities and social worlds and independently identify normative messages, and then the interviewer followed up with more targeted probe questions. See the Appendix for more details about how the study was conducted.

This book's focus is broad in terms of the communities it gathers information about, but it is narrow in other ways. Because I analyze the social influences that interviewees talked about, two interesting and important contexts are left out: U.S. society as a whole, and the media. Interviewees' stories are clearly shaped by these societal-level factors, but they don't usually see this subtle influence themselves. Instead, they are focused on the people and institutions who are trying to control their behavior in their everyday lives. Other fascinating work has investigated dominant cultural frames about teen sexuality in the United States, historical changes in the cultural and structural contexts that shape teen sexuality in the United States, and the national-level policy battles that have shaped what teens learn.[79] Most interviewees didn't bring up media influences, and when the media did occasionally come up, it was often seen as being in conflict with community messages against sex and pregnancy. Interviewee Bethany said, "I think that pop culture really shapes teenagers' ideas about sex because they see on TV that the popular kids have sex. And they have to try to figure out in their own lives what they want to believe about it." Bethany contrasts what happens on TV with teens' "own lives" and suggests that young people are actively filtering media influences to make their own decisions about which messages to listen to.[80]

Some readers may be surprised that a high-risk potential consequence of sexual behavior, STIs (also called sexually transmitted diseases [STDs]), doesn't come up very much. Interviewees were clear that most girls and boys were focused on avoiding pregnancy, and concerns about STIs were secondary at best. As interviewee Helena put it, "pregnancy is like a very real thing, while having an STD, you know, everyone doesn't have to know if you have an STD." For girls in particular, a norm violation will be a public "real thing" if they carry a pregnancy to term, but they believe they can treat an STI without facing social exclusion. Of course, this is not always true, as some of the most prevalent STIs, such as human papillomavirus (HPV), are chronic or untreatable.[81] Pleasure and desire are also rarely mentioned in interviewees' accounts of high school sexuality. Those who had sex during high school rarely articulated clearly *why* they were motivated to do so. This missing "discourse of desire" among teens, especially girls, has been analyzed by others.[82]

Finally, I am not able to discuss four groups of teenagers. The first is younger teens, most of whom are not sexually active. While I didn't set out to exclude the younger teenage years, interviewees focused on the interesting last year or two of high school when many teens were becoming sexually active and starting to question the messages they heard from adults. Second, the experiences of sexual minority teens are not well represented. While a handful of interviewees identified as not completely heterosexual, they described a near-total silence during high school around the experiences of sexual minority teens.[83] Social norms didn't acknowledge these experiences, and teens who had them tended to stay quiet. A few interviewees talked about how marginalized sexual minority teens felt when the messages they heard didn't apply to them. A different study would be needed to do justice to the experiences of high school students belonging to sexual minorities, and luckily a burgeoning body of research is doing just that.[84] Last, two types of communities were not well represented in the interviews underlying this book, perhaps because of the demographics of the state in which the university was located. Although quite a few interviewees came from urban communities dominated by people of color, almost none came from minority-dominated communities in rural areas. Nor were communities dominated by non-Christian religions well represented, even though some interviewees came from non-Christian backgrounds themselves. Both of these groups would add important diversity for understanding norms about teen sexuality.

OVERVIEW

What are the norms about teen sexuality communicated to young people when they are in high school, how do people and institutions try to make them conform, and how do they respond? College student and teen parent interviewees described multilayered social worlds with complicated sets of norms and nuanced attempts to make sure teens behaved the way norm enforcers wanted them to. Interviewees talked about norm communication and social control coming from their families, peers, schools, and communities.

From all of these sources, teens tended to hear one of two primary rationales, or explanations for why the group's norms are appropriate. The practical rationale says that sex and risky sexual behavior seriously threaten young people's futures. It also links sexual restraint to maturity, saying that teens should be responsible and smart and should have self-respect. Different communities' norm sets interpret this rationale in different ways—in some, being sexually active while using contraception carefully is a tolerable (although not preferred) option, but in others, only virginity is acceptable. The moral rationale is dominant in more highly religious communities and says that sexual behavior among unmarried teens is morally wrong. The "even greater sin" of abortion is an increasingly important part of the moral rationale, leading to interesting new conversations and norms in many places.

This book is organized from the perspective of a teenager's social world as my interviewees described it, starting at home and moving outward (Fig. 1.1).[85] For each social actor—parents, peers, schools, and communities—I discuss the norms they communicate to teens about sexual behavior, how they are communicated, how they try to control teens to make sure they conform to the norms, and the consequences this control has.

Chapter 2 is intended for readers who are interested in social science *theory*, norms and social control, and social inequalities. I preview and integrate the book's findings about norms and social control to articulate the overarching theoretical processes that happen when people and institutions communicate about teen sexuality and try to influence young people's behaviors. The norms and social control around teen sexuality laid out in the following chapters add up to a dynamic picture that involves a lot of conflict, strategies, and counterstrategies between teenagers and those who seek to control their behavior. Social inequalities and control over resources are important for shaping normative climates, who gets controlled, and how it happens. The conceptual tools laid out in this chapter wed classic ideas about

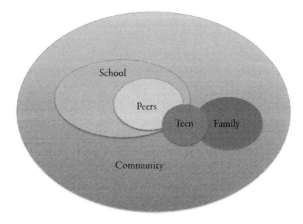

FIGURE 1.1 Teens' perceived social worlds for sexuality messages and social control

norms and social control with newer perspectives that emphasize social inequalities, conflict, and change.

Chapter 3 addresses norms and social control in *families*. Parents and siblings often have the most opportunities to communicate sexuality norms to teens. Older siblings can be important role models, and parents have both physical and legal control over their teenage children. But communication and control around teen sexuality are loaded topics in most interviewees' families. Parents use cautionary tales about other teens' problematic behavior to communicate how their teenage child should behave. They make (often quite serious) threats about the bad things that will happen if the teen doesn't comply. But conversations about the teen's *actual* sexual behaviors are quashed by a "conspiracy of silence" between parents and teens. Many parents choose to assume that their teen is not sexually active rather than seeking accurate information, and teens are usually too frightened by their parents' threats to volunteer information. This situation often results in less support for teens who seek to have sex responsibly. Parents' efforts to physically restrict opportunities for sex among teens can lead to struggles with the teenager and disruptions to the family system.

Chapter 4 focuses on social relationships with close friends and same-age *peers*. Friends and peers communicate the same rationales to teenagers, but an additional message about "being normal" comes up in many groups—especially toward the end of high school, sex with careful contraception in a committed romantic relationship is accepted in many but certainly not all peer groups. The norms communicated by peers are complicated because they regulate not just teens' actual sexual behaviors (which tend to happen in private) but also the public portrayals of those behaviors (which may be very different than what is actually happening) and metanorms about how to treat people who break these rules. Sanctioning peers appropriately is important because it can give others the impression that you are conforming to those rules yourself.[86] So it may be no surprise that the social exclusion of teenagers who are suspected rule breakers is widespread. That exclusion is often based on rumors and innuendo—public portrayals of teens' sexual behaviors that tend to be biased against girls and lower-income and minority teens—rather than on facts about what teens actually did. The ubiquity of social exclusion makes sense because peers don't have legal or physical options for controlling one another's behavior. But teens' interactions within the fairly closed social network of high school make social exclusion an effective strategy that contributes to the exodus of many pregnant girls from their schools and friendship groups. Friends and peers can sometimes provide a more supportive environment for sexual activity, which is particularly important when adults disapprove. But even this somewhat safer social space is fraught with reputational risk, especially for girls, whose behaviors are usually held more strictly to normative standards than those of boys.

Social networks of teens are often centered in *schools*, which are the focus of Chapter 5. Many high schools have social divides along racial or socioeconomic lines that are reflected in the academic tracking of students. These schools often see hostility arising between groups on the basis of perceived differences in their norms about teen sexuality, but having a variety of normative climates also gives some teens options for finding a group that will accept their behavioral choices. Other school environments are more cohesive and dominated by a single social group, which limits teens' options for finding a group to accept them and generally leads to higher levels of social control. But beyond being a site for peer interaction, schools are also formal social institutions, usually overseen by a board of community members, with legal control over students and an educational charge to teach them about sexuality. Schools have agendas for shaping teens' sexual behavior, which tend to reflect the broader community's agenda. They have the means to communicate this agenda to teenagers and sanction those who disobey. This has made many schools a site of conflict about what information should be communicated to students and how.[87] Struggles usually center on the school's explicit agenda for sex education, but the hidden agenda, which is less constrained by legal restrictions, may be just as powerful. An important part of many high schools' hidden agendas is to silence talk about teen sex and pregnancy and make these behaviors as invisible as possible. Some private schools may expel pregnant students, but public schools cannot. Instead, many public schools in larger or better-resourced districts use the "carrot" of special off-site programs for pregnant and parenting teens to convince such girls to transfer. In combination with the "stick" of schoolmates socially excluding pregnant girls, this strategy is often effective, bolstering the impression that teen pregnancy doesn't happen in their school and furthering the social exclusion of pregnant girls. Schools in which pregnant girls tend to stay enrolled (which often serve populations with lower SES) face metanorms that sanction them by questioning their academic standards and commitment and assuming that the schools endorse teen pregnancy.

The broader *community* is the focus of Chapter 6. Schools are the most important social actor for communicating community norms, but other people and social institutions—such as religious organizations, nonprofits, and healthcare providers—are also involved. Many interviewees had no trouble articulating the messy and sometimes internally inconsistent sets of norms about teen sexuality in their communities. I lay out the sets of norms in different types of communities and discuss how they vary by religion and SES and relate to teens' behaviors. Norms in the set target different links in a chain of behaviors that starts with heterosexual intercourse and ends with teen parenthood. But the set also includes norms regulating public portrayals of these behaviors and justifications for why a person behaved as he did, as well as metanorms about how to sanction teens who violate sexuality norms. This norm set is held together by an overarching rationale that explains why the norms in the set are appropriate. The communities my interviewees described can be divided into those with a moral versus a practical rationale, which tends to depend on the importance of religion in the community. Each of these rationales gives rise to an internally contradictory norm set that makes sense after understanding the underlying rationale. The communities' norm sets are further divided by SES, which tends to affect the prevalence of teen sexual behaviors perceived by interviewees. I call these four community types "it could be you" (lower SES and less religious), "be careful" (higher SES and less religious), "it's wrong" (higher SES and more religious), and "it's wrong, but" (lower SES and more religious). The norm sets described by interviewees from these community types are different from each other, but in none of them is teen sex or pregnancy encouraged. Metanorms in the community regulate how people are supposed to respond to teens who have violated norms and shape those young people's experiences and future prospects. Besides working to influence sex education, community members try to communicate with and control teenagers by providing access to teens for organizations (such as churches or reproductive health clinics) whose goals fit the community norm set. Community members also socially exclude and materially sanction teenagers, especially pregnant and parenting girls, who violate their norms.

After this ever-widening set of social contexts has been explored, I turn to *teens' strategies for negotiating norms and social control* in Chapter 7. How do teens respond to the normative pressures around them? Young people see the complicated norms and social control that target them, but they don't passively accept them. Their dependence on adults and institutions for resources that are necessary for securing their futures makes teens more easily controlled. But they still exercise a lot of leeway over their own behaviors, particularly in the realm of sexual behavior, where you can often get away with doing something and publicly acting like you haven't done it. Because young people generally see the stakes of violating dominant norms about their sexual behaviors as too high to risk, their viable options are to conform to those norms or privately violate the norms but try to minimize sanctions. Teens who have internalized social norms (most younger teens and some older teens) tend to choose the first option, and those who no longer want to conform (many older teens) choose the second. Depending on which of these options they select, teens can use different strategies like finding reference groups whose norms match their behaviors, collaborating with other teens to hide their norm violations, or working to justify to themselves and others that their behavior is less problematic than it may seem. For example, many young people who want to engage in sex collaborate with peers to shape a perception of teen sex as "normal." But most of them still try hard to hide their sexually active status from parents and other adults. Reserving sex for committed relationships in which both partners have their reputations at stake, using contraception very carefully, and discouraging public talk about their sexual behavior are common strategies. Sometimes these strategies involve working alone, but other times teens band together or enlist the help of adults.

Chapter 8 concludes the book and discusses its broader implications for understanding social norms and teen sexual behavior and developing effective policies. How do all these norms, social control, and negotiation strategies around sexuality matter for teenagers' lives? As part of human development and the transition to adulthood, people's early sexual experiences matter for physical and mental health and future socioeconomic prospects. Sanctions from violating norms also matter because they can affect teens' interpersonal relationships, resources, and opportunities for the future. The college student and teen parent interviewees seemed certain that the norms and social control they experienced had shaped their lives, even after they had moved on to new social environments. Despite the best intentions of the people and institutions who try to communicate sexuality norms and control teens' behavior, their control has unintended consequences because it often strengthens the negative repercussions of sex and pregnancy without effectively curtailing those behaviors.

2

THEORIZING ABOUT NORMS AND SOCIAL CONTROL

U.S. TEENAGERS NAVIGATE their sexuality in complicated social worlds. They hear strong messages from the people and institutions around them, who try to make teens behave in ways that align with their norms. Because sex, contraception, and abortion aren't public behaviors, though, teens have some leeway to push back against norm enforcement and behave in the ways they want. Norms, social control, and human agency are well-established concepts in the study of groups,[1] but the first two have fallen out of favor in recent years and the third is the subject of scholarly debate.[2] Understanding culture has become an important goal in sociology, but there is less focus on norms and social control as ways that culture can shape people's lives. Much of the work on norms and social control processes is being done in the laboratory and outside of sociology,[3] leading to calls to expand research on normative processes.[4] Experimental research isolates causal relationships, but more focus is needed on the ways norms shape behavior outside the lab. I use a particularly relevant social issue—teen sexuality—to detail complex normative environments and investigate how U.S. teens navigate them, shedding light on how normative processes play out and what makes norms effective or ineffective. In real life, these processes are messy and inconsistent, involving many more strategies than just conformity, norm violation, and sanctioning. I show that norm enforcers do more than just sanction, and teens do more than just comply or deviate. Teen sexuality is especially interesting for studying these issues because it's publicly disputed, visible as a social "problem," includes private acts, and involves age norms proscribing behaviors that, when done by older people, are often welcomed and encouraged.

This chapter addresses influential critiques that have been leveled at sociological conceptualizations of norms, calling into question the overly stable view of culture of which traditional understandings of norms are considered a part.[5] The first of these critiques is that researchers haven't documented how related norms work together, some in conflicting ways and some not. Second, understandings of norms ignore or minimize social inequalities. Third, conceptualizations of norms don't incorporate social conflict. Fourth, little is known about how norms change.[6] Classic ideas about social norms describe a static, self-sustaining system that upholds the current social order, applies similarly to everyone, and reduces conflict and change. Newer sociological work on culture has focused on inequalities, conflict, and change but rarely engages norms directly.[7] I argue that scholars need to expand ideas about norms to address these important critiques and incorporate advances from sociological work on culture that has been done in the intervening years. The following sections articulate how this book's norms perspective can address each of these critiques in turn.

Throughout this book, I work to make sense of complex normative contexts and the strategies interviewees describe through which norm enforcers and norm targets negotiate norms. *Norm enforcers* are people or institutions who seek to control the behavior of others to bring it in line with group norms. *Norm targets* are the people or institutions whose behavior is being regulated. Both strategize individually or collectively to bring norm targets' behaviors in line with their goals. This chapter brings those threads together and provides organizing structures for understanding them. The result is a set of theoretical statements that may be useful for understanding social phenomena beyond teen sexuality. The first part of this chapter lays out concepts and theoretical arguments about norm sets and the strategies of norm enforcers and norm targets. The second part uses the case of teen sexuality to show how this theoretical perspective on norms incorporates ideas about social inequalities, conflict, and change.

SETS OF NORMS

CHAINS OF BEHAVIORS

One of the main insights of this book is that norms about teen sexuality regulate many different behaviors and seem internally inconsistent even within the same community. Teens hear mixed messages such as, "don't have sex, but use a condom," or "shun teen parents for having committed the sin of having premarital sex, but praise them for not having committed the sin of abortion." These inconsistencies make sense once one starts thinking about teen sexuality norms as regulating a chain of closely related behaviors and belonging to norm sets.

Teen parenthood lends itself well to thinking about sets of norms because it is part of what I call a chain of behaviors that can lead to parenthood: teen sex, contraception, pregnancy, abortion, and childbearing (Fig. 2.1; see Chapter 6).[8] Different norms target different behaviors in this chain, and each is important to study.[9] Like many other interviewees, Brooke (who comes from a wealthy conservative suburb and whose story is described in greater detail in Chapter 6) heard normative messages targeting this entire chain of behaviors. Norm enforcers in her community communicated a norm against teen sex, a norm promoting contraception but only once the norm against sex has been violated, a strong norm against teen pregnancy, competing norms for and against abortion, and a strong norm against teen parenthood. Decisions have to be made about each behavior in this chain before someone becomes a teen parent, so norms' influence on every link in the chain matters—but it's important to remember that other influences besides norms also shape people's behaviors.[10]

I argue that studying the norms that regulate such related behaviors *together* is key for understanding normative processes around teen parenthood, just as it is important for understanding many other human behaviors. Each of the behaviors in this chain is highly contested in our society when teenagers engage in it, and norm enforcers try to control teens' behaviors. Societal stigma is often greater for the latter links of the chain. Pregnancy itself is the behavior that is least under the control of the person experiencing it—whether or not an act of heterosexual intercourse without contraception leads to pregnancy is somewhat up to chance. So

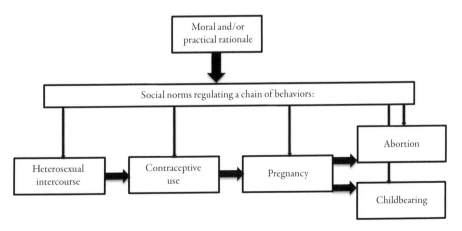

FIGURE 2.1 Social norms that regulate a chain of teen sexual behaviors

although communities' norm sets may discourage teen pregnancy and parent-hood, related norms may target more predictable behaviors in this chain like sex, contraception, and abortion.

Although a lot of research studies only one behavior in this chain, the chain should be examined as a whole to better understand normative processes around teen sex-uality. Norms regulating different behaviors that seem inconsistent start to make sense once they're analyzed as a norm set undergirded by a rationale. For example, the moral rationale strongly discourages both teen abortion and teen parenthood. Since encouraging each of these behaviors could help prevent the other, the two norms seem inconsistent. But when the importance of both the anti-premarital sex and anti-abortion norms to the moral rationale is understood, the discouragement of both these behaviors makes sense. Sexual abstinence until marriage and opposi-tion to abortion are core values in many conservative Christian belief systems, so norms against teen sex and abortion are often strong when teens are being taught the moral rationale.

SETS OF NORMS

When targeting related behaviors, norms come in *sets* that include multiple norms and metanorms (which regulate appropriate sanctioning of norm violators). This book describes norm sets at the meso or group level (see Chapter 6 for more details), but macrolevel societal norms also influence people's behaviors.[11] As Brooke's norm set shows, social norms about teen sexuality do not happen in isolation. Instead, multiple norms simultaneously regulate several related behaviors (teen sex, contra-ception, pregnancy, abortion, and parenthood). Scholarly research on social norms tends to study a single norm by itself, which does not reflect the reality interviewees describe. Some researchers have pointed out that norms can be interconnected, call-ing them "systems of norms" or "bundles of norms."[12] Similarly, I define a norm set as *multiple norms, which can compete with or reinforce each other, that regulate the same behavior or closely related behaviors.* For example, in other research I found that many parents of pregnant teenagers must negotiate a set of competing metanorms regulating their sanctioning of their daughter. One of these norms encourages nega-tive sanctions against the daughter because of objections to nonmarital teen child-bearing, but a competing norm discourages negative sanctions against the daughter because of parents' moral duty to support their children.[13]

These competing social pressures create a space for people to actively negotiate norms because they have a choice about how to behave.[14] But the options are not necessarily attractive ones. In the example, the pregnant teen's parents are in a dou-ble bind because they will be violating a metanorm whether they choose to support their teenage child or sanction her. Ethnographer Gary Alan Fine talks about how this understanding of norms reflects real life:

> The normative structure presumes interpretive options, linked to the existence of a cultural tool kit. In responding to a particular interactional context, individuals select from among a set of possibilities. It is rare that a single behavior is judged to be the only appropriate option. This is particularly true in those situations in which formal, established rules do not exist or are ambiguous.[15]

I argue that these "sets" of normatively acceptable "possibilities" result from sets of related social norms that together regulate actual behavior, public portrayals of behavior, emotions, and sanctioning of norm violators (Fig. 2.2). Underlying all these norms and metanorms is one or more cohesive rationales that explain why the norms have the content they do. When thinking about teens' social worlds in this way, the mixed messages they hear about sexuality make sense.

It's important to understand that norms within a set can conflict, and conflicting norms can still be part of one or more cohesive underlying rationales for why each norm in the set is appropriate. Inconsistencies within a norm set may help explain why there are often contradictions among people's stated attitudes, their behaviors, and their public portrayals of and justifications for these behaviors.[16] For example, Isaac's account of his highly religious community in a rural area (see Chapter 6) includes conflicting norms regulating teens' behaviors (don't have a baby, but don't

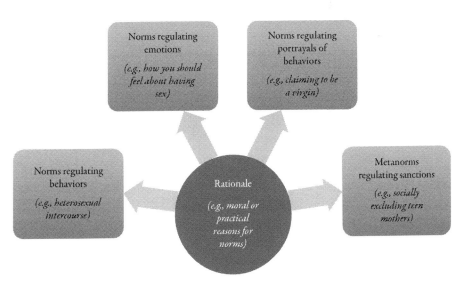

FIGURE 2.2 A set of norms regulating teen sexuality

get an abortion either) and conflicting metanorms regulating sanctions of norm violators (you should negatively sanction teen parents because teen parenthood is morally wrong, but positively sanction teen parents because they chose parenthood over an abortion). The first pair of norms is regulating related behaviors in the same chain—teen childbearing and abortion. The second pair of metanorms is regulating sanctioning of the same behavior—teen parenthood.

Rationales underlying sets of norms

One or more rationales undergirds a norm set. A rationale is a group-level norm specifying the appropriate reasoning people should apply when socially evaluating a topic, such as teen sexuality. A rationale justifies why a particular norm or set of norms is appropriate—it is the *acceptable reason why a behavior, portrayal, emotion, or sanction is encouraged or discouraged.* As Figure 2.2 shows, rationales regulate the appropriate reasons you should have for how you're supposed to behave; how you're supposed to feel; how you're supposed to portray your behavior, feelings, and sanctions to others; and how you're supposed to sanction violators and communicate norms. A rationale is the accepted reason in a group for encouraging or discouraging a behavior, emotion, sanction, or portrayal—so even if you follow the rules and behave the right way, you can be sanctioned if you aren't doing it for the right reason.[17] Because it provides an understanding of why a norm should be followed, communicating a rationale is particularly important if you want the norm target to *internalize* the norm, thereby self-regulating her own behavior.[18]

For example, our society has a norm that you should not litter. But it also has a rationale for that norm: You should not litter because it dirties our environment. If someone refrained from throwing trash out his car window only because the window was broken and couldn't be opened, he would be conforming superficially to the behavioral proscription of the anti-littering norm, but not adhering to its rationale. He could face negative interpersonal sanctions if people found out he would be willing to litter if only his car window would open. Traditional norms theory expects that as long as people conform to the behavior prescription, they won't be negatively sanctioned. But I argue that conforming to the rationale can be at least as important as conforming to the behavioral norm. This makes rationales complicated because rationales are themselves norms—but they are norms about how to *think* about a particular behavior rather than about how to behave. In this way, rationales are a lot like Arlie Hochschild's idea of "emotion norms" or "feeling rules," which are norms regulating how you are supposed to feel emotionally.[19] I extend this idea to norms about how you are supposed to *think*.

So in this expansion of the definition of norms, social norms regulate how you are supposed to behave, portray your behaviors to others, sanction violators, feel, or think (through rationales).

In the case of teen sexuality, conforming to the rationale in a norm set is important, sometimes even more important than conforming to behaviors. For example, teens who have sex without using contraception can sometimes reduce or avoid sanctions by calling these behaviors a "mistake." By doing this, they demonstrate that they accept the rationale labeling the behaviors as wrong, suggesting that they would not normally behave in this way and don't plan to repeat the behavior. In fact, a teen who makes that kind of "mistake" may be considered *less* worthy of social sanctions than a teen who hasn't actually had sex or forgotten to use contraception, but who tells people that these behaviors aren't wrong and she might engage in them in the future. This is because the former teen is conforming to the social group's rationale, and the latter one is not.

As Chapter 3 shows, rationales provide a cohesive logic to what at first glance might seem like an inconsistent set of norms about behaviors, emotions, sanctions, and portrayals. For teen sexuality, religion is pivotal in determining a community's rationale (see Chapter 6). Depending on the importance of conservative religious denominations, communities tend to subscribe to either a practical or a moral rationale underlying norms about teen sexuality. For example, the practical rationale expects community members to think that teen sex is bad because it can expose teens to negative consequences, such as pregnancy or sexually transmitted infections, that can compromise their futures. Contraception is good because it reduces the risk of many of these outcomes. Pregnancy is very bad because it threatens a teen's future, and abortion is tolerable because it removes that threat. Teen parenthood is the worst of all because so many negative consequences are expected to occur. There are also conflicting metanorms (norms about how to enforce norms) in the practical rationale: People should disapprove of teen parents because they endangered their own futures, but they should also provide support to improve teen parents' future prospects.

The moral rationale relies on distinctions between right and wrong that arise from religious teachings instead of threats to young people's futures, but it similarly provides a coherent logic to the seemingly inconsistent norms in the set. Premarital sex and abortion are sinful, and teen parents should be both sanctioned for having violated the anti-sex norm and praised for having conformed to the anti-abortion norm. Some interviewees, especially those like Brooke who come from high-SES, highly religious communities, perceive that both moral and practical rationales underlie their norm set.

Norms regulating behaviors

Early ideas about social norms focused on how norms regulate behavior. Conceptions of norms have typically focused on a single behavior, such as a norm proscribing cigarette smoking or a norm against littering. More recently, scholars have talked about systems of competing norms that regulate the same behavior. Michael Hechter and Karl-Dieter Opp use the example of a baby crying on an airplane.[20] A norm compels parents to try to quiet the child, but another norm discourages others around them from quieting the baby. Depending on whether you're the baby's parent, then, you are expected either to try to keep the baby quiet or to refrain from doing anything to quiet the baby.

Thinking about norms in sets is complex because it allows not only for multiple norms regulating the same behavior, but also for norms that regulate closely related behaviors. In the case of teen sexuality, as Brooke's case shows, a set of norms regulates the chain of behaviors leading from sex to contraception to pregnancy to abortion or parenthood. In the airplane example, a set of norms and metanorms is shaping related chains of behaviors, such as the sanctioning of the parents by flight attendants and fellow passengers and the parents' leeway to "bend" in-flight norms about standing up or going to the bathroom. Like I have described for teens' sexual behaviors, these behaviors are closely related and regulated by the same overarching rationale—in this case, a rationale that gives parents the sole authority and responsibility to control their children as much as possible in public places, allowing them some latitude from following typical rules in order to accomplish this goal and holding them partially but not completely responsible for their infants' behavior.[21]

Norms regulating emotions

As Arlie Hochschild first noted, social norms don't just regulate how we're supposed to behave—they also tell us how we're supposed to *feel*.[22] Emotion norms (or feeling rules) have been well developed as a concept that works in much the same way as norms about behavior. In the realm of work, Hochschild and others have argued that employers expect not only specific behaviors of many employees, but also specific emotional displays. This is particularly true for people like sales clerks and flight attendants, who are supposed to be cheerful and act friendly, but also bar bouncers and bill collectors, who are supposed to be unfriendly or act unwelcoming.

In this example and others, norms regulating emotions tend to go hand in hand with those regulating behavior. Past research suggests that there are powerful and complex processes involving emotion norms about romantic relationships in adolescence.[23] I didn't ask interviewees about emotion norms directly because it can be hard for people to identify how their emotions depend on others' judgments of them or on their internalized judgments of themselves. But emotions came up over and over in the interviews anyway. When discussing teen sexuality, interviewees talked a lot about potential or actual disappointment and anger among adults. These emotions engendered fear in teens—both fear of negative consequences resulting from adults' emotional reactions and fear of those reactions themselves. As Brooke said, "There was definitely an element of fear involved, of what your parents would do. . . . A fear of being judged if you did get pregnant."

Researchers have found that "moral emotions" are part of the link between norms and behavior.[24] There has been a lot of attention paid to the negative moral emotions of guilt, embarrassment, and shame, all of which are prominent in interviewees' discussions of teen sexuality norms. Negative emotions such as fear, anger, and blame can result from seeing others violate norms.[25] Brooke highlighted blame in describing her community's reaction to teen pregnancy: "There was always kind of the judgmental, 'Whose fault was it? Who do we blame?'" More recently, the positive moral emotions of gratitude and pride have been included, both of which were present in the interviews. Brooke described her friends' sense of pride when reacting to a pregnant girl: "'I can't believe she's having sex.' . . . We wouldn't have gotten into that situation." People who violate norms are supposed to experience negative moral emotions, and people who follow norms should experience positive ones. These emotions act as internal regulators and can drive people to conform to a social norm.[26] People who watch someone else violating a norm feel empathic embarrassment, which can influence their own future behavior.[27]

The interviews illustrate norms for how teens are supposed to feel when they behave, portray their behavior, or sanction people in different ways. Children learn to anticipate moral emotions like these and link them to specific behaviors.[28] A teen who has unprotected sex or gets an abortion is probably supposed to feel guilty, embarrassed, and ashamed—more so in some communities than others, depending on the norm set. But a teen who is abstinent or who has successfully avoided pregnancy may feel proud or morally superior to others. All of these dynamics are present in the interviews.

Norms regulating portrayals of behaviors

Besides regulating actual behaviors and emotions, norms in a set can seek to control how people *portray* their behaviors and emotions to others (see Chapter 4).[29] Qualitative cultural sociology has made great strides in understanding how people talk about their behaviors.[30] This perspective asserts that social norms don't shape actual behavior as strongly as previously thought.[31] Instead, social norms influence how you talk about, or justify, the behaviors you've already decided to engage in.[32]

It's an important insight that people may decide to behave however they want, but then try to avoid negative sanctions by justifying their behavior after the fact. These justifications make use of tools from a person's available cultural toolkit. My perspective on norms supports these ideas but also suggests that norms attempt to shape people's actual behaviors. Although the work on justifications has focused on justifications for behaviors, people also work to justify and portray their emotions to conform to norms.

Regardless of how public a behavior or emotional display is, people have the opportunity to try to justify it after the fact.[33] Politicians who cry, say something foolish, or are caught making rude comments over an open microphone are pressed to justify their non-normative behaviors or emotions after the fact. The same behavior can result in different sanctions and different perceptions of norm violation depending on how that behavior is justified. This goes back to the idea of a rationale. If someone calls his behavior violating a norm a "mistake" or expresses regret, as many of our interviewees did when discussing their experiences with unprotected sex, he has conformed to the rationale underlying the norm, though not the norm itself. That person is likely to be sanctioned less strongly than a norm violator who does not express her agreement with the rationale.

But an even better way to avoid sanctions is to conceal the norm violation completely, denying your association with a stigmatized group.[34] This is a feasible option when a behavior is private or only witnessed by a small number of people who are unlikely to disclose the norm violation, as is sometimes the case with sexual behavior and intimate partner violence. Brooke said that parents in her community actually *expected* teens to portray their behavior in ways that did not necessarily reflect reality. Their message was, "If you're going to do it [have sex], be safe and don't tell me about it." Brooke said this portrayal norm made teens' behavioral norm violation "easier to deal with" for parents. Concealing a norm violation is also possible when the situation is in the past and someone is portraying her past behavior to new people who can't check whether she's misrepresenting the truth. Early in U.S. history, some men who had deserted the military or had been discharged dishonorably could create new portrayals of themselves as honorably discharged veterans if they moved to a new place. This became more difficult to do as government recordkeeping and public access to these records improved.

The possibility of concealment makes private behaviors different from public ones in terms of social control. When people have an opportunity to behave privately in a way that violates a norm while portraying their behavior as conforming, they have more leeway to do what they like and still avoid sanctions. In fact, this leeway may be directly encouraged, as in Brooke's case. This encouragement solves a problem for parents in Brooke's community. If their teen violates a norm against sex but doesn't experience negative consequences such as pregnancy, then as long as she doesn't disclose her norm violation, the parents are neither forced to levy potentially harmful sanctions against their teenager nor compelled to leave an acknowledged norm violation unsanctioned.

Metanorms regulating sanctions

Metanorms are norms about how you're supposed to enforce norms (see Chapter 4).[35] Sanctioning norm violators takes time, energy, and sometimes resources. So why would anyone bother to do it who isn't personally harmed by a norm violation? Consider the example of someone talking on a cell phone in a movie theater. No particular person is harmed most by that disruptive behavior, but people sitting nearest that person are the most likely to feel social pressure to sanction the chatty moviegoer, even if they would personally prefer to stay out of the situation. The metanorm prescribes mild sanctioning of the norm violator by glaring at or shushing her, but not stronger sanctioning such as physical violence. People near the violator are held more accountable to the metanorm than those farther away. This dynamic is probably stronger when the people involved aren't strangers—sociologist Christine Horne has found that the social pressure to sanction is stronger in more cohesive social groups.[36] Brooke described metanormative processes around the sanctioning of pregnant teens and their families in her community: "There's a lot of judgment and rumors floating around, and [as a parent] you don't want your kids to be prey to that. And you don't want yourself to be prey to that." Brooke's final sentence shows that parents of teens face metanorms that make them "prey to" social judgment if they don't sanction appropriately when their child violates a norm.

Metanorms tend to go hand in hand with behavior norms and emotion norms. When there are social rules about how people are supposed to behave or feel, there also tend to be rules about how someone who breaks those rules should be treated. But as they have been described in the past, metanorms are a fairly narrow concept. I suggest an expansion of the idea of metanorms in two ways. First, the sanctioning that is the focus of a metanorm can refer to the violation of not only a norm that enforces behavior, but also a norm that enforces an emotion or the public portrayal of a behavior or emotion. For example, several interviewees suggested that teen mothers and fathers who publicly express pride about being a parent—or even teen parents who appear in public with their children, which interviewees interpret as an expression of their pride—should be negatively sanctioned by the people around them. Second, the concept of a metanorm can be expanded to include norms about how to *communicate* a norm to others. This usually happens before someone has violated a norm, and it can be more effective social control than waiting to sanction someone after he violates the norm. In this book, there are clearly metanorms regulating how parents and other adults are expected to communicate norms about teen sexual behavior to teenagers. This can include communicating expectations for behavior, the rationale behind those expectations, and the sanctions a teen can expect for violating the expectations. In Brooke's community, in order to avoid damaging social judgments, parents were expected to shut down direct communication about their teens' sexual activity and, as she said, "keep it on the down low." Thus, there are two kinds of metanorms: metanorms about how to communicate a norm, and metanorms about how to sanction a norm violator.

THE CONTEXT OF A NORM SET

A set of norms is a group-level phenomenon situated within a social context. As the previous chapter's description of teens' social worlds as they perceived them shows, multiple social groups—such as families, teen peer groups, schools, and communities—usually make up the social context of a set of norms. This context has three important aspects that shape how the norm set influences norm outcomes: related norm sets, norm enforcers, and norm targets.

Related sets of norms are distinct from the set of norms regulating teen sexuality, but they also play a role in shaping sexual behaviors, portrayals, emotions, and sanctions. I focus mainly on one norm set that is related to the teen sexuality norm set—norms around socioeconomic attainment—here, but the set of norms about parenting is another example. Norms around socioeconomic attainment affect how the teen sexuality norm set plays out, particularly in terms of sanctioning. The practical rationale says that teen sexual activity and parenthood should be discouraged because of potential damage to a teen's future. This future is often expressed in educational and career terms. Claudia articulated these concerns among community members when describing their reaction to a teen mother: "How is she going to support a baby? How is she going to get her own education and take care of a family?" Alexis talked about her father's concern for the success of her future filmmaking career as a major driver of his communication and norm enforcement around teen sexuality. These expectations about education, career success, and income are norms because they communicate how young people are expected to pursue education and work, and those who do not follow those rules face social and institutional sanctions.

How does the related norm set about socioeconomic attainment play a role in teen sexuality behaviors and sanctions? Sanctioning of teens by parents, schools, and communities is an important part. In Brooke's community, parents expected teens either to remain sexually abstinent or to ensure that their sexual activity was free of negative consequences and kept secret from parents. This set of expectations avoids putting parents in a double bind: If they are faced with the knowledge of their sexually active teen's norm violation, they'll have to either sanction the teen in a way that may jeopardize her socioeconomic attainment or be seen by the teen as people who will not punish the teen when she violates their social rules. In Brooke's case, these sanctions weren't directly related to threats to her socioeconomic attainment. She said that her parents never "sat me down and were like, 'If you ever get pregnant, we're kicking you out of the house.'" Instead, social sanctions like gossip and exclusion can threaten a teen's reputation as "good," resulting in fewer educational and socioeconomic opportunities.

These shared expectations of silence around teens' actual sexual behaviors and the related focus on teens' public portrayals of their behaviors solve problems for everyone. They let teens behave how they like without negative sanctions, as long as they are careful and have a bit of luck. They also allow parents to follow norms that prescribe their support of their teen's socioeconomic attainment, even if the teen is secretly violating norms against teen sexuality. If this normative prescription around socioeconomic attainment did not exist, parents and other adults might be harsher in their sanctions and focus more on controlling teens' actual sexual behaviors.

Parents' support often, but not always, extends to a teen pregnancy. Many of the teen parent interviewees said their parents were very disappointed by their violation of a strong norm against teen parenthood, but they continued to offer material support so that the teen could get an education or build a career. Schools, in contrast, rarely go this far. As Chapter 5 shows, high schools often encourage pregnant girls to leave or provide less support for their education than they did before the pregnancy. This difference between families and schools likely reflects family members' interdependence in terms of resources, especially in lower-income families. Their children's socioeconomic success is crucial for their futures, even if a child has violated a strong norm against teen parenthood. By choosing to support the teen rather than sanctioning him, parents are prioritizing the socioeconomic attainment norm set, or the resources that may arise from the teen's socioeconomic attainment, above norms regulating teen parenthood.

It's clear that both norms around socioeconomic attainment and resource dependence shape sanctioning dynamics around teen sexuality. Teens' own behaviors and portrayals are similarly shaped by these dynamics, as I discuss in Chapter 3. The practical rationale implicitly draws on norms about socioeconomic attainment in justifying *why* certain teen sexuality behaviors, portrayals, emotions, and sanctions are appropriate. Without understanding this related set of norms, it would be impossible to understand U.S. teen sexuality norms.

Two other important aspects of the teen sexuality norm set's social context are *norm enforcers* and *norm targets*. They can be people or institutions, and sometimes the same person or institution can be in both categories—for example, in Brooke's community, teens both are targets of sexuality norms and enforce norms for each other. Norm enforcers and norm targets are social actors who individually or collaboratively strategize to control the outcomes of the norm set (behaviors, portrayals, emotions, and sanctions). In line with current views of culture, norm enforcers and targets deploy the norm set strategically to achieve their own goals. But what are those goals? *Norm targets' goals* can be described simply. Norm targets are trying to act according to their own preferences. If they have internalized the norms of their social contexts, those preferences will be in line with what the norm enforcers want. For example, throughout high school, Brooke felt that it was morally right to abstain from sex and remained a virgin. But if norm targets want to act in ways that violate norms, as many or most teens do by the end of high school, their goal is to engage in this behavior while avoiding negative sanctions.

At least in the case of teen sexuality, *norm enforcers' goals* are more complicated. This is partly because of the strong socioeconomic attainment norms described above, which constrain enforcers' ability to sanction a teen harshly if they care about the teen's future socioeconomic success. The ideal situation for a norm enforcer is one like Brooke's, in which the norm target has internalized the norm and behaves as the norm enforcer wants (e.g., abstains from sex). The next best goal is for teens to comply behaviorally to the norm set without having internalized the norm. Some interviewees did this for at least part of high school, motivated by fear of social sanctions and other negative consequences. If a teen is going to violate norms by having sex, the best option from a norm enforcer's point of view is for it to happen secretly while the teen conforms to portrayal norms by seeming sexually abstinent. This avoids the necessity of sanctions and keeps other teens from seeing that their peers are violating norms. If the norm violation becomes known, for example through a visible pregnancy, then it is best for public sanctions to be levied against the teen by norm enforcers. The worst outcome from a norm enforcer's perspective is for a teen to violate sexuality norms both in her private behaviors and public portrayals, without being known to have faced negative sanctions. This situation would likely teach other teens that they do not need to follow norms. Giving a school award to a pregnant teen, a seemingly rare decision made by Bethany's school to which she objects strongly in Chapter 5, is an example of this dynamic.

This hierarchy of goals for norm enforcers is clear in the following chapters. For example, Chapter 5 shows that most schools try to teach teens norms and rationales so they'll internalize those norms and understand the negative consequences that happen to those who violate them. Schools' silence around sexuality outside of sex education class seeks to prevent the sexual activities of teens who are violating norms from becoming known. If violations do become public knowledge, as they are for visibly pregnant girls, the girl may be informally encouraged to leave. This serves the dual purpose of making her norm violation invisible and showing that the school sanctioned her (even though it is illegal for a public school to expel a pregnant girl, many students view pregnant girls disappearing from school as a deliberate sanction on the school's part). As this example shows, norm enforcers and targets engage in complicated strategies to achieve their goals.

NORM ENFORCER AND NORM TARGET STRATEGIES

This chapter focuses on two key theoretical ideas about norms. The first, discussed above, is that norms about teen sexuality come in sets that can seem inconsistent until the underlying rationale is considered. The second is that a better understanding of norms' effectiveness in a given situation can be gained by weighing the available norm enforcer strategies against the available norm target strategies. Table 2.1 presents these strategies and norm outcomes. But it's important to note that other factors unrelated to norms also shape people's behaviors.

NORM TARGET OUTCOMES

Although it's important to understand the different norms in a set and the rationales underlying them, the individual-level phenomena these norms seek to regulate should also be considered. These "norm target outcomes" are chains of closely related behaviors, emotions, portrayals of behaviors and emotions, and sanctions. The norms and metanorms in a set are intended to influence these outcomes, but they may or may not succeed. Success or failure depends in large part on the strategies of norm enforcers and norm targets, who are trying to control the norm outcomes. Norm enforcers' and targets' strategies may reinforce each other or conflict. The most effective kind of social control happens when a norm target internalizes a norm.[37] When that happens, the norm target outcomes tend to conform to the norm set. This "soft power" form of social control for regulating teenagers' sexuality can be quite effective, but many American parents exercise "hard power" instead.[38] In this more explicit but less effective "hard power" type of norm enforcer strategy that is the focus of Table 2.1, greater efforts are directed at controlling a teen's norm outcomes than at convincing the teen to internalize the norm and self-regulate.

As later chapters show, younger teenagers from all sorts of communities have usually internalized the norms, metanorms, and rationales that they have learned from

TABLE 2.1

Norm enforcer and norm target strategies to control norm target outcomes

Norm Enforcer Strategies	Norm Target Strategies (If Motivated to Violate Norm)
Limit potential for violation	*Facilitate violation*
Decrease privacy of behavior	Increase privacy of behavior
Decrease opportunities to violate	Increase opportunities to violate
Emphasize negative consequences	*Reduce negative consequences*
Outcomes (problems violation will cause)	Hide behavior
Sanctions (problems sanctions will cause)	Justify behavior
Minimize positive consequences	Emphasize positive consequences
Change relationships to discourage violation	*Change relationships to facilitate violation*
Increase dependence on norm enforcer	Seek independence from norm enforcer
Limit reference groups/norms	Expand and choose reference groups/norms

Norm Target Outcomes

Behaviors

Emotions

Portrayals

Sanctions

their social contexts. They behave, talk, and feel in ways that conform to community expectations. But as teenagers grow older, more and more peers are behaving and talking about sex in new ways that violate community norms. Although peer groups don't usually create a conflicting norm in the sense that teenagers who refuse to have sex are socially sanctioned by peers, a new social space is opened up in which teens who want to be sexual can do so without facing as many peer sanctions. Friends often help each other by creating physical opportunities for sex and maintaining public portrayals of each other as not sexually active (see Chapter 7). When this happens, the norm enforcer goals of parents, school, and community are in conflict with teens' norm target goals, and teens' strategies to achieve their goals may be aided by friends. Teenagers' private sexual behaviors and emotions are no longer regulated by soft power but become a battleground over which teens and adults fight for control. Sociologist Amy Schalet points out that this dramatized "conflict" metaphor, in which adults and teens are expected to struggle over teens' sexuality, is a common cultural frame in the United States, but not in some other developed countries.[39] In the Netherlands, parents instead continue to use soft power by adjusting their social norms to acknowledge the appropriateness of their teenager's sexual activity as long as it happens in socially approved ways—in a committed relationship, with effective contraception, and without disrupting the family system or the teen's life. Teenagers are expected to internalize these norms and self-regulate to adhere to them. Although a few of my interviewees talked about specific parents they knew who approached teen sexuality in this way (some of whom were European), it was rare in any U.S. community in my study.

NORM ENFORCER STRATEGIES

In line with an active view of culture that expects individuals and institutions to take action in pursuit of their interests, I expect both teens (norm targets) and the people and institutions surrounding them (norm enforcers) to deploy a variety of strategies to meet their goals.[40] These strategies are not necessarily conscious; cognitive psychology has shown that unconscious drivers of behavior are very powerful and are influenced by cultural phenomena like social norms.[41] I consider the framework laid out here to be complementary to some other theories of human behavior such as the theory of planned behavior or the theory of conjunctural action.[42] This is almost certainly not a complete list of the strategies used by the people and institutions in this book. Other cases besides teen sexuality and other contexts besides the United States will have even more norm enforcer and norm target strategies to add. Not all of the strategies in Table 2.1 are available in every situation, and the availability and success of different strategies can help explain whether the outcomes ultimately conform to norms or to teens' preferences. Norm enforcers' and norm targets' strategies are often in play simultaneously, but one will outweigh the other in shaping norm outcomes.

Limit potential for violation

A particularly effective strategy for norm enforcers is to structure the norm target's social environment so that it is difficult to violate a norm. Decreasing the available opportunities for violating a norm is one option. For a behavior like Internet "trolling" (posting offensive, usually anonymous, online comments), norm enforcer institutions might enact anti-trolling measures such as moderating and removing particularly offensive comments. Individuals might refuse to let known trolls stay in their online groups. Together these actions reduce opportunities for trolling. In the case of teen sex, limiting the availability of contraception, abortion, and informative sex education are strategies some norm enforcers use to make (at least trouble-free) teen sexual activity more difficult.

For behaviors that are performed privately, norm enforcers can also restrict opportunities for norm violation by limiting privacy. Sexual behavior typically requires private time and space. The coming chapters show individual and institutional norm enforcers trying to restrict opportunities for teens' privacy and teens collaborating to strategize opportunities within these constraints. As Finn and others discuss, parents give teens curfews and set rules that remove teens' privacy when they have opposite-sex friends at home. To counteract these strategies, teens may leave the house and try to find places to have sex in cars, or wait to have sex at home when their parents aren't around. Law enforcement, community members, and after-dark closures of public spaces work to restrict teenagers' options to evade parents' control of physical opportunities for sex.

Emphasize negative consequences

While the first category of norm enforcer strategies involves manipulating the social environment so that norm violation is more difficult, the other two categories have to do with socially discouraging norm violation. Communicating norms in such a way that the negative consequences of norm violation are both clear and credible is a less direct form of social control, but it can be effective. Norm enforcers often communicate the problems that the norm violation itself will cause (see Chapter 3). Those espousing a practical rationale emphasize the problems sex and pregnancy can cause for teens' socioeconomic attainment and future relationships. Those who favor a moral rationale may underscore moral and religious consequences of teen sex, such as damnation or a loss of self-respect.

Norm enforcers can also emphasize, rather than the problems caused by the norm violation itself, the problems caused by the negative *sanctions* the norm target will face. The coming chapters show that these sanctions range from being kicked out of the house, to being encouraged to leave school, to social exclusion among peers or in one's religious community. If norm enforcers can point to *cautionary tales* in the community—other teens who have violated norms and actually received these sanctions—then this strategy carries more weight.

This dynamic encourages the sanctioning of teens who are known to have violated norms in order to set an example for others. The experiences of teen mothers who are regularly sanctioned by strangers on buses, in medical offices, and walking down the street show that this strategy is commonplace. These sanctions aren't productive for regulating teen mothers' behavior—after all, they can't undo their childbearing. Rather, they're likely meant to be effective at showing other teenagers the sanctions they will face if they violate such a strong norm. Some have argued that this is the point of the popular reality shows focused on teen mothers. In the online magazine

Everyday Feminism, Raquel Reichard asserts, "Just about every episode of the MTV reality show *16 and Pregnant* has a scene where the new mom is 'reminded' that her pregnancy or baby has 'robbed' her of her social life and ends with her talking into a web cam, expressing her regret for not waiting to have a child."[43] Although my interviewees didn't bring up media as a crucial communicator of the messages they heard about teen sex, perhaps because media messages are often received subconsciously, media may reinforce the messages they hear in their community, making strong norms seem widespread.

Finally, norm enforcers can minimize evidence of any positive consequences of norm violation. This strategy is clearly seen in this book. Discussion with teens of sex bringing pleasure or promoting emotional closeness in a relationship, for instance, is essentially nonexistent in families, communities, or sex education curricula. Norm enforcers try to keep teens ignorant of the benefits of sex by reducing their access to information that portrays it in a positive light. Thus, norm enforcers try to block teens' access to pornography (for this reason among others) but show them the notorious "STD slide show" that many interviewees describe.

Change relationships to discourage violation

Another way to socially discourage norm violation is to structure the norm target's social relationships in ways that dissuade such behavior. First, norm enforcers can work to increase the norm target's dependence on them. Social exchange theory focuses on power in social relationships and defines power as the ability to control someone's behavior—and such control is at the heart of struggles between norm enforcers and norm targets.[44] In social exchange theory, power is created by dependence. People who really need something that another person has will have less power than the person who controls that resource. In the case of teen sexuality, most school-age teens are in a very dependent position, both in terms of material resources and social relationships. Their parents have legal control over their bodies and provide most of the resources they need to survive and create a promising future, so they are highly dependent on parents. Schools, and to a lesser extent other community institutions, also hold the keys to teens' future socioeconomic success. With so much of social life at this age revolving around school, many teens are highly dependent on their schoolmates because social exclusion from this group leaves them with few options for friendships. Because of this strong dependence on others, high school-age teenagers tend to be more motivated to conform to norms than they will be a few years later.

Norm enforcers can also try to structure norm targets' social relationships so that they rarely see norm violation and have few options for alternative reference groups that may communicate competing norms. Among my interviewees, this strategy worked best in isolated rural areas, where group cohesion and homogeneity were high and opportunities for contact with alternative social groups were very limited. In other communities where diverse norm sets do exist, norm enforcers must be more strategic in controlling the norms being communicated to teens in their social relationships. To do this, many norm enforcers' strategies mimic isolated communities by trying to cut off social contacts with alternative norms. In hybrid communities with multiple norm sets, race and class divisions are stark as the higher-status group with stronger or more morally motivated norms about teen sexuality works to minimize contact with the lower-status group. Not just teens, but adults and schools, may seek to reduce this intergroup contact.

Limiting alternative social groups may also promote the second strategy in this category, reducing the number of targets who are seen as "getting away with" violating the norm. The ideal way to do this is to make the violators invisible. Some schools with particularly strong norms against teen parenthood take this tactic with pregnant teen girls, working within the constraints of legal protections to move them out of the school or into a special program that limits their interaction with mainstream students. If norm violators cannot be made invisible, another strategy is to sanction them publicly so they can become a cautionary tale providing evidence of the norm's strength.

NORM TARGET STRATEGIES

When a teenager has internalized adults' norms about teen sexuality (like the younger teens in my U.S. data or teens of any age in Amy Schalet's Dutch sample), her norm outcomes (behaviors, emotions, public portrayals, and sanctioning) tend to be socially approved. But in the situation this book describes that is common in the later high school years in the United States, many teens seek to violate norms despite the social control they are experiencing. In that case, they need to strategize toward the goal of behaving as they like without facing sanctions. Because that goal is in conflict with norm enforcers' goals, teens' strategies tend to conflict with the norm enforcers' strategies. See Chapter 7 for more details on teens' strategies.

Facilitate violation

While norm enforcers try to limit the norm target's potential for violating, norm targets who want to violate the norm will work to structure their social environments in ways that facilitate norm violation. Increasing opportunities to violate norms is an important strategy. For example, creating opportunities to escape monitoring by norm enforcers (whether adults or institutions) can enable norm violation. Holding parties without adult supervision can help teens escape monitoring by adults, but they are still heavily monitored by each other, and casual sex at parties (at least for girls) is rarely condoned by the peer groups my interviewees described. Instead, time spent in an empty house or on a trip either alone with a partner or with close friends may be more effective at avoiding the monitoring of adults, institutions (such as schools or religious organizations), and peers.

With private behaviors like sexuality, teens have greater potential for successful strategies because a person's public portrayal of her behavior can be different from her private behavior. To counteract norm enforcers who seek to exercise social control by minimizing privacy, norm targets work to maximize it. The more private a behavior is, the more control the target has over his public portrayal of the behavior, allowing him to behave as he likes without facing sanctions. This situation weakens norm enforcers' control over behavior, which is why adults and institutions in this book work so hard to limit teens' options for sexual privacy. Maximizing privacy is another reason why teens often avoid the "me having sex talk" and cultivate conspiracies of silence around sexuality. Disclosing sexual behavior to peers is a risky strategy because of reputation, but collective action among close friends can broaden a teen's options for keeping her behavior private from adults.

But there are disadvantages when private behaviors are uncoupled from public portrayals. Unfounded rumors can damage the reputations of people who aren't violating a norm (for example, a norm against having sex with multiple partners) because their conformity to the norm can't be publicly proven. This is how so many of the teen mothers ended up with unfair reputations as promiscuous and slutty. Stereotypes that are gendered, raced, and classed come into play in labeling a girl (or more rarely a boy), and because sexual behavior is private, she has no way of rebutting the accusations. So although interviewees didn't address this directly, to me it's clear that increasing the privacy of teens' sexual behavior is a double-edged sword for teens.

Reduce negative consequences

Teens' strategies of increasing the privacy of sexual behavior can serve to hide the behavior. Hiding behavior that violates a norm is an important way in which a norm target can reduce the negative consequences associated with norm violation. Teen sexual behaviors, which are usually private, are more easily hidden than other behaviors like mowing a lawn or running a red light. As in Brooke's case, many parents collaborate with their teens to make it more feasible to keep sexual activity hidden.

This helps parents avoid levying damaging sanctions on the teen but also avoid facing metanormative sanctions for refusing to sanction the teen.

If hiding the behavior is unsuccessful, a teen can work to justify the behavior to others by demonstrating her conformity to the rationale underlying the norm. The most straightforward way is denial of responsibility by calling the behavior a "mistake," an option that is differentially available to teens depending on their gender, class, and race. For teen parents who have violated a strong norm, emphasizing that they agree with their community's rationale is a strategy to minimize negative sanctions. A teen mother can try to claim the moral rationale, for example, by pointing out that she didn't get an abortion. Logan talked about how his family and religious community viewed this strategy positively: "Abortion is kind of like, just compounding the mistake [of unintended pregnancy]. So if you get pregnant, you're [supposed to stay] pregnant." Girls who stay pregnant in Logan's community are allowed to call their premarital sex and pregnancy a "mistake," presumably facing less negative sanctions than those who are known to have had an abortion. More commonly, teen parents try to emphasize their adherence to the practical rationale by talking about their socioeconomic success. Adriana's response to people who sanction her is, "I still go to school." Teen fathers often talk about being saved from a life of crime by their children.

The final strategy norm targets engage in to reduce negative consequences of norm violations is to emphasize the positive consequences of sexual behavior. Behaviors that social norms seek to control tend to have "upsides." Sex and drinking can be fun, refusing to leave tips to restaurant servers leaves you with more money, and so on. Sexual desire can be a strong motivation to violate norms. Even though norm enforcers seek to limit information about the positive consequences of teen sexual behavior, norm targets can try to find alternative sources of information to supplement these messages. Interviewees talked about having asked close friends or "safe" adults for information about sex when they were in high school. Because alternative information is pretty easy to find, the norm target strategy is often stronger than the norm enforcer strategy in this case. Later in high school, peers often start talking about sexual desire and sexual activity being "normal." Believing that others are violating a norm can increase the likelihood that people violate a norm themselves, perhaps because the normality of the behavior is seen as a positive consequence.[45]

Change relationships to facilitate violation

Just as norm enforcers can try to structure norm targets' social relationships to make norm violation more difficult, norm targets can work to create social relationships that enable norm violation. As norm enforcers seek to increase the resource dependence of norm targets on them, norm targets can try to reduce that dependence. I didn't see this strategy as much among my main interviewees, perhaps because their parents often had a lot of resources for which the teens were willing to exchange dependence. But among the teen parents, who came from socioeconomically disadvantaged families and communities, the "carrots" of current well-being and future success that parents, schools, and communities could dangle to make teens willingly dependent weren't always as tempting. Making the decision to reduce dependence by becoming financially independent, moving out, or leaving school wasn't as scary when dependence didn't provide as much of an upside to begin with. Many teen parents at least initially tried to take such dependence-reducing steps, for example by moving in with someone else, as Adriana did for a while. Sometimes that strategy worked and they became more self-reliant in their resources and social contacts, but sometimes they ended up in dire straits and willingly returned to their families' and schools' social control.

Expanding one's available social groups to create alternative normative contexts is another norm target strategy that can work against norm enforcers' efforts to constrain alternative normative messages. By decreasing the consensus about a single norm set in one's social context, a norm target can choose which norm he wants to conform to among multiple options. For example, sociologist Amy Wilkins has written about young people who seek out subcultures—like Goths, born-again Christians, and Puerto Rican wannabes—to develop identities in groups that provide some alternatives to mainstream norms about youth sexuality.[46] A group can also work together to create an alternative normative context. This is what teens did during their older years at many of my interviewees' high schools, framing sexual activity as "normal" and helping each other evade adults' social control. This is a group-level strategy among norm targets rather than an individual-level strategy. Chapter 7 includes many examples of teens strategizing collectively about their sexuality because groups often have more power than individuals to enact strategies.

If all else fails and a teen can't avoid negative sanctions, she can try to push back using alternative identity strategies. Teen parents do a lot of internal identity work to minimize internal damage from people's negative social reactions. For Nicole and Christian in Chapter 7, reminding themselves of their strong identities as good parents helps minimize the damaging effects of social sanctions. This internal process of "narrative repair" can be quite powerful.[47] As I heard from the teen parent interviewees, teens who are socially ostracized at school can also create alternative identities outside of school with other friendship groups or with an older romantic partner.

Weighing the success of norm enforcers' strategies used on a norm target against the success of the norm targets' strategies tells us something about how effective normative control is likely to be. Norms are ineffective when they result in norm target outcomes that don't conform to the norm set, and they are effective when the outcomes conform. For example, if norm targets are in a social context in which they hear a strong and consistent normative message proscribing a behavior, attaching serious sanctions to its violation, and making the behavior sound not fun, and in which their privacy to engage in that behavior is strictly controlled, their norm target strategies are likely to be less successful than the norm enforcers' strategies. Their behaviors are likely to conform to the norm set. In contrast, if norm targets have a lot of freedom to choose among alternative normative contexts, are not dependent on norm enforcers, don't perceive serious sanctions for norm violation, and have leeway to behave one way and portray their behavior another, their behavior is less likely to conform to the norm. This helps explain why there is sometimes a weak link between norms and behaviors.[48] Although I use behavior in this discussion, the same processes may apply to the other norm outcomes of emotions, portrayals of behavior, and sanctions.

It can be complicated to judge the effectiveness of a norm. For example, Brooke says that in her community, most teens were having sex, but few parents knew about it and few teens were getting pregnant. Thus, parents thought teens were conforming to their norms, and teens successfully avoided sanctions. This situation is ineffective in terms of the anti-sex norm controlling teens' actual sexual activity, but it is effective in terms of teens' public portrayals and their avoidance of damaging sanctions and some other negative consequences of sex.

NORMS AND SOCIAL INEQUALITIES

Throughout this book's description of norms and social control around U.S. teens' sexuality runs a strong thread of social inequality. As group-level phenomena, normative processes can validate people's social identities, contributing to inequalities.[49] Power and inequalities also profoundly shape normative processes.[50] Norms and social control are tools of power, and they both reflect and create social inequalities. Norms themselves are different depending on who you are, often benefitting more advantaged teens. A minority teen having sex with a longtime partner may be judged more harshly than a White teen, or a girl judged more harshly than a boy. Social control is also applied unequally.[51] The same behavior, such as having unprotected sex that could result in a pregnancy, can be interpreted as either a major norm violation or a "mistake" that isn't a true norm violation, depending on who that person is. There are also inequalities in who has the means to conform to the normative standards to which they are being held. For example, for this generation of teens, effective contraception methods and the healthcare needed to prescribe them were both quite expensive. And there are inequalities in who gets to apply social control and what strategies they can use. In Brooke's case, high-status religious groups "promoted abstinence" and engaged with teens in an attempt to control their behavior. Taken together, all of these processes show that norms and social control both reflect existing social inequalities and actively strengthen them. This research answers a call for more work on how social status shapes the consequences of norm violations.[52]

Gender is the most obvious factor that makes the content or strength of teen sexuality norms vary for different people.[53] A social norm is only a norm if the social rule has sanctions attached to it—if people don't care enough about your behavior to sanction you for behaving wrongly, it isn't a norm. Chapter 4 shows that some of the people in boys' social contexts aren't prepared to sanction them if they have sex. This is true for some girls, but not as many. Norm enforcers generally communicate stronger norms against teen sex and pregnancy to girls than to boys, and they promise girls stronger sanctions if they don't comply.

As the stronger threatened sanctions against girls suggest, social control is also applied unequally to different people. Peers' social exclusion of pregnant and parenting teens, or of teens who are rumored to be promiscuous or to have had an abortion, usually extends only to girls. Much of the time when interviewees discussed teen pregnancies or births at their schools, they talked a lot about the mother but didn't even know who the father of the child was. This suggests that he didn't face many social sanctions from peers.

Much has been written about inequalities in the social control of sexuality.[54] Besides holding women more strictly than men to sexual standards, communities also tend to "rig" the system to more strictly control racial minorities and people with lower SES.[55] Bodily purity and abstinence are values that can be used strategically to heighten boundaries between higher- and lower-status groups.[56] If people from the latter groups don't adhere to the stricter normative standards, it is taken as proof that they deserve their lower-status position in society. Chapter 3 shows that social norms and their underlying rationales link teen sexuality to socioeconomic success, intelligence, and morality. The practical rationale judges teens who have unprotected sex as stupid and bound for failure. The moral rationale deems teens who have premarital sex or an abortion to be immoral sinners. Both of these rationales assign deeply seated personal flaws to teens who violate sexuality norms that label them as undeserving of success.

The puzzle that makes this reasoning particularly interesting is that, as Brooke noted of her community, most teenagers *do* violate sexuality norms by the end of high school. Because this happens, people exercising social control have the opportunity to choose whom to sanction. They can excuse the temporary "mistakes" of some teenagers while holding others deeply accountable for their norm violations. Lillian pointed to this process when she said that girls in her low-income community and girls in a wealthy White suburb start to have sex at about the same ages, but she thought the privileged people "talk all this shit about how you think they're [girls in the low-income community are] having sex and doing all this shit when they're young." To her, this is a double standard that excuses wealthier White girls for the same behavior that condemns lower-income minority girls. Ethnographic research supports Lillian's impression.[57]

Publicly portraying oneself as sexually restrained is part of what labels a teen (especially a girl) as deserving of success in life, particularly socioeconomic success. There are differences between the practical and the moral rationales' definitions of sexual restraint—for the former, it is preferably virginity but may implicitly be consistently "careful" sex, while virginity is the only accepted standard for the latter. As long as a privileged teen is very careful to hide signs of sexual activity, she can usually successfully portray herself as sexually restrained, regardless of the community's rationale. This focus on public portrayal is what creates the conditions that allow some teens to get away with norm violations while others are strongly sanctioned.

But the cultural system around teen sexuality is even more rigged than that. Girls who "look like" teen mothers in terms of race, ethnicity, or class are often considered guilty of a lack of sexual restraint, *even when there is no objective evidence to support that assumption.*[58] Julie Bettie's ethnography of a racially and socioeconomically heterogeneous high school found that both teachers and peers automatically assumed Latinas and girls on less rigorous academic tracks were sexually active and destined for teen motherhood. In contrast, college-bound White girls actively constructed an image of themselves as sexually restrained by minimizing makeup and strategically selecting the color and cut of clothing, and teachers and peers generally bought into that image. In actuality, Bettie found few differences in the sexual behaviors of these groups of girls. I presume that boys sometimes face similar raced and classed stereotypes about their sexual restraint but that the consequences aren't as severe.[59]

Many teens (especially girls) who are known, or even unfairly suspected, to be sexually unrestrained are considered undeserving of socioeconomic success because they have put themselves at risk of becoming teen parents. The specter of teen parenthood is highly visible in our society, leading to a common perception that the teen birth rate is on the rise when it has actually decreased sharply in the past 20 years.[60] Interviewees from all social groups received consistent messages that becoming a teen parent would ruin their lives. Decades of research from across the social sciences has debunked this myth—on average, becoming a parent has a fairly small negative effect for a teen's future, but there is no effect for some people and some life outcomes.[61] This myth may be so persistent despite a lack of evidence because it allows people to apply the label of "failure" to teens who don't conform to sexuality norms.[62] By having a baby, as about one in seven teen girls in the United States does, a teenager is seen as giving up much of her claim to socioeconomic mobility (if she comes from a lower socioeconomic background) or her right to a middle-class life (if her socioeconomic background is higher).[63] As Lee SmithBattle writes, because of her perceived lack of sexual restraint, a teen mother is seen as having committed "the sin of . . . not planning and rationally choosing her future."[64] From these perceptions come the many vitriolic judgments of teen parents (especially mothers) that interviewees expressed and recounted.

The strong normative focus on teen pregnancy and parenthood serves another purpose: It maintains the focus on public portrayals of sexual behavior rather than on sexual behavior itself. The worst social and material sanctions against teen sexuality are reserved for girls who are visibly pregnant or have children. Knowing that the most severe sanctions aren't going to happen until that point gives teens normative leeway in their private sexual behaviors. They can often get away with having sex as long as they are careful about using contraception. If they don't use contraception, girls' risk of pregnancy from a single sex act is quite low.[65] And as a last resort, if they end up pregnant, abortion is a legal option, though parental consent laws and accessibility may make it more or less feasible in different areas. The stakes are lower for boys, who are unlikely to be sanctioned unless their female partner becomes pregnant and carries the pregnancy to term. And even then, sanctions are less severe for boys.

The class and race differences in teen childbearing are much starker than differences in teen sexual activity.[66] This may be because of the resources needed to be sexually active while avoiding childbearing. Especially in the pre-Affordable Care Act era when my study was conducted, contraception can be quite expensive, particularly the most reliable long-acting/hormonal forms. Abortion is often prohibitively expensive for lower-income girls, especially once transportation costs are factored in since 87% of U.S. counties do not contain a healthcare facility that performs abortions.[67] What all of this means is that socioeconomically privileged and White teens, especially boys, are more able to avoid the severe sanctions that come with teen parenthood. Less privileged and minority teens disproportionately end up sanctioned and labeled as deserving of failure in life.

But as this book shows, these social control processes are actively countered by teenagers' strategies. Most teen parent interviewees had expended considerable time and energy creating new identity strategies to push back against people's judgments. These strategies look different depending on the rationale in the teen's community. Teens pushing back against a moral rationale say that their choice not to have an abortion makes them moral people who deserve success. To push back against a practical rationale, teen parents talk about how much harder they are working at being socioeconomically successful than their childless peers are, or than they themselves were before becoming parents. This hard work makes them deserving of socioeconomic success. Besides the examples of these strategies given in the book, there are many others throughout the teen parent interviews.

This kind of identity work can be successful for protecting a teen from internalizing negative social judgments, but it may be less useful for changing the minds of the people who are doing the sanctioning. My interviewees suggest that lower-SES communities do give some credence to the moral and practical claims the teen parents are making, although norms against teen parenthood are still strong.[68] Older people in Annika's isolated mining town sometimes praise teen mothers for refusing to get an abortion, and people in Lillian's urban neighborhood exhort teens to be kind to teen mothers because "you could be in that situation." But my teen parent interviewees from communities like these are clearly not forgiven for their violation of sexuality norms. They face stigma on a regular basis and often feel powerless to prevent people from judging them. Higher-SES communities lend even less legitimacy to teen parents' claims. Because people from these communities are more likely to be gatekeepers for the socioeconomic success of teens from lower-SES families (such as teachers, school administrators, and leaders of community organizations), this lack of forgiveness may have important implications.

Although most research on social norms tends to focus on within-group dynamics, the intergroup dynamics around teen sexuality norms are fascinating and important for understanding social inequalities. Teen sexuality is a highly salient social dividing line in a way that not all normatively regulated behaviors are. It is often used to justify and strengthen intergroup boundaries. Higher-status groups make negative assumptions about the sexuality of teens from lower-status groups, perhaps to label them as undeserving so that their low likelihood of socioeconomic success feels justified. Whether there were multiple social groups within their own community or they were just talking about other people outside their community, interviewees tended to focus attention on differences between their own group's norms about teen sexuality and those of other groups, which were used to justify metanorms regulating differential sanctioning of teens. The importance of teen sexuality for intergroup relations may be part of what makes Americans view it as such a serious social problem.

But the negative sanctioning of low-status groups around teen sexuality isn't limited to teens themselves. Higher-status people also tend to perceive that the lower-status group isn't appropriately sanctioning sexually deviating teens, which allows them to think of *all* the members of that community as violators of a metanorm about the regulation of teens' sexual behavior. This can give rise to negative stereotypes about the deservingness of success of *everyone* in the lower-status group. Rochelle, who came from a racially divided low-income community, focused primarily on the racial divide when talking about teen sexuality norms. She spent at least as much time judging the whole Latino community for inappropriately sanctioning teen mothers as she did talking about the teen mothers themselves. When I asked how common teen pregnancy was in her high school, she immediately transitioned to repeating her earlier story about the Latina students who allegedly said, "Oh, let's have a party in the hallway, you're pregnant!" To Rochelle, this lack of negative sanctioning by peers and adults seemed to be as problematic as teen motherhood itself.

Both within and between social groups, norms can be a source of conflicts and inequalities. Norm enforcement is contested both by teenage norm targets and by the different people and organizations that seek to influence teens' behaviors. Interviewees' representations of normative processes can seem chaotic, but there are identifiable patterns and predictable processes. These processes represent dynamics of *power*, conceptualized by sociologist Vincent Roscigno as "the constitutive interplay of structure, culture, and action" created by interpersonal interactions and people's invocations of structure and legitimations of social inequalities.[69] In this perspective, norms and social control are manifestations of power.

Taken together, the stories in this book show that social inequalities are fundamental to understanding normative processes around teen sexuality in the United States. People's place in the system of social inequalities affects their behavior, but it also shapes how that behavior is interpreted, what messages they hear about it, and how people react to their behavior. These reactions have very real consequences for young people's lives. Sanctions are applied selectively to teens in ways that tend to privilege higher-status people, and more privileged teens often have the opportunities and the means to be sexual while publicly portraying themselves as sexually restrained. But the very few[70] higher-status teens who violate strong norms by becoming parents potentially face quite negative sanctions.[71] Almost none of my teen parent interviewees came from these privileged groups, and there were few cases the college student interviewees could think of. But a few examples in the coming chapters suggest that higher-status parents sometimes follow through on their threats of extreme sanctions in this situation.

NORMS AND CONFLICT

Earlier sections have laid out strategies and counterstrategies in the struggle between norm enforcers and norm targets over teens' behaviors, portrayals, emotions, and sanctions. This active way of looking at normative processes addresses one of the major critiques of existing conceptions of norms because it incorporates conflict between normative prescriptions and individual agency.[72] This section lays out other ways conflict can be incorporated into normative processes.

Conflicts over control of people's behaviors, emotions, and sanctions are inevitable unless norm enforcers are successfully able to use soft power to convince the norm target to internalize a norm. When that happens, conflict doesn't arise because the teen does what both she and the norm enforcers want. Chapter 4 shows that this is typical of younger teens, most of whom are not yet motivated to be sexually active. But as soon as targets become motivated to deviate from a norm, their preferences come into conflict with those of norm enforcers. Sometimes this conflict is overt, like the sanctioning of those who violate a norm through social exclusion or resource withholding. In Brooke's community, pregnant girls were "judged" and gossiped about severely enough that the prospect of this judgment instilled fear in teens and their parents. But sometimes the conflict can be covert, operating under the surface without anyone acknowledging its existence. The struggles between teenagers and adults over access to information about the upsides of sexuality and over the privacy of teens' sexual behaviors are good examples. The conspiracies of silence most parents and teens collaborate in minimize open conflict about teens' sexual behavior, but teens are aware of the covert struggles happening beneath the surface. Alexis called it a "denial thing." Patton emphasized that "there were signs" that parents could see about their teens' sexual activity, but he said "they didn't want to know what their kid was doing . . . It was maybe too much for them to think about or face."

But conflict between norm enforcers and norm targets isn't the only kind of struggle going on. Besides these conflicts over teens' behavior, emotions, portrayals, and sanctions, there are conflicts over the content of norms themselves, who exercises social control, and what strategies they use to exercise it. I describe such conflicts in Chapters 5 and 6, and research on struggles for control of sex education lays them out in greater detail.[73] In higher-SES communities, parents are considered appropriate channels of social control, but in lower-SES or minority communities, parents are often not trusted to communicate the right norms or enforce them thoroughly. Alana talked about this in a way that discredits the influence of any parent from a divorced family, making teens in divorced families sound like orphans: "The poor minority kids who were having the babies . . . you know the statistics. Most of their parents were divorced. So it's not like they had their parents to help them." As I discuss in Chapter 6, questioning parents' legitimacy as norm enforcers can strengthen school administrators', teachers', and community organizations' efforts to control teens.

There's a general rule underlying this dynamic: People with more power and status are seen as more appropriate norm enforcers. But when the same person is both a norm enforcer and target, people with more power and status are also held to a less strict standard for their own behavior—which means they can behave in ways that conform less to norms while actively holding lower-status people to a stricter standard.[74] I saw this dynamic among some interviewees, who actively sanctioned lower-status teens for their (usually assumed rather than verified) sexual behavior while excusing their own and their friends' verified deviant behavior as "mistakes." Rochelle's vitriolic portrayal of the Puerto Rican teens in her community as sexually deviant, while simultaneously not condemning her White peers (who, she later admitted, engaged in similar behaviors) for their actions, is a good example. But some lower-status teens, like Lillian in her tirade against the "way nastier" wealthy teens who judge the sexuality of people like her, fight back against these stereotypes. So even among relatively powerless teens, conflict over norms and social control is widespread.

HOW NORMS CHANGE

A final important criticism of traditional ideas about norms is that we don't know how norms change, even though there is evidence that they do.[75] The case of teen sexuality in the United States can shed some light on this question, though my data are limited by their short retrospective horizon. We know that norms about teen sexuality are different than in previous generations—for example, in many communities, teen girls who have carefully protected sex within a heterosexual romantic relationship and who don't talk a lot about their sexual activity can avoid severe sanctions now, but they would have been judged harshly several decades ago.[76]

Conflict is one of the main ways that change in norms occurs. Interviewees talk about a change happening among teens over the course of their high school years. Most of them start out having internalized the norm sets their communities communicate. By the end of high school, many interviewees still personally agree with those normative messages, but many more have begun to adopt a critical stance that questions the norm against teen sex while continuing to internalize the one against teen parenthood. As has been shown, a growing number of teens who question the norm against teen sex creates a change in the normative context that has implications for teens' behaviors and the effectiveness of adults' social control. This is the result of collective action taken by people who individually question a norm.[77]

Conflict can also lead to change when new, related norms enter a norm set or existing ones become stronger within a set. The most obvious example from this book is the rapid growth in the importance of anti-abortion norms described by interviewees from highly religious communities. When I was a teenager in a rural low-income community in the 1990s, both the anti-abortion norm and the anti-teen parenthood norm were present in the norm set and supported by the moral rationale, just like today. But their relative importance was different—sanctioning unwed teen mothers was paramount, and I don't think it would have occurred to many people to praise them for having refused to get an abortion. Finn talked about how this norm changed in his highly religious, higher-income community during the time he was in high school, the result of a movie about teen pregnancy that linked teen pregnancy to abortion spurring conversations among teens and between teens and parents. He suggested that the community has arrived at a new norm about how to talk publicly about the issue—praising teen parents for not having had an abortion and discouraging abortion for teenagers—but he also thought teens' actual abortion behaviors in private and their parents' suggestions about how to resolve pregnancies might not yet mirror the norm change.

Sociologist Janet Jacobs and I have also written about the change in norms over 20 years that she saw in the low-income minority communities served by a school for teen mothers.[78] Norms against teen parenthood became stronger over this time and shifted from having a moral rationale to a stronger practical rationale. We linked this change in norms to the worsening financial circumstances of low-income and minority families in an era of rising income inequality. Families now communicate to teens that they need to succeed in life so they can be financially independent and support their family members. Like others in the United States, families view teen parenthood as socioeconomic failure.[79] They anticipate correctly that in the short term, teen parents will usually not be financially independent and will need lots of resources from their already overextended family members. Although many teen parents initially think they can establish financial independence, few manage it in the short term. Families' expectations of longer-term failure aren't supported by research evidence looking at earlier cohorts of Americans, but this research has not permeated popular conceptions of the impacts of teen parenthood.[80] It's hard to tell what the longer-term implications of early parenthood will be for today's teenagers growing up under conditions of greater inequality and uncertainty.

As this example suggests, changes over time in the content and importance of norms in a set can be the result of changes to the rationale underlying the norm set. That rationale is responsive to changing cultural and material circumstances. The practical rationale underlying norms against teen sex, contraception, and pregnancy is dependent on the socioeconomic circumstances of the teens who are the targets of these norms. If conditions worsen or become more uncertain, as they have in recent years, the practical rationale may strengthen or change. As Finn described above, changes in the moral rationale happened as the anti-abortion movement became an increasingly visible component of the "religious Right's" moral discourse.[81]

Another important way norms can change is when norm targets' options for violating a norm or norm enforcers' alternatives for preventing norm violation change. Social upheavals in the gender system and in medical control of fertility have influenced the social control of sexuality in the past several decades.[82] Since its introduction in 1960, the birth control pill has given women the option of having heterosexual intercourse while keeping the risk of pregnancy low.[83] The legalization of abortion in 1973 further expanded women's control over their own fertility. Both of these changes affected the normative climate of teen sex.[84] For girls, having sex used to come with a high risk of publicly portraying oneself as sexually active because of the higher likelihood of pregnancy with no legal option for abortion. After these two new developments, both boys and girls could keep their sexual behavior more private and reduce potentially negative consequences, which I have identified as a norm target strategy that helps people evade social control.

Another important change is the introduction of Title IX in 1972. Title IX protects against a broad set of gender discrimination practices in institutions that receive public funding, and it includes protections for pregnant and parenting teenagers.[85] Although violations still occur, it is illegal for public schools to expel these students or force them into alternative educational programs. The law has thus restricted schools' options for physically and socially controlling pregnant and parenting teenagers. Instead, as Chapter 5 shows, many schools apparently use a variety of complicated workarounds in their attempts to make teen pregnancy invisible.

In general, these three major changes—the pill, the legalization of abortion, and Title IX—have limited norm enforcers' options for preventing teens' violations of sexuality norms. I argue that the first two trends leading to the increased privacy of sexual behavior have made teens' public portrayals of their behavior a more important focus of norms in recent years. As Brooke said, because of these societal changes that have made it possible to be sexually active without becoming visibly pregnant, parents have the option to ask their teens to "not tell me about it" if they violate sex norms. Social control can still influence public portrayals, even if it has a harder time influencing private behaviors.

Finally, norms can change if the power dependence relationship between the norm enforcers and the norm target changes. Societal trends have increased the dependence of many teens on their parents, although rising inequalities may not make this true of all teens. Young middle- and upper-class people have become financially dependent on their parents for increasingly long periods, giving rise to the label of "emerging adulthood" for a new, socially classed life phase in the late teens and early 20s.[86] Rising college costs have outpaced inflation, making it very difficult to pay for one's own higher education without parental support.[87] The decreasing value of the minimum wage has reduced the financial independence of working teenagers,[88] and high unemployment rates among young people and those with less education have reduced employment options for other teens.[89] At the same time, the average age at first marriage has risen steadily for decades and is now in the late 20s for U.S. women and men.[90] These trends have made many teens more dependent on their parents while lengthening the period of time during which their sexual activity may not be socially approved.

To sum up, in the past few decades the privacy of sexual behaviors has increased, especially for girls. This has broadened teens' possibilities for being sexual without publicly violating norms and has decreased norm enforcers' control over teens' behaviors. Schools can no longer legally sanction pregnant and parenting teens as severely as in the past. But macroeconomic trends have increased teens' dependence on adults, both in their current lives and into their foreseeable futures. Listening to the interviews, I see that these trends seem to have resulted in many communities' norms focusing on planned, "careful" teen sex that avoids public portrayals of oneself as sexually active. This is true of Brooke's community, despite its political conservatism. Having sex is discouraged, but in many communities adults are resigned to seeing this decision as ultimately controlled by the teenager and difficult to influence. But because most teens are now so dependent on adults, they are still at least as scared as they were in the past of *publicly* violating norms about teen sexual behavior. If they can pull off "careful" sex successfully and discreetly, though, they are safe from sanctions. This situation gives teenagers greater control over their sexuality, even in more religious communities that morally condemn premarital sex and abortion.

CONCLUSION

Grounded in the real-life dynamics around social regulation of teen sex and pregnancy in the United States, this book provides new conceptual tools for understanding norms and social control and how people navigate these social pressures. This chapter has distilled the theoretical ideas so that they can be useful to people in thinking about other social norms and other settings. The coming chapters more fully develop how these dynamics play out in interviewees' families, peer groups, schools, and communities.

I have argued that we can better understand what makes social norms effective or ineffective if we expand our ideas about norms in several ways. One group of conceptual tools I have developed has to do with multiple norms. Sometimes norms occur in sets, within which norms can conflict or work together. These sets of norms regulate not only behaviors, but also emotions, public portrayals of behaviors, and metanorms. Seemingly contradictory norm sets can be understood by considering the rationale underlying them. Norm sets can be influenced by related norm sets in the same social context.

A second group of conceptual tools developed in this chapter relates to the strategies of norm enforcers and norm targets as they deploy norm sets in an attempt to control targets' behaviors, portrayals, emotions, and sanctions. These strategies involve the well-developed processes of conformity, norm violation, and sanctioning. But they also engage new ideas about how norms are communicated—including metanorms about norm communication to which norm enforcers are held—and how the social environment of relationships and resources in which normative processes play out is manipulated.

This expanded understanding of norms and social control results in a less static view of these processes, one in which norms are being used as tools by social actors to achieve their goals, in which conflict between norms and between social actors is common, and in which norms and behaviors can change quickly. This perspective on norms relates them strongly to social inequalities. Norms and the strategies of norm enforcers and targets are created and constrained by social inequalities. But they are also tools of power through which people can gain or maintain social advantages and keep disadvantaged people powerless. This complicates our understanding of what it means for a norm to be effective. A norm might be effective if people's behaviors conform, or if portrayals and sanctions conform, or even if there is only a weak link to these outcomes but the norm is effective at maintaining the advantages of powerful people and institutions.

An important question is whether these patterns and processes apply to norms that regulate other types of behavior besides teen sexuality. This chapter is meant to generate ideas based on the case of teen sexuality that can then be explored using other cases of norms. I don't have the data to know whether or in what circumstances these theoretical ideas apply to other kinds of norms, so future research using other cases should examine how the theoretical framework can be expanded or refined. For example, norms about homosexuality and marijuana use are changing rapidly in our society, and they are both private behaviors that can be kept separate from public portrayals. Research on adults' medical marijuana use suggests that many of the same normative processes described in this chapter do apply, but adult marijuana users feel quite comfortable openly questioning norms against medical marijuana consumption in an attempt to change those norms.[91] The same is not true for teens questioning sexuality norms. Using the perspective laid out in this chapter, this difference is not surprising because of adults' lower dependence on norm enforcers compared to teens, their greater options for behaving as they like in their own homes, and their opportunities for changing their social relationships to facilitate marijuana use. It would be interesting to study normative dynamics in cases like these in greater depth using this book's lens.

The comparison case my data can begin to address is sexuality norms regulating college students. Many college student interviewees in the first phase of interviews spontaneously compared their communities during high school to the normative climates they were experiencing in college. In the second phase of interviews, my research team asked everyone to compare sexuality norms in their high school to those in college. The differences we saw made sense within this chapter's theoretical framework. College students at this study's largely non-commuter "party school" campus, the same type of higher education setting that has been researched by sociologists Elizabeth Armstrong and Laura Hamilton,[92] live in a very peer-oriented social world. Students are not under near-constant surveillance from teachers and administrators as they were in high school, and their parents and home communities have no physical control over them and don't know what they're up to. This makes social control from adults less relevant, allowing young people to be more open about their sexual behavior in their everyday lives.[93] Of course, norms about this behavior are still gendered, classed, and raced, but both girls and boys are held to much less strict standards than they were in high school.[94] In this context, young people are usually not sanctioned for being sexually active as long as they are consistently "careful" (interestingly, a term that applies to contraception, but not to drinking or sexual violence). There are also more opportunities for casual sexual activity, and the structure of college life may facilitate that kind of sexual behavior.[95] College students' sexual behavior seems to be more heterogeneous than it was in high school, suggesting that norm target strategies reflecting young people's diverse sexual goals may be more successful. Even if young people violate their peer group's sexuality norms, the university is so big and heterogeneous that other friends with different norms can often easily be made.

In this setting with far less social control, interviewees feel they have more power over their own lives and believe that more models of sexual behavior are accepted. And most of all, they no longer feel nearly as afraid. Many still worry about pregnancy or STIs but feel better equipped to handle these risks, despite still engaging in plenty of risky sexual behaviors. But many college students and their parents still participate in the same "conspiracy of silence" around their sexual behavior. The strong financial dependence of most (at least in this setting) college students on their families ensures that whatever they do in college, they don't flaunt their sexual behaviors at home to avoid possible sanctions. This comparison between high school and college sexuality norms suggests that the theoretical ideas laid out here may be useful for thinking about other cases of social norms.

3

"DON'T ASK, DON'T TELL"

Sexuality Norms and Social Control at Home

PARENTS PLAY AN important role in communicating and enforcing norms about teen sexuality. Many interviewees even said their parents were the greatest social influence on them.[1] Alexis and her family illustrate the ways in which this communication and enforcement of norms can happen.

Alexis grew up in a beautiful commuter town in the Rocky Mountains with a wealthy population and highly ranked schools. Although there are plenty of differences from one family to the next, Alexis's family is pretty typical in terms of what norms about sexual behavior are communicated and how they are communicated. Alexis told us:

> I think parents are the biggest driving force . . . even if your school is teaching abstinence-only [sex education], the parents themselves can still go to the child and say, "Well, this is what's really happening." I feel like for a lot of parents, sex ed[ucation] becomes a way out of that responsibility of teaching their child those things, just because it is awkward for them. But really at the end of the day, at least for me, my parents were my biggest social influence. Like, that's where I got most of my views on how society works, and how I fit into society, and what society would think of me.

Alexis thinks a lot of parents don't talk with teens about sex as much as they should, but parents still communicate the bigger picture of norms about how to be a "good" teenager. Sexual behavior is an important part of that picture, even though different parents have different norms about it. Parents are typically the family members with the greatest opportunity to control teenagers' behaviors. They have legal authority over their teenage children and sometimes over their children's bodies. For example, parents regularly set curfews and house rules, "ground" teens who disobey them, and authorize their teenage children's medical care. Interviewees were very sensitive to this power hierarchy and its effects on communication between parents and teenagers.

Other family members often came up in interviews as well. Similarly aged siblings' and cousins' experiences frequently shape interviewees' sexual behaviors and their communication with parents. If an experience is bad, it serves as a cautionary tale for teens. Things that aunts, uncles, parents, and other relatives did when they were teenagers serve the same purpose as cautionary tales. Grandparents come up as standard-bearers for traditional morality, communicating stricter norms about teen sex and pregnancy and often reacting badly if teens break these social rules. But parents are far and away the most important family influence on the interviewees.[2]

Among different reference groups, families are physically closest to teens and have had an influence on them for the longest time.[3] Many parents feel a responsibility to communicate and enforce community norms about teen sex, but at the same time they want their teen to make it through adolescence with a bright future. These goals sometimes conflict. Parents often have—or at least report having—inaccurate information about their teen children's sexual behavior.[4] Bethany Everett and I found in a national study that among teens who'd had sexual intercourse, a majority had parents who believed they were virgins.[5] These parents tended to communicate less with their teens about sex and contraception than the parents who had a more accurate picture of their teen's sex life. Even though teens and parents usually want to communicate about sex, that communication doesn't often include concrete information about what the teen is doing.

What are parents communicating? A national survey found that 93 percent of adults want teens to be taught not to have sex until after high school, but at the same time, 73 percent think teens should also be getting more information about contraception. Although there seems to be some consensus about what to say, 82 percent believe parents "often don't know what to say" when they talk with their teens about sex.[6] All of this adds up to a highly charged and confusing situation when parents try to communicate sexuality norms to teens. Indeed, sociologist Sinikka Elliott found that parents are anxious and confused about managing their teens' sexuality.[7] Here, I discuss young people's perceptions of their interactions with their parents and the norms their parents communicated, which may not be the same as parents' own perceptions—in fact, parents may think they're communicating openly about sex.

But I argue that because the young person is the one engaging in sexual behaviors, that person's perceptions of family influences are particularly important to understand. Of course, teens don't always believe what their parents tell them. Chapter 7 shows how teens actively react to parental communication and control. Finally, it's important to note that although the interview questions weren't limited to heterosexual sex, interviewees' responses were. Parents' silence around non-heterosexual sex appeared to be near total.

NORMS COMMUNICATED BY FAMILIES

Some families (like Alexis's) are more open and forbearing about teen sex and pregnancy than others, but regardless of what behavioral prescriptions they communicate, they use one or both of two *rationales* to explain why the norms they are communicating are appropriate. Most interviewees didn't hear both rationales from their parents. Rather, different families and communities emphasize different rationales or their combination in ways that tend to reflect their socioeconomic and religious composition. Many teens internalize the rationales they hear and use them to explain decisions about their own behavior and judge the behavior of others. Eventually some of them question aspects of these rationales when deciding to become sexually active, but almost nobody we spoke with rejected them entirely during high school.

THE PRACTICAL RATIONALE: "RUINED BY HAVING A KID"

The *practical rationale* focuses on the potential of teens' sexual behaviors to undermine their futures and their efforts to become mature adults. This rationale has four main parts: problematic sexual behaviors can ruin your life, they are irresponsible, they are stupid rather than smart, and they show that you lack self-respect. It is important to note that the practical rationale can be used flexibly to justify different norms in a set, such as a norm against teen sex, a norm encouraging contraception, or a norm encouraging abortion if a teen gets pregnant. In the most common use of the practical rationale, a teen can demonstrate that she has praiseworthy, adult qualities and cares about her own future by abstaining from sex, or barring that, by practicing "safe" sex (i.e., using reliable contraception).

Alexis's father focused his communication about teen sex on the first aspect of the practical rationale, about the *future*, by telling her how "disappointed" he would be if she got pregnant because she would be placing her promising future in jeopardy.[8] Alexis said this was "mostly because he has more job ambitions right now for his family. . . . He would be disappointed because he really, like in my case, he just really wants me to be successful as a filmmaker. And I would think that if I did just have a baby and started being a mom, that probably would put any filmmaking ambitions on hold, if not cancel them altogether." Alexis also thought that like her mother, he would be "disappointed in himself for not preparing me enough to prevent a teenage pregnancy."

This focus on the teen's future is the most widespread aspect of the practical rationale. Teens from many social classes, religious backgrounds, and geographic areas—especially girls, in part because families think they would bear the responsibilities of a teen pregnancy—hear a clear normative message that having sex can mess up their futures. Like many parents, Alexis's father left some wiggle room about whether Alexis should abstain from sex or use contraception carefully, as long as she avoided getting pregnant. A pregnancy (or for boys, a sexual partner's pregnancy with the financial and social responsibilities it can entail) is seen as the main threat to the teen's future. Interestingly given teenagers' high levels of risk, STIs, even HIV/AIDS, are not usually a focus.

In her wealthy, White, liberal community, Claudia learned about the effect of teen sex on her future from hearing her parents talk about other girls in her community who had babies. She said, "It was always like, 'Wow, what is she going to do? How is she going to support a baby? How is she going to get her own education and take care of a family?'" Her parents' normative message about the future highlights the negative consequences they expect a teen pregnancy to result in: a compromised education because having a child would disrupt schooling, financial problems because of the expense of having a child, and problems with family life. Claudia's parents, like most others, never communicated any upside to teen sex or pregnancy.

Spencer, a boy from a wealthy suburb in a large Western city, links the strong "future" message from parents in his community to the families' wealth:

All of our [private] high schools cost like $20,000 a year to go to, which was ridiculous. And these parents would put so much money into all of these kids' different after-school activities, whether it be sports or acting or any of that stuff, that it almost seems like the parents would not let that [teen pregnancy] happen. And ingrain that into everybody's head from the day they were born almost that—well, not the day they were born, but from the day they understood that possibility [teen pregnancy] existed—that it was just not acceptable because of the amount of time and the effort that these parents were putting into these kids and the dreams and the aspirations, that all these kids that I knew had put on them by their parents. They would just not allow it.

In Spencer's community, families have made expensive investments in teenagers' futures, and in return teens have an obligation not to "blow it" by having a baby. If a pregnancy happened, Spencer told us the families he knew had a backup plan to avoid negative consequences for the teen's future: "If the girl were to get pregnant, she would almost 100 percent get an abortion."

Joel comes from a working-class family in a mixed-income community in another large Western city. This makes his upbringing very different from Spencer's in terms of SES, but the practical rationale being communicated about teen sex focuses on the future in ways that are still pretty much the same. Joel says parents are worried about teens having pregnancies. "They [parents] didn't want their [the teen's] whole life to get altered, because they saw their kid's potential. They didn't want that to get ruined by having a kid." Joel told us that if he wanted to live with a girlfriend and have sex before marriage, his father would say: "What are you doing? You know, you have so much more to do. This isn't what you should be spending your time on. You need to get good grades." As in Spencer's case, families in communities like Joel's see their teenagers as a major investment in the future, a potential route to achieving the "American dream" for the family. Yet in many lower-income urban communities, the backup option of abortion is not as widely available or accepted, even though religious views against abortion don't always play a big role. Joel said, "There's still kind of a bad view on abortion maybe. In my school you don't just get rid of them and your life's going to be fine now. But it [abortion] costs a lot of money, which is another big problem. Students don't have access to those kinds of funds, so I know only a few . . . that would have had the funds to go and do that." This is ironic since having a baby costs much more than an abortion, but it echoes cultural messages about personal accountability in which teens are taught to bear primary responsibility for their mistakes.

Like Alexis did when she called teen sex "rebellion . . . like drinking as a teenager," many interviewees say their parents talked about teen sex as one of many problem behaviors that could compromise their child's future. The focus of the practical rationale on the teen's future fits neatly with this way of thinking about teen sex as one of several problematic distractions that can mess up a teen's life. This narrative sidesteps moral implications to focus on practical ones.

Many of our interviewees believe parents' linking of sexual behavior with the child's future is limited to high school age. When the interviewer asked Alexis if you can become old enough to be allowed to have premarital sex, she was clear:

> Yes, eighteen. . . . It probably wasn't an exact age, but yeah, there came a point, with my parents, where it didn't really seem like they would care anymore.

Especially with my sister, before she graduated high school and before she turned eighteen, there was very much the attitude that either they thought she still wasn't having sex or that they didn't really want her to, even though I knew she was. And then afterwards it didn't really matter, and her boyfriend could sleep over without any problem, and we would joke about her getting pregnant. . . . But it wasn't really a, "well, you shouldn't be doing this," sort of mentality after she turned eighteen. And with me, too, the talks about being responsible shifted to fiscal responsibility and jobs, instead of, "well, use a condom if you're gonna have sex," sort of talks.

Many interviewees feel that the norms about sex their families communicated in high school are very different from the ones they hear now that they are older. Alexis's parents, like many others, dropped the rationale's link between sexual behavior and the child's future once their teens finished high school, even though it's often irrational because its logic still applies: If their children are attending college, they still have few financial resources to support a child, so a pregnancy would still be harmful to their futures. In this way, parents from all walks of life use the practical rationale's focus on threats to the teen's future strategically and selectively during high school.

The second aspect of the practical rationale that teens hear is about *responsibility*: Responsible teenagers don't have sex, or if they must have sex, they do it in responsible ways. Alana, who came from a socioeconomically and racially diverse urban community, says that in high school her religious mother communicated a consistent norm against teen sex: "She did have the whole 'no sex before marriage' [norm]. . . . Every weekend when I would go out with my friends, she would say, 'Don't do anything stupid. Don't do anything I wouldn't do. Be responsible. I hope you're not fooling around.'" Some parents add the somewhat contradictory norm that teens should not have sex, but if they do, they should be responsible by using contraception carefully. For example, in a wealthy resort town, Lucy's dad told her, "If you're going to be having sex, you need to be responsible in doing that." Gavin, who grew up in a wealthy, "very liberal" community, spelled out the rarer and more permissive message he received about what responsible sex means: "Sex is okay as long as it's responsible. You know, you're not out there giving people pregnancies and STDs."

Many parents' practical rationales extend beyond teen sexuality to emphasize competing responsibilities that should be more important than sex if a teen is behaving in a mature way. In her mostly White, middle-income small town, Isabella's family's focus has "always been more education-oriented, or to have other responsibilities and to get yourself prepared to have a family. Rather than doing it in high school. . . . Like having a career, being able to provide [financially] for a family. Completing other goals, or definitely finishing school, going to college, having a significant other to help raise the child." These competing responsibilities highlighted by Isabella's family are traditional markers of adulthood, and they are asking her to focus on achieving these markers rather than having sex and risking pregnancy.

Talk about responsibility is particularly interesting because it is used in contradictory ways in communicating norms about teen sex and pregnancy. On one hand, teens who don't have sex or who use protection are praised for being responsible. Yet on the other hand, teen parents are condemned because their situation requires them to be *too* responsible. Alexis described teen parenthood this way: "I don't think that a lot of teens have the world experience to know what it means to be a parent . . . Being a child yourself and then bringing another child that you're responsible for into the world, especially if you're not prepared for it or if you don't have the support that you need . . . it would probably really suck for you." Similarly, Mackenzie said, "Teenagers aren't really mature enough to handle the responsibility of a pregnancy. . . . Teenagers aren't really responsible enough to have kids." The perplexing message many teens receive, then, is that they should behave responsibly by not having sex (or barring that, by having protected sex), so they can avoid having to behave much more responsibly if they have a child. This confusion makes more sense when considering the different kinds of responsibilities that are considered normative or non-normative for teenagers, especially in predominantly White, middle-class settings. Teens who put off transitions to adulthood, for example by postponing sex, are being appropriately responsible. But teens who make these transitions early or put themselves at risk of early transitions are seen as "growing up too fast" and taking on inappropriate levels of responsibility for their age.[9]

This means that teen parents are labeled as irresponsible because they behaved immaturely by taking on a non-normatively high level of responsibility at a young age. Teen parents are sanctioned for having had irresponsible sex. Haylie said that in her ethnically diverse, low-income city, she and her friends "obviously knew that you need to use contraception not to get pregnant. And so we just never really understood how the accident happened, how they were able to get pregnant if they were being responsible." Beyond irresponsible sex, teen parents are considered irresponsible for giving up the prospect of a good future (a theme discussed above). Claire describes the rationale used by parents to discourage teen pregnancy in her large Southwestern city this way: "It's a blessing to have a child, but at the right time. And how irresponsible of you to get in this situation so young when you're given so much opportunity." Teen parents' irresponsibility is often bolstered by bringing up their other supposed "problem behaviors" as evidence of their irresponsibility. John told us that in his mostly White, fairly conservative suburb, teen parents were seen as "the kind of kids who were less responsible. . . . Like they were more the do-a-lot-of-drug types, not really care about school." Camryn said that in her very conservative, racially diverse Southern town, "Teen pregnancy was the ultimate sign of irresponsibility, basically."

The practical rationale also links mature, responsible sexual behavior to *intelligence*. Interviewees talk a lot about teen sex, contraception, and pregnancy as being either "smart" or "stupid." Above, Alana's mother linked teen sex both to irresponsibility and "being stupid," which is her code phrase for having sex. In contrast, being "smart" means avoiding penile–vaginal intercourse or using contraception consistently. In his middle-income, conservative suburb, Parker told us, "I think initially most families are disappointed in their kid [if the teen has sex], but once they realize their virginity is gone, it's over and done with. I think from then on they want them to be smart about it. Safe sex. Practice safe sex." Many interviewees told us their families had communicated this kind of potentially confusing two-stage normative message to teens, in which the ideal behavior is to abstain from sex, but "smart" sex is a tolerable alternative. This kind of sex is often talked of as "careful." But Dylan's parents in a conservative large city communicated a more permissive norm that boys sometimes heard: "Do what you're going to do, but be careful."[10]

Interviews with the secondary sample of teen parents show clearly that teens who violate norms about sex and contraception are indeed labeled as "stupid" by their families and communities. When Amanda thought about telling her boyfriend's mother about their accidental pregnancy, "we were like, 'She's going to smack you and yell at you. It's going to happen. She's going to call you stupid.'" When they told her, "She just looked at him and goes, 'I don't think it's the smartest thing you've done.'" Adriana's older brother reacted similarly to her teen pregnancy: "He was really mad. He wanted to beat my boyfriend up. He was talking stuff like, 'You're stupid for being pregnant!'" In fact, probably the most common negative reactions faced by the teen parents my research team interviewed were having their intelligence and maturity questioned.

A final aspect of the practical rationale, and a particularly important one for girls, is the link between sexual restraint and *self-respect*. Mature people are supposed to behave in responsible, smart ways that show they respect themselves; for many teen girls this includes not having sex. Bethany said of herself and her friends, "We all came from parents who taught us pretty much the same values: to respect your body, or respect yourself and be careful. And I'm pretty sure we were all taught not to have sex." "Respecting your body," if you are a teenage girl in many places, means abstaining from heterosexual intercourse. This theme is often present for boys but not emphasized as much. Growing up in a large Western city, Chloe internalized this rationale communicated by her parents. She said her parents' emphasis was "mostly don't have sex, not don't get pregnant." She went on to talk about how important her parents' influence was on her decision to remain a virgin until just before entering college. Chloe told us:

> I can say that my parents had a huge influence on it [the decision not to have sex]. . . . I take their opinion and their values to heart and have always tried to make them proud and have just always tried to have a good relationship with them. So had I not had that, and not had the type of friendship that I had with them, I think that my relationships with guys would have been a lot different. I don't know, I just don't think I would have respected myself so much.

Like her parents, Chloe equated respecting herself with remaining a virgin throughout high school, although it is interesting to note that immediately afterwards she followed peer norms and started having sex to avoid the stigma of being what she called "the college virgin."

The practical rationale communicated by many families stresses that teens need to show responsibility, intelligence, and self-respect by adhering to the family's norms about teen sexual behaviors. The irony of the practical rationale is that parents encourage teens to prove that they have adult-like levels of maturity by avoiding behavior—such as drinking and sex—that adults regularly engage in.[11]

THE MORAL RATIONALE: "THIS IS WRONG"

Besides the practical rationale, the other common explanation underlying the norms about teen sexuality that parents communicate is the *moral rationale*. Many families communicate an ideal of abstaining from teen sex but supplement it with a more pragmatic norm about using contraception if a teen does have sex. In many interviewees' families, this second norm is not present; rather, having sex at all, regardless of contraceptive use, is a problem. This may be solely for moral reasons, or a moral rationale may be supplemented by the practical rationale's reasons for why teen sex is inappropriate. The moral rationale is usually directly tied to religious beliefs, although not all religious teachings subscribe to the moral rationale. Dylan contrasted the practical and moral messages being communicated in his conservative large city: "From the parents' perspective it varied really diversely. I feel like my parents told me, 'We understand that you're going to do this [have sex], but keep your consequences [from being negative].' But other parents' talks were like, 'You don't do this, this is wrong, religiously, morally. If you did this it would completely destroy our family.' So it really varied." Lucy talked about her "conservative" friends' parents in her wealthy resort town, whose "family belief" about teen sex was "that it was wrong and they shouldn't be doing it." Charles elaborated that people in his ethnically diverse, middle-income city saw teen pregnancy as "immoral" because "women are seen as a slut even after just one time [having sex].... Having sex is seen as not the right thing to do." Bryce tied the norms in his "Catholic environment" within a middle-income small town more explicitly to religion: "We were taught that premarital sex and pregnancy outside of wedlock is against God, and therefore wrong."

The moral rationale about teen sexual behavior focuses on sex and abortion rather than on contraception, which is largely missing from this rationale's focus. Teen sex is immoral, but abortion is, in Makayla's words, "really wrong." I discuss this complicated norm set in Chapter 6. For now it's enough to realize that many teens who do not hear a moral rationale, like Alexis in the example described immediately below, still wrestle morally with abortion. Alexis and her mother and sister debated the morality of abortion in a "What if?" example of her sister getting pregnant, even though her parents did not communicate a moral rationale about teen sex.

DIFFERENT COMMUNITIES, DIFFERENT NORMS

As I discuss in Chapter 6 (see Table 6.1), the practical and moral rationales are communicated by different social actors in a teen's community, including families. The SES and level of religious influence in the community are important drivers of the rationales and norms held in that community. More highly religious communities tend to communicate the moral rationale, while less religious communities communicate the practical rationale. This is why Claudia and Julie from the beginning of the book, both of whom came from middle-class communities, described being taught very different norms about teen sexuality: Their communities differed in the salience of religion. Communities that are both wealthier and more religious are complicated, tending to communicate the moral rationale in public while families also espouse the practical rationale privately. Community religious influence, via the dominant public rationale, shapes teens' public portrayals of their sexuality. Teens in communities with a public moral rationale are often more careful to present themselves as sexually abstinent. But teens' actual sexual behaviors—as perceived by the interviewees—are largely shaped by the community's SES. Teens from more advantaged communities are less likely to have sex or get pregnant and engage in fewer risky sexual behaviors. Families play an important role in these dynamics as normative mouthpieces of the community, as independent social actors in communicating norms that may differ from those of the community, and as enforcers of norms.

HOW NORMS ARE COMMUNICATED

EXPLICIT COMMUNICATION: HYPOTHETICALS AND "THE SEX TALK"

Family members deploy different rationales when communicating a variety of different norms about sexual behavior to teens, all of them discouraging teen heterosexual intercourse and pregnancy and some encouraging contraception. (Sex acts other than penile–vaginal intercourse, including those between people of the same gender, are apparently not even acknowledged.) But *how* do parents communicate these norms? The actual sexual behavior of the teen in the family is almost always a taboo topic, so parents use a variety of strategies to get their message across obliquely without having what Veronica calls "the 'me having sex' talk."

Rather than providing the kind of "open, honest" information that most teens say they would like to get from their parents, most parents of our interviewees stayed at an abstract level when communicating norms about sexuality.[12] Like many other parents, Alexis's mother used hypothetical situations to communicate what the consequences of sex could be and promote contraception. Alexis usually only talked about sex with her mom, and they didn't approach the topic head on. Alexis's mother tended to bring up sex by talking about:

> hypothetical situations in which really weird things happen. So when we always, not always, but when we had those talks of adolescent-hood and stuff, then she would say things like, "Yeah, and if you ever got pregnant then your dad and I would totally help you out. And if you wanted to get an abortion, okay, we would help you with that. But if you wanted [to have the baby], then you know we would help you with that, too, and it wouldn't be the end of the world or anything. But here's ways to prevent it, and you should do those instead."

Alexis's mother was more open and tolerant about sex, contraception, and pregnancy than most of our interviewees said their parents were. But even she used a roundabout way of communicating through "What if?" scenarios. Hypothetical situations have the benefit of letting parents make clear how they would react to a pregnancy without having to acknowledge that their teenage child might be sexually active. Alexis's mother is a real exception in terms of describing a mild reaction to Alexis's hypothetical pregnancy. Many other parents used hypothetical situations to emphasize how dire the consequences of teen pregnancy would be and how negatively they would react.

This approach, though abstract, was actually the most direct of the common ways of communicating norms. Other parents used broad euphemisms, like Alana's mom above telling her, "Don't do anything stupid." Her follow-up statement, "I hope you're not fooling around," is more direct than what many other parents said, but again it is a statement of the mother's general expectations rather than useful information about how to avoid sex or its risky consequences, such as advice on how to say "no" in sexual encounters or how to use contraception carefully. The few parents who give more concrete information about sex or contraception communicate it at an abstract level rather than in the context of a teen's current sexual activity. For example, Patton told us that while growing up in a wealthy, liberal city, "I know that personally my parents had a pretty open dialogue with me about having safe sex *way before the thought of me having sex was in consideration*" [emphasis added]. In this way, parents can be more concrete in their communication while avoiding the taboo topic of their teen's actual sexual activity.

Parents' and teens' avoidance of direct communication about the teen's sexual behavior is often mutual. Many teens fear the prospect of detailed communication with parents about their own sexual behavior. In fact, interviewees often mentioned it as one of the main reasons they tried to avoid sex or pregnancy. Noelle said it was "a huge scare for teenagers, having sex." Brooke said she avoided sex in her high school in a wealthy conservative suburb because "there was definitely an element of fear involved, of what your parents would do. . . . I think you're always influenced by what your parents think." Similarly, my interviewees who ended up becoming teen parents felt acute fear about telling their families. James asked his girlfriend to tell his mother about being pregnant because "I thought I was going to get kicked out of the house or something, or get beat up by my mom. . . . I was just scared of my mom."

Concrete exchanges between teens and parents about what sexual behaviors the teen is currently or is considering engaging in are common in some other countries such as the Netherlands, but certainly not in our interviewees' families.[13] This may not necessarily be a matter of parents' personal preference, but rather a strategy for maintaining the teen's and family's reputations in the community. For instance, Brooke said that in her wealthy conservative suburb, "there's a lot of judgment and rumors floating around, and you don't want your kids to be prey to that. And you don't want yourself to be prey to that. So I think parents really kept it [their teens' sexual behavior] on the down low." In Brooke's case, that meant that teen pregnancy and sex was "not something we [she and her parents] really talked about. . . . It's not like my parents ever sat me down and were like, 'If you ever get pregnant, we're kicking you out of the house.' " Instead, teen sex "was always just a hushed subject. . . . It was just, 'If you're going to do it, be safe and don't tell me about it.' It was just easier to deal with if you [parents] didn't have to hear about it." Without concrete advice from parents, teens like Brooke may make sexual decisions that are less wise than they could have been.

Explicit talk about sex and contraception is more common among siblings than with parents. Mackenzie told us, "I mean, I usually go to my sisters more for issues like this, because they are going to be less judgmental than my mom." Siblings can more easily communicate more concrete information about sex and contraception, but they also serve as role models. Alexis watched her sister become involved in a serious romantic relationship in high school and knew she had become sexually active. Discussions like "me and my sister talking about whether or not we would keep a child if we had it" were a source of hypothetical decision making that shaped her own life. Yet siblings are also a source of social control, and teens care a lot about their siblings' reactions. Alexis said her sister and brother "would make fun of me" if she got pregnant. Teen parents talked in their interviews about siblings' (often brothers') reactions to their pregnancy being a source of grief for them. For example, Cristina's brother "was really mad, because he's very overprotective, my brother."

GOSSIP AND CAUTIONARY TALES:
"WHAT HAS SHE DONE WITH HER LIFE?"

Besides abstract talk and hypothetical situations, talking about other teenagers who have gotten pregnant is another common way parents communicate norms about sex, pregnancy, and contraception. This talk is almost always about girls—boys' sexual behavior isn't judged nearly as harshly. Parents talk about other teens to their teenage children in two interconnected ways that communicate norms about sexuality: gossip and cautionary tales. Engaging in gossip about other teenagers lets parents communicate both the rules about teen sexual behavior and the bad things that happen to teens if these rules are broken. Gossip is an effective social control tool—people who expect that group members will gossip about them are more easily socially controlled by their group.[14] Claudia told us about her experiences in a wealthy, White, liberal community:

> I think my parents are really not okay with it [teen pregnancy]. I heard them talking about a girl that I played soccer with, and she went to school near me. And I guess she got pregnant, and that was even after high school was over. And my mom responded really negatively to it, and how she made the "eek" face, and kind of like, "Oh, God, what has she done with her life?" kind of thing. . . . It was always like, "Oh, God, can you imagine having to do that at this age? Can you imagine having to be stuck with that person?" . . . I don't think I ever heard it [teen parenthood] being spoken about in a positive light.

It was always, "Wow, what is she going to do? How is she going to support a baby? How is she going to get her own education and take care of a family?"

Claudia's parents seem to be making careful use of the opportunity to gossip about a pregnant girl (the child's father is invisible) in order to talk about the ruined education, financial future, and romantic relationships they think will result from having a baby at that age. By asking, "Can you imagine?" they turn the story of the pregnant soccer player into a hypothetical scenario to scare Claudia. For the community, this kind of gossip serves the dual purpose of frightening teens and negatively sanctioning pregnant girls who have violated a norm.

What I call *cautionary tales* don't serve the same dual purpose, because they aren't about an ongoing situation in the community. Instead, these stories are told to the teen for the purpose of communicating norms about sexual behavior and its negative consequences. Often these stories come from within the family. Ivy told us about her experiences in a low-income rural area:

> Well, my dad did sit me down. And he just kind of told me—and this was actually just before I met the child my aunt had when she got pregnant, she gave her up for adoption and we met her a few years ago—my dad sat me down before when he was telling me, so I would know what was going on. And he told me what happened with his sister, and basically said that kind of behavior, AKA [also known as] sex, that causes you to get pregnant, was not acceptable at all in our house. And that he would have no problems sending me away. He is pretty scared with what happened to his sister because it had a big impact on his life and his relationship with her. . . . My mom was more like, every time you have sex, just assume you are going to get pregnant, so you better be married because then somebody will be able to take care of your kid. So that was the sex talk I got. If you are going to have sex, you are going to get pregnant, and just assume it. And you better be able to take care of it financially and everything like that. Never any talk from my dad beyond that.

Ivy's parents used a family cautionary tale to communicate a strong message against premarital sex and justify it using the practical but not the moral rationale.

Similarly, Chloe's family in a large Western city told her, "Don't have sex." She said, "I had been raised to, you know, save myself for the person I loved or marriage or whatever." Unbeknownst to her mother, Chloe's father used a family cautionary tale to underscore this message: "My dad told me he knocked up a girl though in high school. . . . The girl he got pregnant, I think, just kind of told him and then . . . really didn't have any communication. . . . I don't think my mom knows."

Cautionary tales don't always come from within the family. Nadia's mother worked as a nurse in a large Western city and would bring home cautionary tales from the hospital. "I mean, my mom hasn't really said much about it, but she'll make little comments on the side, like, 'Some girl was sixteen, and I delivered her baby today. And you know, if that were to happen to you . . . I would support you about that, but I don't think it's a good thing at all.'" These cautionary tales served as a main form of sexual communication between Nadia and her parents. Nadia told us, "I know my parents would not have been open about me telling them that I was sexually active."

SILENCE: "DON'T ASK, DON'T TELL"

Given the awkwardness of communication between parents and teens about sexuality, it may not be surprising that both parents' and teenagers' most common way of dealing with the topic is *silence*. Not just awkwardness, but shame about sexuality prescribed by emotion norms, may be reasons for this silence. Silence is used in two different ways. The simpler way is that parents tend to express their disapproval of teen sex and pregnancy by not talking about it—the fact that the topic is taboo makes it clear that it is unacceptable.[15] As Noelle said of her community based around a Catholic school, "It's just kind of understood. We don't really talk about teen pregnancy very much. And if we do, it's kind of more like if someone we know got pregnant. It's kind of like looked down upon." Noelle is saying that although her family and community are generally silent about teen pregnancy, she still understands that they disapprove. As in the examples above, this condemnation tends to be communicated through gossip about teens who broke the rules. Lots of interviewees reported "just knowing" that their families discouraged teen sex and pregnancy, even though family members didn't usually talk about these topics.

Beyond staying quiet about teen sex and pregnancy, parents tend to be silent about the reality that two thirds of teenagers are heterosexually active by their senior year of high school, a statistic that is reflected in my college student sample and that most of the interviewees confirmed in the case of their own communities.[16] Yet this is not something most parents discuss with their teenagers. Noelle said, "Most people were having sex in high school. It was pretty casual." She went on to say that although "it was just one of those things where you just didn't really talk about it, I think that a lot of parents knew what was going on." Here, Noelle is describing the second, more complicated use of silence as an active conspiracy maintained both by parents and teenagers, a "strategic ambiguity."[17] Parents and teens working together to keep parents ignorant of teens' sexual behavior is very common. In Noelle's community, parents "didn't want to directly know about it [their teens' sexual behavior]," so "definitely a lot of the parents were left in the dark." Patton talked more about how the *conspiracy of silence* worked in his wealthy, liberal city:

> I think that some parents probably turned their head because they didn't want to know what their kid was doing. I think that if the parents were involved in their kid's life, I'm sure that there were signs that they would see. That if you were talking to your kid and kind of knew what was going on, that they would probably have some suspicion that that was happening. But I don't know that a lot of parents wanted to know what their kids were doing on the weekends necessarily. Even as a pretty tight-knit community, I think that it was maybe too much for them to think about or face.

Alexis summed up the conspiracy of silence this way: "It's a denial thing where they just look the other way . . . like a 'don't ask, don't tell.'" I write later in this chapter about the (sometimes elaborate) strategies parents and teens engage in to maintain this conspiracy of silence.

Some parents make it clear that they will only engage in the conspiracy of silence up to a point, and if a pregnancy occurs, they will break the silence to help the teen. Because boys don't bear the brunt of pregnancies, this means parents don't usually have to break their silence with sons, but they may have to with daughters. Growing up in an ethnically diverse, low-income city, Haylie describes general silence from her parents on the topic of teen sex and contraception. The interviewer asked her, "So do you think their main message was don't have sex, or was it contracept if you're having sex?" She replied, "I think it was contracept if you're having sex. But, you know, they never really encouraged me to have sex, or wouldn't talk about it a whole lot." But Haylie's parents also taught her to engage in a conspiracy of silence—up to a point: "I think my parents were just teaching me to be responsible, you know, not to put yourself in that situation. And to talk to us if anything happens." Her parents communicated that Haylie was on her own unless "anything" (presumably a pregnancy or maybe an STI) happened, at which point she should consult with them. But Haylie might have benefitted from their support sooner than that.

Opening up to parents if negative consequences occur is a risky strategy for teens because not all parents are willing to put the teen's norm violation aside in times of crisis. Larena, who went to a low-income high school in a large city, broke the conspiracy of silence during a pregnancy scare: "When I told my parents, because I thought I was pregnant, they said, 'How dare you? Your body is your temple. Premarital sex is totally against everything we believe. We don't want you to be like how we were when we were younger.' Just a lot of shame." Larena received neither emotional nor practical support from her parents, even though she says they implied that they had themselves not lived up to the normative standard to which they were holding Larena.

As the most widespread strategy for communicating messages about teen sex and pregnancy, silence is particularly important. It solves problems for both the teen and the parent. If they stay quiet on the topic of sex, teens can engage in behavior that parents disapprove of without having to face condemnation. At the same time, parents can maintain ignorance about teens' potential violation of the norms they have communicated. But this leads to perhaps the biggest problem of all: If parents don't know that their teen is having sex, they can't help the teen avoid potentially risky consequences of sex such as pregnancy or STIs. Like most interviewees, as teenagers Alexis and her siblings went to great lengths to avoid talking to their parents about their own sexual behaviors. When Alexis's sister started to have sex, "she had to go get birth control pills and buy condoms and stuff on her own because she was seventeen. She didn't want to go to our parents, obviously. Because who wants to go talk to their parents about, 'Yeah, I'm having sex'?" Alexis believes teens thought of sex as "rebellion in that you can't tell people, really, that you're doing it, but people will know a lot of the time. . . . People being parents." Alexis's family isn't unusual in being uninformed about their teenage children's sexual activity. She guesses that about "60 or 70 percent" of teens had sex in her high school. When asked if adults were aware of this, she said:

> See, I'm not even sure, because it always seems like adults get this weird double standard in which they forget that they were ever teenagers and experienced the same things. So probably not. I think it becomes, "Well, when we were young we did this, but our kids aren't going to." . . . Or they just don't want to realize it, so it's a denial thing where they just look the other way . . . like a "don't ask, don't tell."

This "denial thing" led to increased risk for Alexis's sister as she tried to negotiate effective contraceptive use while underage.

As I discuss below, many teens are not receiving concrete information about contraception in school or from other sources, so without parental support they may not be able to use contraception effectively. In particular, longer-acting contraceptives— such as birth control pills, hormonal implants, and intrauterine devices—are the most effective at preventing pregnancy but are also expensive and hard to hide from parents. The conspiracy of silence around teens' sexual activity often rules out long-acting contraceptives as a possibility for many teenagers. This is important because the lack of these types of contraception contributes to the high teen pregnancy rates in the United States compared to the rest of the industrialized world.[18]

Not only does the conspiracy of silence keep teens from using contraception as effectively as they otherwise could, but it also keeps them from receiving other information about sex. Amy Schalet found that in the Netherlands, parents explicitly communicate norms to teens about appropriate and inappropriate ways of being sexually active. Appropriate ways in the Dutch context include waiting to have sex until you are in a committed romantic relationship and having sex in safe settings such as a bedroom at home. Sexual activity is also not supposed to interfere with the teen's family relationships or schoolwork. These messages are an important part of the sexual socialization process that cannot be communicated if there is a conspiracy of silence between parents and teens.[19]

HOW PARENTS TRY TO ENSURE CONFORMITY

Parents communicate social norms about sex to teens. But norms have another important component that sets them apart from other cultural messages people hear: They are social rules that must be followed, and people who break the rules are sanctioned. In this section, I describe different strategies parents use when they try to enforce norms about sexual behavior. As Table 2.1 showed, many of these strategies have to do with either communicating the practical and emotional rewards or sanctions that will follow depending on how the teen behaves, or restricting teenagers' opportunities for breaking the rules. Some strategies involve social control through interaction, while others involve physically controlling the teen's body.

SOCIAL CONTROL: "I WAS INFLUENCED"

Threats

Parents often explicitly or implicitly threaten teens when trying to influence their sexual behavior. Parents tend to draw on the strongest threats they can conjure, especially when communicating with daughters. As earlier quotes have shown, teens are often afraid of emotional outbursts or even physical abuse if their parents were to find out that they were sexually active or pregnant. Even though there were plenty of pregnant girls in her low-income high school in a large city, Larena felt sure that her parents "would kick my ass" if she got pregnant. Josiah thought if he got a girl pregnant in his tiny, predominantly White mountain town, his parents "would've been really angry, I'm sure. Just furious." He thinks they would have calmed down and tried to support him after their initial anger. Emotional threats like these were some of the most salient to interviewees, even milder ones like Alexis's apprehension about her father's "disappointment" if she were to get pregnant. Threats of negative emotional reactions from parents are pervasive throughout the interviews.

Beyond family members' initial emotional or physical reactions, teenagers fear being kicked out of the house and cut off from financial support. Above, Ivy told how her father used a story about his sister getting pregnant to communicate that if the same thing happened to Ivy, "he would have no problems sending me away" from her low-income rural home. When she was growing up in a politically moderate, middle-income suburb, Jessica's father told her, "if I chose to have a baby, it would be up to me [her family would withdraw support]. They said that they had two kids and were done." Alana said of her family in a racially and socioeconomically diverse urban community, "My parents even to this day tell me if I were ever to get pregnant, that they're completely cutting me off . . . because we are very religious."

Although being thrown out of the family might seem like the most severe threat a parent could come up with, many teens seem to fear another common threat equally: the threat that the teen could break up her family by violating rules about sex. Dylan said that in his conservative community, parents paired the moral rationale ("Parents' talks were like, 'You don't do this [have sex]. This is, like, wrong, religiously, morally'") with explicit threats to the family's stability ("'If you did this, it would completely destroy our family'"). Larena's story of a pregnant friend in her large city shows how parents often combine a threat to the family's existence with other severe threats, such as being thrown out of the home:

One of my friends is pregnant right now. She told her parents over winter break, and I knew for about three months she didn't go to the doctor or anything. And she expected her parents to get a divorce because of it, because she was always told, "If you got pregnant, I don't think our family would be able to stay together." She had the impression that her father would be the one to be more upset than her mother and that her mom would really support her. And when she told her parents, she actually got the opposite reaction. Her mom kicked her out, so she's looking for her own place right now. Her dad is more supporting—it's her stepfather—but he's more supporting of it. She's barely going to the doctor's now, and she's in her second, almost third trimester. She's sort of had it rough. She had to drop out of school immediately.

As Larena's story shows, these threats are not always empty and can have serious implications for teenagers' lives.

Incentives

Most of parents' explicit efforts to communicate the consequences of rule breaking focus on threats; only occasionally do parents try to outright bribe teens to conform to norms about sex. Larena told us that her parents "bribed me ever since I was really little. I've always been taught, ever since I was seven or eight, not to have premarital sex. And my mom, every time we'd go to the doctor, she'd be like, 'Larena, I know you hear this every time we come, but I will give you $10,000 on your wedding if you wait [to have sex] until you actually get married.' So for me, I was influenced to not have sex. [But it] just ended up happening." Larena's parents' explicit bribery targeted the behavior that concerned them most: preventing premarital sex rather than encouraging contraception. As is typical when parents try to compel teens to abstain from sex, even that sizable bribe was not enough to make Larena follow their rules. She ended up being sexually active in high school.

Most parents in this sample of college students had a major incentive they could offer when trying to ensure that teens didn't break their rules about sex, contraception, and pregnancy: financial support during college. This seemed to be done implicitly and perhaps not even consciously. Parents don't talk about college support as an explicit incentive; instead, they talk about the teen's promising future and how it would be ruined by a pregnancy. But however unspoken it is in power negotiations over teens' behavior, the promise of support during college is a major incentive for the teen to at least appear to follow parents' rules. Kaitlyn is a typical example of the rewards many interviewees could expect if they followed (or at least outwardly appeared to follow) the rules. She said, "My parents pretty much pay for everything. The housing and college. I don't have a job, so they are fully supporting me. . . . They are pretty much paying for all my fun and amazing life." When asked for details, she told us her parents bought her a car and pay for all transportation costs, medical expenses, clothes, food, books, and spending money. The estimated cost of tuition and expenses at Kaitlyn's university was about $20,000 to $40,000 per year depending on state residency, with the higher figure applying to her. Kaitlyn is aware of how hard it will be when her parents take this support away: "They have always supported me, so that if and when they ever stop, it's going to be hard to make the amount of money that they give me right off the bat. It's going to be hard for me to be poor, so I don't know what I am going to do." The power dynamics around this financial support are important for those teens who expect to receive it. Below, I discuss teens whose families could not afford to support them through college and the equally powerful ways finances play into their decision making.

PHYSICAL CONTROL: "SHE GOT GROUNDED"

Removing opportunities for sex

Many parents are clearly willing to resort to serious threats in an attempt to get teen-agers to follow their norms about sexual behavior. But as the legal custodians of their children's physical well-being, parents also have many options to physically con-trol their teens' bodies and limit possibilities for norm violation. A private act, sex requires physical opportunities if it is to remain hidden from family members.[20] The interviewees said that many parents work hard to reduce these opportunities. The more resources a family has, the more likely it is that parents can successfully moni-tor their teens' activities. But as Chapter 7 shows, teenagers recognize the power of this strategy and often band together to resist it more effectively.

Finn talked about one strategy that parents in his conservative Western city could take by keeping the teen at home but without opportunities for sex: "The smarter parents would be, like, 'All right, boys and girls can come over and do stuff, but leave the door open in the room.'" Rules vary from leaving the door open, to keeping one's feet on the floor, to not allowing anyone of the opposite sex into a bedroom. Of course, the success of these rules presupposes that a parent is available in the home at all times, which is not true for many families. Spencer told us that in his high-income community within a large city, "my parents used to give me shit . . . about having girls up in my room . . . but, I mean, such was high school." He also perceived a gender dynamic in this rule: "I think that it's much more acceptable for me to bring a girl into my [bed]room than it is for my sisters to bring a guy into their room. I know for a fact that my stepdad would absolutely . . . flip out if he saw a guy going into one of my little sisters' rooms."

Many parents seem to trust that without opportunities for sex at home, teenagers will have a hard time finding such opportunities elsewhere. Finn said, "We weren't put in very many situations where it [sex] was possible. Like, we don't have cars. If you do have a car, we're on [a military] base and freaked out about the law. . . . You don't have a bed anywhere." Other teens living in civilian communities also talked about the lack of opportunities for sex outside their homes. But the homes of friends are potentially dangerous places from a parent's perspective, so parents sometimes control teens' friendships to prevent the risk of sex occurring when they are together with a particular friend. For example, Julie told us that in her very conservative middle-income suburb, her parents banned her friendship with Mary, a pregnant teen. "They definitely would not allow me to hang out with Mary anymore. . . . They didn't want me to be around her anyway, and that was both a little bit before she got pregnant and then very much afterwards." When asked why they banned the friendship, Julie said, "My mom felt that she was 'White trash' and that I would get into trouble if I spent time with her." In drawing a class-based and moral distinction between Julie and her friend through the term "White trash," Julie's mother is also implying that the friend's parents might improperly monitor Julie and her friend if they spent time together. Julie also talked more generally about a sense in her community that "if girls see other girls getting pregnant, they'll want to get pregnant, too, or something ridiculous of that nature."

When all parents maintain consistent strategies in their homes, teenagers can sometimes be effectively prevented from finding safe places for sex—though this kind of sustained effort at physical monitoring must be exhausting and sometimes impractical for parents. Charles explained that dynamic in his own experience in an ethnically diverse, middle-income city: "It was my first girlfriend. We were in her room, and her dad walked in. And I had to go, and she got grounded." His girlfriend's parents kept them out of "risky" rooms, as did Charles's own parents. He went on to say, "My parents had this rule that I wasn't allowed to be in the basement. I wasn't allowed to be downstairs alone with another girl. So when I did go down there, my dad would get really angry." Charles's example illustrates parents' strategies to curtail opportunities for sex, teenagers' rebellion against these rules, and parents' responses. "Grounding" teens (in other words, restricting them to their bedroom or home for an extended period of time) is a strong form of physical control that should remove all opportunities for sex. But even then, teens may try to sneak away. Joel told us that in his racially diverse urban community, "There was a lot of students getting grounded because they were sneaking out and going to see their boyfriend or going to see their girlfriend. That did happen a lot."

Like the conspiracy of silence around teen sex, the removal of opportunities for safe sex is problematic, especially for girls. Whether parents are encouraging teens to stay under their watchful eyes with an open door at home or relying on active law enforcement and a lack of available beds to keep teens from having sex in the community, preventing attractive opportunities for sex is a common norm enforcer strategy. But this strategy can backfire, resulting in teens creating opportunities for themselves (see Chapter 7) that are less safe from sexual violence or other crime, less planned, and less conducive to using contraception.[21]

Restricting access to contraception

An implicit way interviewees said parents (and, as Chapter 6 shows, communities) physically try to control teens' sexual behavior is by making it harder for teenagers to access contraception. Restricted access to birth control is mostly a necessary consequence of the conspiracy of silence around teen sex, as I discussed earlier. If parents are working hard to assume that their teen is not having sex, then they cannot easily help the teen access contraception. It may be that parents hope teens will give up on the enterprise of having sex if contraception is hard to get. But this strategy does not often have the intended effect—interviewees told us that many or most teens in every community in the study had sex by the end of high school anyway. Lucy described how in her wealthy, geographically isolated resort town, the conspiracy of silence led to a lack of reliable contraception among teenagers, but not often to a lack of sexual activity: "I didn't know too many girls who were on [hormonal] birth control. So it was mostly abstinence and condoms. . . . If they were under 18, they would have to talk to their parents about it, which I think would have been the problem because they would be scared to talk to their parents about them having to be sexually active." Relying solely on condoms increased girls' risk of pregnancy compared to other contraceptive options.

Madelyn talked about teens' efforts to get around their parents' withholding of contraception in her LDS/Mormon-predominated city: "I knew a few girls who went to [a reproductive health clinic] and got the pill . . . on their own. Those were usually the girls who had been dating a guy for a year or something, and they didn't want their parents to know." In Madelyn's community this strategy was available because there a reproductive health clinic, but in other communities it would be more difficult. But even in this case, the girls waited until they were in a lengthy sexual relationship to access long-term methods of contraception. This lack of reliable contraceptive access from the start might have put them at risk for pregnancy earlier in their relationships.

Providing contraception for nonsexual reasons

Judging from interviewees' stories, many parents seem to understand the serious risk involved in maintaining the conspiracy of silence: not being able to help the teen avoid negative consequences of sex. Sometimes alone and sometimes in consultation with other parents, many parents came up with an innovative strategy to prevent pregnancy while avoiding the appearance of condoning or even acknowledging the possibility of their teen's sexual activity. This strategy was giving their daughter birth control pills for nonsexual reasons. It is surprisingly common for parents to put their teen daughters on birth control pills for reasons other than contraception.[22] These reasons include acne, menstrual cramps, and irregular periods. This often happened in communities and families with higher SES.

Our research team asked Noelle what kinds of protection sexually active teens were using in her community based around a Catholic school. She said, "A lot of the girls were on the pill. People would start early, for cramps or to clear their face [of acne]. So they didn't have to have the conversation [about heterosexual intercourse] with their parents if they're already on the pill. . . . A lot of the moms would start their kids on the pill early for their period or cramps or stuff, so it [their teens' sexual activity] really just didn't come out." Noelle links this off-label use of birth control pills to protecting the conspiracy of silence. Describing parent–teen communication in her very conservative middle-income suburb, Julie talked more about how this use of the pill can benefit both parents and teens:

> Parents . . . were kind of uneasy about approaching that subject [teen sex]. It's one thing to say, "Don't get pregnant. You can get pregnant if you don't use protection." But to be like, "So how's sex going? Are you using protection?" You know. I was on birth control for different medical reasons, and so I think that put my parents at ease, because they knew that I was on birth control, even though it wasn't for sex initially. So I think that kind of took some pressure off. But a lot of girls, like I remember driving someone to [a reproductive health clinic] to get birth control, because her parents couldn't know. So there were some parents that didn't know.

Julie implies here that parents are complicit in this strategy, knowing that their daughters will probably use the pill as birth control at some point.

Teens who know this strategy is available can also use it to avoid pregnancy while having penile–vaginal intercourse and still keep their norm violation secret. Nadia did this successfully in her large Western city: "When I wanted to get on birth control or something, I told my parents it wasn't for that reason, like for sex. It was just to get more regular on my period or whatever. And it wasn't really something that I would directly talk to my parents about. . . . And I think the same with my friends, too." In the same community, some parents offer off-label birth control while others refuse to, and teens work to obtain their own. Isaac told us that in his small, conservative city:

> Every girl was on the pill, it seemed like. . . . Any girl who could afford it or had access to it was on it. . . . The girls themselves, they took care of it in secret almost. And I know the girls talked amongst themselves about how to get it, where it was cheaper, because I know the cost was always an issue. Because some people were getting it without their parents knowing. Also, a lot of girls were, I knew a lot of girls whose parents bought it for them, for the reasons that it prevented cramps and things like that. It minimized the impacts of a period.

Isaac's example illustrates how much easier and more reliable birth control is when parents provide it, compared to teens using it on the sly.

In a very few cases, parents explicitly put their daughters on the pill as a method of contraception. Rochelle said of her experiences in a low-income, small Northeastern town, "Yeah, my mom made me go on the pill. And this is, like, before I was even having sex. I just brought it up, and she was like, 'Okay, if you're even thinking about it, just in case.' . . . They weren't like, 'Do it!' [have heterosexual intercourse], but they understood." Rochelle contrasted her experiences, which she viewed as unusual, with those of her peers: "I don't think that many girls were on the pill . . . Well, they might've been on the pill, I'm not sure. But I don't think it was for sex, though. I think it was for [regular] periods because at that time of your life you're so off."

Whether initiated by parent or teen, birth control pills are a powerful way to control teen girls' bodies in order to avoid pregnancy, though not sex or STIs. Its popularity as a parental control strategy suggests that, like most teens, many parents are more worried about pregnancy than about other perceived negative consequences for which many teens are also at high risk, such as STIs or abusive relationships.

HOW EFFECTIVE IS PARENTS' NORM ENFORCEMENT?

Many parents bring out their most powerful weapons when attempting to control teens' sexual behaviors. But do they succeed? On one hand, parents' attempts to enforce rules about teen sex aren't very effective. Most teens have penile–vaginal intercourse by the end of high school in nearly all the communities interviewees talked about, as well as in national statistics.[23] On the other hand, teens tend to wait until quite late in high school to initiate sex, and the average age at first intercourse has risen somewhat.[24] But still, parents' nearly universal message against sex during high school usually isn't shaping teens' behavior in the intended way.

There are apparent exceptions in which parents and other social actors successfully convince a lot of teens to abstain from sex. In his wealthy Rocky Mountain suburb, Liam estimated that "about half" of teens had sex by the end of high school. He said:

> I think that it wasn't the fear of pregnancy. It was the fear of sex itself that prevented people from having sex. . . . Some people had religious reasons. Some people wanted to save themselves for marriage outside of religion, just to remain pure, that glorified image of the pure girl. Everyone's saving themselves. . . . People were more scared of the institution of sex than they were of the results of it being pregnancy.

But this is the exception more than the rule. Many more interviewees told us that teenagers are afraid of pregnancy more than sex.

Even though most teens start having sex by the end of high school, especially in communities and families with higher SES, parents' control efforts are pretty successful at motivating teenagers to avoid pregnancy. Reducing opportunities for sex is also likely to lessen the frequency of sex even among sexually active teens, which decreases pregnancy risk. Isaac told us about the messages teens were receiving in his small conservative city and the ways those messages shaped their decision making:

Abstinence was certainly promoted among a lot of parents. And even those parents that weren't considered religious. But abstinence was a big deal. It's not that people, the community, didn't want students to get pregnant, so therefore promoted contraception.

It was more promoting abstinence?

Yeah. I would say there wasn't very much active promotion of abstinence; however it, was just . . . Generally, "Don't get pregnant. I don't care how you do it. I'm not going to give you condoms. You're not supposed to get pregnant when you're seventeen."

Yeah. Okay, do you think most teenagers like you in your community started having sex by the time high school ended?

Yes. I would probably say 85, 80 percent were sexually active to some degree.

Do you think the adults either in school or parents in the larger community knew that their kids were having sex?

No. If you asked them, they would probably give you a number like 20 percent. . . . Students like me, my friends, maybe those that were also similar to my [relatively higher] socioeconomic status and, you know, pretty similar results as far as grades, were very, very, very, very careful to not get pregnant. . . . The termination of the pregnancy, people saw the results from that, the emotional results in girls. And then they also saw how quickly people's lives changed if they decided to carry the pregnancies all the way through. So those were . . . for many people it was pure fear of that, true fear of that.

Okay. Do you think that most teens like you who were having sex in high school were using contraception, or were they practicing abstinence, or what's your take on that?

Contraception was rampant.

Isaac's narrative ties together several of the themes discussed here. He says parents communicated an anti-sex norm without "active promotion," they remained silent about contraception and engaged in a conspiracy of silence about teenagers in the community being sexually active, and they succeeded at instilling "pure fear" in teens of the negative consequences of pregnancy. Teens did not conform to norms about sex, but they worked hard to avoid pregnancy. In Isaac's community, like many others, parents' efforts at physical and social control ended up as part success and part failure.

MANAGING NORM VIOLATIONS

DEALING WITH PREGNANCY: "GET THIS TAKEN CARE OF"

Parents do their best to enforce norms against teen sex and pregnancy, and they threaten dire consequences if teens break the rules. But what actually happens when norms are violated? Here, I focus on teen pregnancy because it is apparently rare for parents to find out about their teenager's sexual activity unless there is a pregnancy scare. I combine interviews with college students and teen parents to answer this question.

Many teens who violate norms by becoming pregnant work to hide this fact from their parents. For example, Isabella helped her friends in a mostly White, middle-income small town use "Plan B" medication to eliminate potential pregnancies so they would not need to tell their parents: "A couple of times, . . . I got the morning after pill for a girl who didn't have . . . an account with [a reproductive health clinic], I guess. So, I would get it for her. I mean, it's so easy to do that how can you not, really, if you're even worried about it at all?" Ella, the mother of a one-year-old, told us, "When I found out I was pregnant, I was scared. . . . I was in eighth grade. . . . I still haven't told them [my parents]. . . . They know I have a baby, but I haven't said, 'Mom, I'm pregnant. Dad, I'm pregnant.' I didn't actually go up to them and say it." Her family has not been very supportive materially or emotionally. Although Ella's case is extreme, many teen parents waited as long as possible before revealing their pregnancy to family members.

Not telling parents can have negative consequences, as in Veronica's case in her affluent, White suburb of a very large city. After Veronica started college, she had unprotected sex with her boyfriend and felt that she could not afford to buy a "morning after pill." Because she had never "had the 'me having sex' talk" with her parents, she did not tell them about her pregnancy and chose to abort it (which presumably cost substantially more than the "morning after pill"). She now regrets the abortion: "I guess the lack of information I had about abortion . . . I guess really led to me making a bad decision." Communicating openly with her parents might have led to a more satisfying decision-making process for Veronica.

Many other teens feel they can't manage pregnancy or parenthood without telling their families. When their teenage child reveals a pregnancy, parents may choose to do damage control by hiding the pregnancy from public view. This involves either abortion or sending the teen away during the pregnancy and giving the baby up for adoption. Alternatively, the parents can discourage abortion, making the pregnancy public, and the teen can become a parent with or without family support. In my data as in national statistics, both abortion and carrying the pregnancy to term are common solutions, but adoption is not.[25]

In many families, keeping the teen's norm violation private is paramount. A friend of Josiah's in his tiny, isolated mountain town decided together with her mother that she would get an abortion: "So she told her mom, and her mom drove her. And she [the mother] says . . . 'It's okay, honey. We'll get this taken care of.'" This mother was supportive, but many other parents are not, so telling parents about a pregnancy entails taking a great risk. For example, Henry talked about a friend in his conservative Southern city who told her parents about her pregnancy: "She left town for a while after she had the abortion. Her dad made her live with her mother in Florida. He was very ashamed of the situation." This father did damage control to hide his daughter's pregnancy, but he still kicked his daughter out of the house as a sanction for her norm violation. As I have discussed, parents' ability to throw teens out of their homes is a powerful type of social control. It is noteworthy that Henry's friend had an abortion despite being from a Catholic school and community in which, as Henry said, "abortions are bad. And at the same time they're not supposed to be having an abortion, but they're also not supposed to be having sex. So it's sort of a tricky topic." In this case, the desire to abort the pregnancy privately overwhelmed religious considerations.

Jessica's experiences in a politically moderate, middle-income suburb show how many parents try to control teenagers' decision making about pregnancy. She first told us that when she told her parents about her pregnancy, "They reacted in a very supportive manner," and her mother told her that she had gotten pregnant at age 18 herself and aborted the pregnancy. At first, her mother's reaction was "a big weight off my chest." However, she soon realized that her parents' support was only valid if she decided to abort the pregnancy:

> Well, growing up, my parents . . . had discussed with me that if I were ever to get pregnant, what I would do. And they always said that if I had gotten pregnant, that I should be able to financially support my child, myself and my child. And therefore, if I couldn't financially support myself and my child, then I shouldn't be having a baby. If I did choose to have the baby, they would financially stop supporting me. I would have had to move out, and be on my own. . . . It was never *really* an option to have it at the time, but at the same time, I do want to be a mom, and I think that I can be a great one. . . . I just kinda thought that it was the best decision for myself and for the child.

Although Jessica framed the abortion as her own choice, her parents' threats of banishing her and cutting her off financially clearly shaped her perception of what was the "best decision."

Sometimes parents literally try to take over the decision making about a pregnancy. Dashiel and his girlfriend had an unintended teen pregnancy, and his girlfriend wanted to have the baby while her mother wanted an abortion:

> Her family, honestly, they didn't want her to have the baby. We went to [a reproductive health clinic]. They tried to get her to have an abortion. But honestly, I think the person who was supposed to do it, she had asked my girlfriend, did she want the baby or not? And my girlfriend told her, "Yeah." So the doctor told my girlfriend, "It's not up to your mom whether or not you get an abortion. This is your body. So if you don't want to have an abortion, I'm not gonna make you have an abortion." What she did was, she got my girlfriend's mom a pregnancy test and told her, "*You're* not pregnant."

If the doctor had not intervened dramatically to make the point that it was Dashiel's girlfriend, and not her mother, who was pregnant, the girlfriend's mother would have succeeded in forcing an abortion against the girl's will. Similarly, Pedro's girlfriend's family was "trying to talk her into putting him [his son] up for adoption, if not having an abortion. I completely disagreed with it. She did, too, but her family kept on pushing her and pushing her." At the abortion clinic, she decided to carry the pregnancy to term. Unlike in Jessica's case, the parents' attempts to control these decisions were unsuccessful.

DEALING WITH TEEN PARENTHOOD: "YOU'RE A BABY YOURSELF"

Once teenage girls find out they are pregnant, the stakes over parents' control of their decision making become even higher than they are for controlling teen sex and contraception. Many teens face extreme negative sanctions from their parents if they make a non-normative choice about abortion (which choice is seen as non-normative varies between the practical and moral rationales). Because family members' desire for control over teens' decision making is often framed in terms of protecting the teen's future, it is ironic that these negative reactions themselves have the potential to cause great damage to the girls' futures. How do these family dynamics continue if the pregnancy is carried to term and a teenage girl or boy becomes a parent? Interviews with teen parents provide some sense of this, but keep in mind that their socioeconomic background is different from most of the college student interviewees.[26]

Pregnant teenagers are scared to tell their parents. Charlotte, who became a mother at age 15, is a typical example because her parents' reactions were negative, but not as negative as she had feared:

> I was just keeping it [the pregnancy] in me for a really long time, because I was scared. I didn't know what to do, and then one day I just couldn't take it anymore and I called my mom. She was the first one I told. . . . On the phone right then, she was really nice and supportive, because I was crying and all that. And then she wasn't too mad. She just didn't really talk to me for a couple weeks, because she just needed time to get used to it. . . . And then I finally told my dad, and he was the last person to find out. . . . He was pretty upset. That's why I decided to tell him last.
>
> *Why do you think he was upset?*
>
> I don't really know. I guess because he didn't really know where I was at in my life. . . . So he was probably just upset by the fact that I was so young, and then all these other people knew, and he was the last one.

Charlotte's boyfriend's parents were even angrier. After several months, Charlotte's mother "decided that she was upset about it again," but both families "came around" after the birth. Charlotte told us, "As soon as the baby comes out and they see him, they're like, 'Oh, how cute,' and they forget everything else." This thawing of negative reactions after the birth is common.

When they react negatively to an impending birth, families tend to take action in ways that have problematic consequences.[27] The first, very common action is to withhold needed resources or provide more contingent resources. Amanda's situation is typical. She had a child at age 16, and she and her boyfriend now get by on his income of less than $750 per month, limited help with groceries from food stamps and WIC, and Medicaid health insurance for mother and child. Amanda's father is dead, and her mother "can never help me out." She is still paying her mother back for the $2,000 medical bill for the birth. Her boyfriend's parents let them live in their basement rent-free and provide free childcare, but his mother "is just awful to deal with" according to Amanda. His mother sells the young couple's belongings when she needs money and won't give Amanda's daughter solid food because feeding her takes time away from the other children she watches (whose parents pay her). Amanda knows that "if she gets another kid [paying for child care], my daughter gets kicked out." This situation is common in that some family members are giving a lot of support while others are not, but also in that the tenuous support can be taken away at any point. Because she doesn't know how long they will have childcare, Amanda has trouble making plans for her further education.

The second common action families take is to treat the teen badly. This kind of reaction is an informal sanctions for violating a norm. Ella, the teen mother who didn't tell her parents about her pregnancy, faced scornful reactions from many family members. Her older sister said, "You're just a little girl that's pregnant in denial." Ella's mother told her, "You're too little to have a baby. You're a baby yourself." She was excluded from family dinners out because there wasn't "enough room for her," and her "other family members were like, 'You're going to get fat!'" In the interview, Ella was upset about this negative treatment. Support from her boyfriend's family is even more problematic, as members of the two families are in rival gangs and try to shoot each other on sight. Ella's case is more extreme than most, but all the teen parents my research team interviewed faced interpersonal sanctions.

Finally, families try to exert control over the couple relationship between the parents of the baby.[28] Sometimes this results in trying to keep the couple together but more often in pushing them apart. Pedro, who became a father at age 16, said, "Her [his child's mother's] family really don't like me. . . . They were always telling her that she shouldn't have this Black baby because she's White, stuff like that. . . . Sometimes I think they try to test me to see what I would do in certain situations." He went on to tell a story about her family asking him to book a hotel room and walk eight miles each way to see his son for half an hour. They were "mad that I did it. . . . They want me to be a failure, I think. . . . They've threatened me with court, they've tried to get me to sign over my rights [as the father]." Pedro and his son's mother have indeed split up, although they "are trying to get back together."

Each of these actions some families take when reacting negatively to teen parenthood—withholding resources, imposing interpersonal sanctions, and controlling the couple—has negative consequences for young parents. Because these parents usually have few resources of their own, negative consequences for them translate directly into negative consequences for their young children. Although family reactions aren't usually as severe as the teenagers thought they would be, families enforce norms against teen pregnancy in ways that matter for teens' and their children's futures.

CONCLUSION

This chapter told teens' side of the story of how their parents and family members communicated and enforced norms about teen sexuality, viewed with the benefit of hindsight so they have some distance from the situation and can be more philosophical about its implications. Young people see parents as important communicators and enforcers of norms about teen sexuality. Their norms tend to reinforce the normative messages teens are getting from their schools and communities, and they are justified using one or both of the practical and moral rationales. Parents and teens are motivated to keep silent about the teen's actual sexual behaviors, so hypothetical situations, gossip, and cautionary tales are important ways of communicating indirectly. Parents use emotional and material threats, as well as control over the teen's body and contraceptive options, to try to enforce norms. But even so, most teens have sex while still in high school.

Interviewees' parents are trying to manage two goals that sometimes come into conflict: communicating and enforcing messages about how teens are supposed to behave sexually, and ensuring that their teen has a bright future. Chapter 2 discussed how these related norm sets influence each other. Whether the sexuality norms they're communicating are practically or morally undergirded, these goals can be hard to reconcile. Most parents use indirect techniques, like cautionary tales or gossiping about other teens, to communicate norms—but they stop short of giving much concrete advice about how to negotiate sexual situations or access and use contraception. Many parents are doing a reasonably good job of communicating norms, but they're falling short on ensuring the teen's bright future because many teens aren't learning enough about how to avoid sexual risks. Parents and teens also tend to collaborate in a conspiracy of silence around the teen's own sexual behaviors, which has the advantage of letting parents believe teens aren't violating norms about sex even when they are. But this conspiracy of silence also means that parents can't tailor their communication about sex to the teen's actual situation and needs. This jeopardizes both of parents' goals because their messages are less targeted to the teen's situation and they are less able to advise the teen on how to avoid sexual risk. Many parents use threats to motivate teens to conform to their expectations for sexual behavior. But if parents are ever called on to make good on those threats, they will hurt the teen's future prospects. Parents are in a bind: They are expected to be the enforcers of norms about sexual behavior, but that enforcement can be damaging to young people. So in many cases, they try to stay ignorant of what their teen is up to, even as they implicitly try to control the teen's behavior through threats and by limiting access to contraception and opportunities for sex.

How do teens view their parents' communication and enforcement? Interestingly, many seem sympathetic to their parents' dilemma. They usually participate in the conspiracy of silence around their own sexual behavior, even though many would prefer to be getting concrete information from their parents. Many teens internalize their parents' norms and believe their threats of enforcement—even when those threats seem empty, like when parents threaten divorce if their teen gets pregnant. This internalization creates a strong sense of fear among most teens. Fear certainly motivates many to avoid the appearance of being sexually active, but not even fear can stop most teens from having sex by the end of high school. Why this happens can't be fully understood simply by looking at parents. Close friends and peers need to enter the picture.

4

"WHAT ARE PEOPLE GOING TO THINK?"

The Influence of Close Friends and Peers

ALTHOUGH PARENTS AND other adults communicate norms about sex to teens, friends and teenage peers represent a different social world with its own norms, ways of communicating, and social control. Haylie grew up in a low-income small city in a rural Western area. Her high school served a racially and socioeconomically diverse population, and she says its dropout rate was high. Like many high schools our interviewees described, Haylie's included a disparate set of friendship groups. She said, "There was definitely a sort of divide between the people that were in those [honors] classes and the people that didn't come to school as often or were just struggling or something for various reasons. . . . So there was a separation between the friend groups, I think, because of that." Her group of close friends was "pretty small . . . upper-division, college-bound type of people . . . not particularly religious." As far as Haylie knows, none of them had sex during high school. "My friend group, we'd date people and not have sex with them; I mean, that was just sort of how we did it." A substantial minority of our interviewees remained virgins throughout high school (but not in college), and many of them believe their close friends did the same.[1]

Haylie thinks her friends were an important influence on her decision not to have sex. In her view, "Teens are definitely looking to their friends for advice and approval, more so than [they are looking to] certain adults." Haylie told us, "My decision to not have sex was more based around myself not being ready, and not being in serious relationships in high school, and then my friends also not having sex." Haylie thinks her friends could have influenced her to make a different decision: "I'm the type of person who compares myself to other people, and it's like, 'Well, if they're doing it, then I should be doing it, too.' Then I would worry that there was something wrong with me if I wasn't [having sex], or nobody would like me, or whatever." Haylie would have told her friends, but not her parents, if she had started having sex. "I wasn't very close to my parents in high school. Like if I had a boyfriend, I wouldn't tell them I was dating the boy. . . . If I were to have started to have sex, I probably wouldn't have come to them."

Haylie was "sure" reputation was a big deal in her friendship group, even if negative sanctions for having sex wouldn't have been severe. "In my friend group . . . if one of us started having sex and told the other people in the group, that would have been sort of a big deal, I guess. But I don't think they would have necessarily judged us or made us feel excluded because of it. It just would have been like, 'Whoa, we're not doing that yet.'" If Haylie had gotten pregnant, she didn't think her friends would have been very supportive. "They would want to be there for me, but wouldn't know how to react or how to help me through it." Reputation and gossip were even greater concerns in Haylie's wider circle of peers beyond her close friends because teens in her school gossiped about each other's sex lives. "You definitely hear rumors about so-and-so were having sex. . . . If someone got pregnant, we'd gossip about it and sort of feel bad for them, I guess. It would be the hot topic for a little while." Haylie thinks teens deciding whether or not to have sex were influenced by gossip: "You know, what people are going to think about this [the teen having sex] if they find out."

Like most other interviewees, Haylie described a peer-oriented social world in which teens negotiate sexual decision making carefully and work hard to keep their behavior private. They—particularly girls—risk social exclusion and a tarnished reputation if they don't navigate a cautious course of action. Because of these concerns, the fear around teen sex and pregnancy that interviewees expressed when talking about their parents was also reflected in their interactions with friends and peers. Some young people think parents' influence is more important than that of friends and some think the opposite, but they agree that friends and peers matter a lot.

Close friends are an important buffer protecting teens from the often more hostile normative environments of peers and parents. Not surprisingly, then, close friends are often very influential for teenagers' sexual behavior.[2] But our interviewees make a clear distinction between *actual* sexual behavior—which is typically private between two partners—and *public perceptions* of sexual behavior—which may or may not reflect private behaviors. Chapter 2 discusses how both actual behaviors and perceptions of behaviors are part of a set of norms. High school peer groups can act like a hall of mirrors at an amusement park, creating skewed public perceptions of teenagers' actual private behaviors and reflecting them back to teens. Many teens go to great lengths to avoid being publicly scrutinized in this way. Another important category besides close friends and more distant peers—romantic partners—is largely absent in Haylie's story because of her lack of an emotionally committed relationship in high school. In this she is typical of my college-bound interviewees, but romantic partners were very important influences in the interviews with teen parents. For the very few college student interviewees who talked about having had a serious romantic attachment in high school, the partner shaped both their sexual behavior and public perceptions of that behavior.

NORMS COMMUNICATED BY PEERS

HOW PEERS ARE DIFFERENT FROM PARENTS: "WORLDS APART"

Chapter 3 lays out the rationales that parents communicate to teens. The same two rationales are also communicated among close friends and within wider peer groups. Interviewees told us about hearing some or all of the following from peers: (1) Sexual behavior may endanger their promising future, is irresponsible, is stupid, and shows a lack of self-respect (the practical rationale) and (2) sexual behavior is morally wrong (the moral rationale).

But there are also important differences between the norms communicated by friends and peers and those communicated by parents. First, there is a lot more variation in the norms about teen sex being communicated by friends and peers. Parents' norms about sex are almost uniformly negative, with essentially no parents telling their teenagers that sex is encouraged. Some interviewees' friends and peers do say this, though. Carter was pretty typical in distinguishing between kinds of sexual behavior that are viewed differently in his wealthy, predominantly White small city. Among teenagers in his community, he says, sex "was promoted more so than it was frowned upon. . . . No one would judge you if you did or did not [have sex]." But in the interview he referred to a girl he knew as "slutty." When asked to explain what he meant, Carter replied, "[My hometown] is a liberal town, so if you sleep with someone, you are not considered a whore. But if you are partying a lot and you're constantly having sex with other people—with random people—sex seems to dominate your life." In Carter's peer group as in many others, sex in a committed romantic relationship is considered okay, but casual sex at parties or with multiple partners is inappropriate.

Not all peer groups consider sex acceptable, though. In Finn's conservative Western city, he said most teenagers were not having sex. "We were always confused because we heard about these schools where lots of people have sex all the time. And we were like, 'What? Aw, they're all sluts. They must all be sluts, whores.' You know. Just the whole school full of whores." Having sex at all earned teens in Finn's school the "slut" label, a gendered term that regulates girls more than boys.[3] But in many schools, different peer groups have different norms about sex—peer norms aren't as uniform as Finn and Carter said they were in their high schools. Logan told us that among his friends in a middle-income suburb, sex was viewed as "something that's [appropriate] within the confines of marriage." But he went on: "I had one friend who played football, and he would kind of switch between our group and the football players [within the same school]. And the stories he would tell, and the things that they did, just like worlds apart, you know." Although there was variation in peer norms about the acceptability of at least some kinds of sex, teen pregnancy was still considered inappropriate in all peer contexts.

A second factor that showed up starkly in interviewees' descriptions of peers' messages about sexual behavior, but not as much in parents' messages, is gender. Sociologists Barbara Risman and Pepper Schwartz discuss how norms about teen sexual behavior became more gender neutral in the 1990s. Sex within committed relationships became more acceptable for both girls and boys, while casual sex was considered unacceptable for both genders.[4] Some of the same dynamic exists in my more recent interviews, but there is a lot of variation from place to place. In many contexts, gender equality in sex norms is still a long way off—but this is sometimes hard for interviewees to see. Like Carter and Finn, interviewees tended to talk about peer norms about sex as if they were gender neutral, but the examples they gave of people who had violated these norms or who were the targets of vicious gossip were almost always girls. This pattern could stem from two possible causes: Either the norms about sexual behavior are different for boys compared to girls, or the norms are enforced more strictly for girls than for boys. The data suggest that both are true, as I discuss below.

Once prompted, many interviewees identified gender differences in the norms about sex that are communicated to girls versus boys. Rochelle is a good example. She thinks most teens in her low-income, small Northeastern town had sex, but they didn't talk openly about it. Instead, people assumed that teens who were in a long-term relationship were having sex. Teens having sex in casual relationships or one-night stands were looked down upon, "especially girls. . . . It was a lot harsher for girls. Like, how do I explain it? There was one girl, she hooked up with two guys randomly, and she was considered the biggest whore in our school." Similarly, Ella told us that in her wealthy, liberal small city, "I think it's different for guys, because no matter what, if a baby happens or not, it's just different for them having sex. Girls are chastised a lot more for being sexually active, while guys, it's not only acceptable, it's expected." Growing up in the same city as Ella, Patton also thought that the gendered double standard for sexual behavior was alive and well in peer messages about teen pregnancy: "It was the girls that were shunned if they were pregnant. And the boys were kind of looked on as, well, it was a masculine thing, so it was okay. . . . I think the brunt of the blame was usually placed on the girl."

The last difference between norms communicated by friends and peers and those communicated by parents has to do with time horizons. Parents focus on the teen's future when discouraging sexual behaviors. Peers and friends talk about the future in the same way, but they also focus on the present. Sex can lead to negative consequences for a teen's future, but it can also bring benefits in the here and now. Besides being pleasurable and furthering intimacy with a partner, sex can create a feeling of being normal and more adult.[5] These benefits may outweigh the risks, depending on how strong norms against sex are. And in some peer contexts, at least for boys, having sex may lead to social approval.

In many of the interviewees' peer groups, the benefits of sex were gendered because it was considered more acceptable for boys. Kaitlyn told us that in her Western community, "pretty much everyone I knew" was sexually active by the end of high school. She felt that peers "definitely" influenced each other's sexual behavior, "I mean, especially from a guy's perspective. Guys always make fun of each other and make fun of the virgin. They make fun of their friends that aren't getting any [sex]. I mean, on the girl's side, once their friends have sex and start experimenting, it starts to be okay. Once everyone is doing it, you think it is okay. You start to think, 'Everyone is doing it, so why am I not doing it?'" This description of peer influences on teenagers' decision making is focused on social approval and here-and-now pros and cons, not on potential future consequences. Among Kaitlyn's peers, boys may feel encouraged to have sex to appease their sexual desire, but girls' sexual desire isn't supposed to be a factor in their decision making—girls are expected to be motivated by a desire to be normal.[6] The benefits of sex among Kaitlyn's peers are there for both girls and boys, but they are gendered and are stronger for boys.

THE NORMS PEERS COMMUNICATE:
"SEEN THROUGH A DIFFERENT LENS"

As the examples above suggest, peers and friends communicate three different categories of norms about sexual behavior that are part of the same norm set: norms regulating the behavior itself, norms regulating portrayal of the behavior to others, and norms regulating teenagers' reactions to people who violate the first two categories of norms. Past research on social norms has identified the first and third categories of norms, but not the second.

First, peers and friends communicate norms about how teens are supposed to behave sexually. As the previous section showed, even these norms can be complicated—for example, sometimes sex within a romantic relationship is considered acceptable by peers but casual sex isn't, or sex is acceptable for boys but not girls. The interviews strongly suggest that teens' actual sexual behavior is often shaped by their close friends' norms.[7] Kaitlyn and others articulated an "everyone is doing it" logic in which norms about sexual behavior in the wider peer group also matter. Interviewees often drew on broader peer group norms when deciding to have sex, but not as much when deciding to stay abstinent.[8]

The wider peer group matters much more for the second kind of norm, which regulates how sexual behavior is *portrayed* instead of the behavior itself. Sexual behavior is usually private with a partner, giving teenagers the opportunity to separate their actual behavior from their public portrayal of how they are behaving—if they can control how their partner portrays the encounter. Lilly, who like most of her close friends in her large urban high school was sexually active within a long-term romantic relationship, described how this public–private split works: "I feel like anybody who did have sex, it was really kept low, like secret. . . . You just didn't talk about it. It wasn't like everyone knew. I mean, people would *assume* if you'd been dating someone for a long time, but no one would be like, 'Oh my God, you're having sex, I can't believe you!'" Lilly portrayed her sexual behavior accurately to close friends, but to other peers she followed norms and didn't admit to having sex. Charles described a similar dynamic for girls among his peers in an ethnically diverse, middle-income city. "There was always kind of the issue like, 'Oh, keep that [sex] behind closed doors,' you know? . . . Nobody expects a girl to be a virgin. Nobody that I knew in high school. But if you did have sex and it was known, you were seen through a different lens, you know? It wasn't always negative, but most of the time it was." Charles is describing a very clear split for girls between the norm about actual behavior (having sex is acceptable) and the norm about how to publicly portray your behavior (being known to be sexually active is unacceptable).

Charles said peers' reaction to heterosexual—but not gay—boys who portrayed themselves as being sexually active was markedly different: "Player. 'Oh, you the shit.' It was like, you hear about them and, 'Oh dude, she's so hot, how'd you get with her?' You know, so it's very different." Among Charles's peers, boys and girls were both sometimes motivated to portray their sexual behavior differently than it actually was, but in starkly contrasting ways. Among his peers, girls were motivated to hide their sexual behavior, but their male sexual partners were often motivated to tell the truth or even exaggerate their sexual exploits.[9] I talk later about how teens work with friends and peers to navigate this social challenge. Some teens themselves saw sexual behavior as private and pregnancy as public, as Claudia said of her wealthy, White, liberal town:

> Well, I think that sex is something that happens privately, and pregnancy is something that happens publicly. So they kind of exist in different realms in our thoughts. So whether or not we say we are okay with it or not okay with it, either in sex or in pregnancy, that behavior really changes whether or not it is something that everyone is gonna know or not. . . . You could say, "I wouldn't mind if one of my friends was pregnant," and you might respond totally differently because you would have to deal with that in a more public setting. And I think that that creates a situation where . . . as far as having sex, you could do what you wanted, but the pregnancy part is, you would probably do what your community would want. See what I'm saying?

Claudia says that by conforming to norms about how to portray their sexual behavior to others, teenagers can privately engage in sexual behaviors without receiving negative sanctions.

Third, peers and friends communicate norms about how to react when someone has violated sex norms. These are called *metanorms*—norms about appropriate ways to enforce norms.[10] Metanorms are an important social dynamic because without them, it often wouldn't make sense for people to waste time and energy sanctioning someone who violates a norm. Metanorms ensure that people who sanction others according to the group's norm are socially rewarded and those who refuse to sanction are sanctioned. Metanorms can be so strong that they can ensure the survival of an unpopular social norm, one that even its enforcers don't agree with. By sanctioning people who violate the norm, people are able to signal their agreement with the norm (even if they privately disagree with it).[11] In Charles's example above, there was probably a metanorm encouraging peers to socially sanction girls who portray themselves as sexually active, and another metanorm prescribing social rewards for boys who convince others they've had sex. Below I expand on how metanorms work in peer groups.

Interviewees described experiencing complex norm sets with one category of norms for what you can do in private, another for what you can tell people you've done, and a third for how to behave toward and talk about people who have broken the rules. Because communication among high school friends and peers is usually more public than communication among family members, the stakes are higher when teens communicate normative messages to each other.

HOW NORMS ARE COMMUNICATED

EXPLICIT TALK ABOUT NORMS: "WE'RE NOT DOING THAT YET"

Teens talk more openly about sex with each other than they do with their parents, but it is still a difficult topic for many of them. Even as college students, interviewees often responded to questions with comments like, "This is awkward." There were other signs of discomfort with talking about sex, even with an acquaintance in the case of the peer interviews in this study. Some interviewees used goofy voices and baby talk, like "preggers" for pregnant and "shmushmortion" for abortion, to ease their discomfort.[12]

Interviewees often said they used indirect ways to talk about sex and pregnancy with friends, as they did with parents. The same tactics are often deployed, such as discussing hypothetical situations or using euphemistic or ambiguous language. Above, Haylie verbalized her friends' hypothetical reaction to news of her sexual activity as a vague, "Whoa, we're not doing that yet."[13] Two other strategies from Chapter 3—talk about other people and silence—are much more common than explicit talk about sex norms. In this way, teens' communication of sex norms is surprisingly similar to parent–teen communication. A common exception to this lack of direct communication is adult-mediated conversations among teenage peers in settings such as religious youth groups and school classes. The topic of the class doesn't need to be sex for conversations to break out, as Annika told us of her low-income small mountain town: "There were so many [conversations about sex], we would have debates in math class or whatever." Annika's school had another common way for teenagers to explicitly communicate norms about sexual behavior without talking directly—through messages on clothing. She said, "We had a lot of those, I don't know if you've seen those sweatshirts, but they say, 'Abortion is homicide.' . . . There was a lot of very anti-abortion stuff in the school, so I think if people did have an abortion they kept it very quiet."

GOSSIP AND CAUTIONARY TALES: "RUMORS SPREAD LIKE WILDFIRE"

Gossip about other teens is often the main way sex norms get communicated among friends and peers. Gossip achieves a dual purpose. Not only does gossip communicate how teens are supposed to behave, portray their own behavior, and sanction others, but it also serves as an important way of socially sanctioning teens who violate norms. I focus here on how gossip communicates norms, and later in the chapter I discuss gossip as a form of social control.

Peer gossip can either encourage or discourage sexual behavior. The latter is more common, but in some communities the former is important as well. In Patton's liberal college town, a pro-sex norm was communicated among peers through rumors that may or may not have been true. He said that in the later years of high school:

> I think that was kind of the myth, that if you were having sex you were one of the cool kids, because those were the kind of rumors that you heard about—the cool kids that were having sex on the weekends. . . . I think it was usually the "in" crowd, the students who were in athletics, and then usually you heard about them being the ones that were going to big parties on the weekends and drinking lots of alcohol, and usually with alcohol followed sex. And that's generally, I think, where that myth was born from. . . . Rumors get spread, and you think it's more widespread than it actually is.

But the same peer group also spread negative rumors about the related behavior of pregnancy. Patton told us, "I feel like looking back, it was probably mostly a lot of rumors that were spread around about whoever it was who got pregnant. I don't feel like there was probably a lot of truthful knowledge being passed around." Patton said pregnant girls were "shunned" in his peer group, although boys who got a girl pregnant did not face negative rumors.

Teen pregnancy is often the main target of peer gossip, serving as a "cautionary tale" to warn teens not to violate peer norms. Pregnancy gossip also communicates norms about related sexual behaviors, like sex, contraception, and abortion. Sophie told of the one girl she knew who ended up pregnant in her predominantly White, middle-income suburb, and "rumors spread like wildfire right when she got pregnant." She summed up the gossip that would start about a pregnant girl: "Probably someone who doesn't have that great of a reputation as far as sleeping around goes. And I guess 'slacker' kind of comes to mind, like school probably wasn't a priority in that girl's life. I don't necessarily see drug use or being totally delinquent, but just an overall maybe less responsible, less mature kid." Even though any sexually active girl could become pregnant, these judgments weren't passed on nonpregnant girls. Makayla laid out the gossip that a previously "popular girl" in her wealthy suburban school faced upon getting pregnant: "It was negative. It was saying, 'Oh, she's a slut,' and 'Oh, she slept around,' and 'Oh, I hear in middle school she had an abortion.' You know, just ridiculous rumors." This gossip is an effective way of communicating norms: a norm against girls' casual sex with multiple partners, another against abortion, and the maturity and future aspects of the practical rationale. Because carrying a pregnancy to term is more common among girls with lower SES, this kind of gossip is also a way to target sex shaming to these teens while sparing their sexually active, higher-SES counterparts.[14] As discussed below, this is a form of symbolic boundary work that gives advantaged teens more leeway from social sanctions.[15]

Boys are much less often part of these cautionary tales because they usually have the option of socially distancing themselves from a pregnant partner. When asked to talk about teen parents they knew in their communities, interviewees almost exclusively brought up girls. They usually knew little to nothing about the baby's father when asked. This pattern implies either that the babies' fathers were already out of high school (which statistics show is often the case) or that they had distanced themselves socially from the pregnancy.[16] Logan contrasted the social sanctioning of pregnant girls with boys' option of detaching from the pregnancy in his middle-income Western suburb: "If a girl ever was pregnant, you know, it was kind of—she wasn't outcast by any means, but she was no longer part of [trails off]. They [the boys who got the girls pregnant] would go on, move on to other girls, rather than keep going out with her." This symbolic boundary work around gender allows boys more leeway to avoid sanctions.

Some communities with lower SES and higher rates of teen pregnancy have a different dynamic. Pregnant girls still face damaging gossip and become cautionary tales for their peers, but there is also a general sense among teenagers that a pregnancy could happen to them. Lillian, who comes from a lower-income urban area, described the alternative view of teen pregnancy there:

> You can say, yeah, it was typically the girl who was a ho [whore]. But really, there were girls who were "hos," quote unquote, and they didn't get pregnant. I remember one certain girl who would make fun of all these other girls because they would get pregnant and because they weren't using protection. And she would be like, "Why don't they just use a condom? They wouldn't be getting pregnant." To me it's like, you know what would be hilarious? When your condom breaks, when *your* condom breaks. You think that your condom breaking is not gonna cause that. It's not just one particular kind of person who's gonna get pregnant. It could happen to anybody. To *anybody*.

This sense of pregnancy as a risk faced by every sexually active teenager sometimes goes hand in hand with a somewhat less brutal peer climate for pregnant girls. In contrast, some interviewees from communities with higher SES seem strangely invulnerable to the idea that their own sexual activity entails a risk of pregnancy.[17] This may be because of the symbolic boundary work in teenagers' gossip that tends not to hold people like them accountable for their behavior.

SILENCE: "DON'T TELL ANYBODY"

Like parents often do, peers can communicate norms through silence. Patton said that among his peers in a liberal college town, teen pregnancy "was kind of pushed into the dark corner—the taboo topic that we don't want to talk about." Patton suggests that shame around sex, which could be prescribed by emotion norms, may underlie the silence. Silence, especially when paired with the social exclusion of girls who violate the norm against pregnancy, is an effective way of sending a normative message. The near-total silence around non-heterosexual sex in the interviews is an example of this dynamic.

Silence serves another useful purpose for teens. Like the "conspiracy of silence" many engage in with their parents, peers and even close friends often share a conspiracy of silence with each other. The most straightforward way to conform to a norm against portraying oneself as sexually active, while still privately having sex, is to stay silent about that behavior. Teenagers do this a lot, even in peer groups that don't actively discourage sex. Although the interviewees didn't talk much about why this happens, I argue it is a strategy to prevent any peers, parents, and other adults who have norms against teen sex from finding out about the teen's sexual activity. Helena, who attended a "very liberal" school with pervasive casual sex, said of her peers: "I think because it was such a small school, they just didn't want to talk about it all [sex] with people, as things go around really quickly. So, yeah, they would just keep their mouths shut about everything." Silence can help ensure that a teen is unlikely to become the target of gossip.

Close friends often help each other stay silent about sexual behavior, either by curtailing discussion of sex within the friendship group or by keeping gossip from spreading outside the group to other peers. Dylan's friends used both of these strategies in a large conservative city:

> Well, the group of friends would know [about their friends' sexual activity]. But most of us, I think, if you were close enough to the person, were pretty good about respecting their privacy. So we wouldn't ask too many questions, and we wouldn't spread stuff. So in the case of that girl [a pregnant friend who was keeping her pregnancy secret], when people were like, "Oh, where is she?" We'd say, "Oh, I don't know, maybe she's sick or has a health issue." It's what she asked us to say.

Madelyn said flatly that in her highly religious city, "You do not talk about your sex life. So no one really knows. Between my closest, bestest friends, we did know each other's sex lives. But that was it." Disclosing sexual activity to a close friend requires a lot of trust in that person's silence.

In peer groups with strong norms against sex, the strategy of keeping sexual behavior private even from one's closest friends is common. In telling us the story of a girl who made the mistake of confiding in a friend, Finn illustrated the social risk teens in his highly religious Western city ran if peers found out they were having sex: "If you have sex with anybody, everybody would hear about it . . . if it leaks. So you don't tell anybody. But everybody did end up telling one of their friends. So that's what this girl did, and everybody in the whole school knows. And then that girl gets this terrible reputation, and then she never lives it down, ever." The boy she slept with was the brunt of peers' jokes until "eventually he started to deny it," exercising a boy's privilege to distance himself from violations of sexual norms. Finn himself may have violated a norm by refusing to enter into this conspiracy of silence. He told us, "I was one of the people who had sex, and I told some of my friends that. And they were a little bit shocked, a little bit proud, or surprised."

As Finn's story implies, a successful conspiracy of silence about sexual behavior requires the silence of both sexual partners, even as the reputational stakes are higher for girls than for boys. This can be particularly difficult because many sex partners of high school students come from within their school.[18] There are often different social pressures for girls and boys—so in a heterosexual encounter in a peer context that is more tolerant of teen sex than Finn's was, the girl may be motivated to keep the sex quiet while the boy is motivated to talk about it.

The typical social settings where teens have sex are different depending on how strong peer norms against sex are. The first is a highly gendered casual sex model, with sex taking place as "hookups" at parties and fueled by alcohol use. Although it is widespread during college, this setting for sex is less common in high school than readers might think.[19] This model of teen sex tends to be more prevalent in peer settings that consider sex appropriate, like Patton's example above. In Finn's conservative city, his unusual group of friends "hated the community" and encouraged sex because it was "one of the things to do with spite [to spite the community]." He said, "One of the things to do was to have sex . . . Friends hanging out at parties, trying to score alcohol . . . 'cause once you got drunk, it was a lot easier to have sex. And it was a lot easier to have fun." Importantly, the "hookup model" of teen sex was only considered a socially acceptable option for a few *boys* in these interviews. Girls only talked about sex at parties when explaining how much it damaged girls' reputations; they had not participated in this model themselves. The hookup model may be rare in high school because of its public nature, which rules out the possibility of staying silent about sexual activity.

The much more prevalent socially acceptable setting for teen sex was the "relationship model." Adrian described what this looked like in his wealthy suburb: "The people that I knew who were having sex were doing it as monogamous as you can in high school. And so not really [worried about their reputations]. It seemed like if you were [having sex in a monogamous relationship], that was fine. I don't know of anybody who had sex with lots of different partners." Now in college, our interviewees rarely described having had a strong emotional attachment to high school partners. Instead, some talked explicitly about high school relationships as a useful way to have sex with a trusted partner who would hopefully be reliable about staying silent and dealing with a potential pregnancy. Lilly talked about her own and her friends' sexual activity in a diverse large city:

> My friends who were sexually active, most of us were sexually active at the same time because we all had got a new relationship at the same time. We waited a really long time, then finally we're like, "Ah well, all right!" Like with us, if we were to have a baby . . . if the guy didn't stay, we'd hunt him down and choke him. . . .
> *Do you think that's why you feel like you waited to have sex in a relationship instead of more casual sex?*
> Yeah, definitely. . . . Anybody who did have sex, it was really kept low, like secret.

Lilly and her friends waited a long time to have sex, trying to ensure that their boyfriends would be reliable in keeping sex and its consequences quiet. They decided as a group when to become sexually active, showing how important an influence on sexual behavior close friends can be.

HOW PEERS TRY TO ENSURE CONFORMITY

Interviewees said that teens are very worried about facing negative sanctions from their close friends and peers. This is similar to their fear of parents' reactions to their sexual activity or pregnancy, but most teens draw a clear line between the normative expectations of their peers by the end of high school and those of their parents. This creates a difficult juggling act for these teenagers, who must work hard to (at least appear to) conform to two distinct sets of expectations for their sexual behavior. It's important to realize that pro-sex and anti-sex expectations among peers are not equally strong. Teens who violate anti-sex norms typically face strict negative sanctions. But if they are in a peer climate that considers teen sex appropriate and they stay abstinent, they don't often talk about people reacting negatively. This lack of sanctions suggests that at least in some places, the pro-sex peer "norm" may not actually be a social norm in the traditional sense, but rather a prevalent behavior pattern that can influence teenagers. This kind of prevalent behavior with no sanctions attached is a descriptive (or statistical) norm, while a prescribed behavior with sanctions attached is an injunctive (or social) norm.[20]

SOCIAL EXCLUSION: "WHAT EVERYBODY IS AFRAID OF"

Negative sanctions around sex are mostly limited to teens who have sex when a peer norm says they shouldn't, or teens who portray themselves as sexually active when a peer norm discourages it. But how do peers sanction one another? Unlike parents and schools, which have a legal right to control underage teenagers' bodies and movements, peers have few options for physical control of each other. Teens' scarce resources and their lack of formal power over same-age peers also limit many options for social control, such as bribes and threats. But as our interviewees' accounts have already shown, there is an effective weapon in peers' and close friends' arsenals: *social exclusion*, the threat of losing status among peers or even being left out of peer interactions. Teens change friendship groups regularly, and they use reputational aggression as a way to seek increased social status as friendships change.[21] These dynamics encourage social exclusion and make it easy for people who are behaving in a different way from their friends to get left behind. Not only the nature, but the physical setting, of teen friendships lends power to social exclusion. High schoolers are generally obligated to spend the whole school day in the company of their peers, and as is typical in the adolescent phase of development, many interviewees described having been peer-oriented people. As research on social norms has shown, exclusion from peer interactions is a particularly effective sanction if you care a lot about peers' approval and spend every weekday with them.[22]

Finn explained what social exclusion looks like in his conservative Western city when telling us how peers from his Evangelical church youth group would have reacted if he had gotten a girl pregnant:

> Oh yeah, all those people would have given me a lot of shit . . . because it's [sex is] so embarrassing. They would tease me, just because they would be like, "Ha ha, you're the kid that did that. Oh, my God!" They would have done all that, I guarantee it. And that's what everybody is afraid of, because they'd seen it happen before in other similar situations. And they knew these people are getting a lot of shit. Or they give you the silent treatment. Either way, it's like total social exclusion. And that's the only the only thing we were worried about. That was our highest priority. . . . I've been in situations like that, and usually I just don't like to acknowledge it. But it's impossible not to, if everybody is teasing you about the same thing, I would imagine it's impossible. It's

just—you get so pissed off you might have to just leave. And that's what happened to a lot of people.

In Finn's account, the teasing or silent treatment can be so severe that teens choose to leave the peer group voluntarily. Leaving the group is an option for a church youth group, but leaving school is more difficult. In this way, many teens can get trapped in the setting where they're being excluded. And as other interviewees said, the brunt of peer sanctions usually falls on girls rather than boys. Madelyn said that in her highly religious city, pregnancy "definitely damaged the girls' reputations more. . . . I think it was because they were sexually active, and then the whole school knew about it. Because I knew other kids that were sexually active, but it wasn't broadcast. Because sex is something you just don't talk about in our high school. So that's why it damaged their reputation." Madelyn implies that sexually active teens who kept their behavior quiet weren't sanctioned. Research on a national sample of teens supports Madelyn's assumption and finds that peer social exclusion is gendered and classed: Girls who have more sexual partners are less accepted by peers, but boys who come from disadvantaged backgrounds have more friends the more sexual partners they have.[23]

Teens' fear of social exclusion is clear in interviewees' talk about which aspects of sexual behavior worry teens and how they work to hide norm violations from peers. Helena told us that in her wealthy resort town, getting pregnant "is the number one thing people [teens] would worry about. . . . Because pregnancy is a very real thing, while having an STD, you know, everyone doesn't have to know if you have an STD." Helena defined pregnancy as a "real thing," and STIs as implicitly not, because of the public nature of pregnancy. She went on to imply that the "everyone" teens were worried would find out about their sexual activity was peers more than parents. Like many others, Jessica said that some peers (including herself) in her politically moderate, middle-income suburb had abortions to keep a pregnancy secret and avoid sanctions: "The community would look down upon them as well if they got pregnant. It reflects being irresponsible, so many kids got pregnant and had abortions. Just nobody knew about it."

How do teens reconcile their emotional attachment to close friends with an assumption that their friends would be willing to socially exclude them? It might be difficult to think of people who would be willing to do that as good friends. Patton's description of how his friends would have reacted if he had gotten a girl pregnant in his liberal college town shows one way in which this can be justified: "I think it would have changed my friendship group. . . . I think it would be really hard for teenage friends to understand what someone was going through if that was their situation. Not to say that they would despise me or not want to be my friend anymore. I just don't know that they would truly understand what was going on and everything that was kind of affecting my life if that were to happen." Even though he's a boy and presumably faces weaker sanctions, Patton thinks his friends would distance themselves. They would do this not through deliberate exclusion, but rather because they just would not be on the same wavelength. In fact, the teen parent interviewees said this is what often happens to friendships after a pregnancy. Given the life changes that becoming a parent entails, making this transition at a different time than most peers makes it more likely that a distance will grow up between friends. But the consequence—social exclusion—is the same regardless of why people claim to be doing it.

METANORMS ENCOURAGING SOCIAL EXCLUSION: "I DON'T WANT TO BE IDENTIFIED WITH YOU"

The social exclusion of peers who violate norms about sexual behavior is a powerful dynamic because peers are often highly motivated to sanction each other. This happens because metanorms (social norms encouraging the sanctioning of others) prescribe the social exclusion of violators. In some social situations, people who refuse to sanction others are suspected of being norm violators themselves.[24] This may be particularly true when people have few social cues to tell them who is actually violating a norm, which is the case for most sexual behaviors. Teenagers need to "prove" that they are conforming to sexuality norms, and one way of doing this is by sanctioning violators. Helena described how this kind of metanorm played out in her "very liberal" school:

> When they [girls in her school] are pregnant, you could definitely see people moving away from them. . . . After the pregnancy, if you didn't know about it, you treated them the same. The people who did know about it were very careful around them, like they have a disease or something. . . . And so I think it was just like, "I don't want to be identified with you because, you know, you're clearly not responsible enough, so I don't want to be seen as your friend." . . . If you're going to do it [have sex], that's one thing, but to do it poorly [not use contraception], that's another.

In Helena's account, people who can be "identified" as the friends of a pregnant girl face the threat of social exclusion. Their strategy for avoiding this threat is to socially exclude the pregnant girl themselves, thus conforming to a metanorm about how to sanction violators of sexuality norms. Lucy said much the same of her wealthy resort town: "I think there would be other friends who are like, 'You're a slut, and

I don't want to be friends anymore.' That's just high school, and that's the reality of it. Some friends are so judgmental, and their image is everything. And they don't want a friend that is pregnant because it reflects the image I am." Lucy thinks a pregnant girl's norm violation is socially "reflected" onto her friends' images unless the friends socially exclude her.

As Helena suggests, the people who are closest to the pregnant teen are under the most metanormative pressure to distance themselves from her. In other words, they have to work hard to avoid having "courtesy stigma" extended to them.[25] Carsen, one of the most vociferously negative interviewees in his statements about teen pregnancy, is a good example. In describing a girl who got pregnant in his middle-income suburb, he said:

> She was the girl that got around [sexually]. [Laughs] Then she was the girl that got pregnant. And everyone said, "Should have seen that one coming," but it was very funny to watch her walk around school being all pregnant-like. It was like, "Ha! You're pregnant!" . . . Because it's like, you are having a baby, you were stupid and careless, didn't know how to pay $3.99 for a box of condoms, or you were just stupid and immature and didn't think about it, or not on birth control, and then you're going to have taxpayers pay for your baby's formula and stuff, when you're out drinking and having a good time still? That's messed up.

Carsen's reaction was surprising given that both his cousin and a "close family friend" got pregnant. This experience seemed to be salient for him. When the interviewer asked how his parents would respond if he got a girl pregnant, he expressed bravado: "Now that my cousin did it, I can do whatever I like." But his descriptions of peer interactions and of his own reactions to peers' pregnancies suggest that he worked hard to distance himself socially from the pregnant girls he was associated with. He drew a symbolic boundary between himself and teen parents by emphasizing the interests of "taxpayers." Carsen's need to conform to the metanorm by distancing himself from norm violators was greater because of his association with his pregnant cousin. In describing how a good friend would react if his girlfriend got pregnant, he said, "Adam with a kid, I don't know. Probably love it, or like [to the girl], 'Hey, meet me by a flight of stairs. Karate for practicing multiple stomach kicks.'" While physical violence against teen mothers is a disturbing undertone in many interviews (for example, it was often brought up as a possible reaction by parents finding out about their child's pregnancy), Carsen was particularly casual about it. His enthusiastic sanctioning of pregnant girls may have helped him avoid courtesy stigma and social sanctions.

Abby said that in her large urban community, teens conformed to metanorms and sanctioned peers in ways that didn't necessarily reflect their own beliefs. When asked how her friends would have reacted if she got pregnant, she told us, "They probably would have been like, 'She wasn't being smart.' They probably would have just assumed that, 'Oh, she wasn't using birth control.' . . . But I think that's ironic, because I mean, they were all having sex." Abby knew that teens who got pregnant were automatically labeled as violators of the norm prescribing consistent contraception, and she knew this wasn't always fair. But that didn't stop her from sanctioning a peer herself using the same logic. Earlier in the interview, she talked about a friend who got pregnant in high school:

> I was supportive of it, [but] I think she should have been using birth control personally. . . .
> *Was she not using birth control?*
> I heard rumors. You know, I didn't even ask her, but I heard rumors that she was not on the pill. And I don't even know if they used condoms. I hope they used condoms, but she wasn't even on the pill. So it wasn't that I wasn't supportive, but I just feel like she should have been on the pill, I guess. I mean, even go to [a reproductive health clinic] and get that stuff.

Even though Abby acknowledged she didn't know about her friend's contraceptive behavior, she sanctioned her friend for presumably not using birth control without making an attempt to find out the truth from her friend. This condemnation was mild compared to Carsen's, but it allowed Abby to claim being "supportive" of her friend while socially distancing herself. Abby's use of metanorms is all the more interesting because she did not always use contraception consistently herself—so she sanctioned others for the same behavior that she herself was engaging in.

SLUT DISCOURSE: "A PREGNANCY IS A PHYSICAL MARKER
THAT YOU ARE A SLUT"

Abby's rhetorical slide into condemning her pregnant friend without knowing the facts was a widespread occurrence in the interviews. Although her particular case had to do with blame over shoddy contraceptive use, several other examples in this chapter involved the more common "slut discourse." For girls, the specter of being labeled a slut is a powerful form of social control, similar to being labeled gay for boys.[26] In many settings, boys can perform masculinity by performing heterosexuality, while for girls it is performing *restraint* from heterosexuality—by not being a "slut"—that is tied to femininity. Because they can appear more masculine the more heterosexual they seem, boys often do not have the same social incentives as girls, which could lead to conflict in their public portrayals of sexual behavior.

Being called a slut often has to do with a girl's disadvantaged class, race, and social status as well as gender.[27] Applying the slut label is like playing a game of "hot potato" in which the way to get rid of the hot potato is to throw it to someone else.[28] Teens, particularly girls, are concerned about their reputations because they want to avoid the slut label. Using the slut label can be an effective way for friends of a pregnant girl to avoid metanorms by throwing the hot potato to her, as Lucy said above: "You're a slut, and I don't want to be friends anymore."

The game of hot potato keeps the slut label from being too sticky—girls are called sluts in particular situations, but it's often hard to point out a single person who is permanently "the slut."[29] Because sexual behavior is private, the slut label is related to public perceptions of behavior rather than the behavior itself. This means that girls who are not sexually active can end up being labeled, but girls can also try to influence public perceptions and refute the label. In my interviews, it's clear that there is one category of girls—pregnant teens—who do get permanently stuck with the hot potato of the slut label, unable to throw it back to someone else. Ella described how this happens:

> *Do you think the teens' behavior was affected by what kids at school thought about teen pregnancy?*
> Probably. I think it wasn't so much the consequence of being pregnant that people were afraid of. It was more like, if I sleep around, then people will think I'm a slut. I think that's what girls were more afraid of, was the fact they'd be labeled a slut more than being pregnant.
> *Why do you think that's a worse consequence?*
> I think pregnancy goes hand in hand. A pregnancy is just like a physical marker that you are a slut. [In] high school especially. You think so much about what people think about you.

According to Ella, because a girl's pregnancy is seen as proof of her having had "slept around" (although it is not actually proof at all), the slut label is unavoidable. This assumption that pregnancy equals promiscuity doesn't square with empirical evidence, including my interviews with teen parents, which shows that a committed romantic relationship is a greater risk factor for pregnancy than short-term hookups.[30] It's telling that Ella thinks the prospect of being labeled a slut was seen as more terrifying than the actual pregnancy, and also that she was describing a "very liberal," affluent city where it seemed like "everyone was having sex."

MANAGING NORM VIOLATIONS

A visible pregnancy is the clearest proof—short of getting caught in the act—that a teen has violated norms against sexual activity and inconsistent contraception. So to avoid social sanctions, girls are motivated to end a pregnancy before it becomes public knowledge. But especially in the many U.S. communities that have strong anti-abortion sentiments, pregnant girls cannot necessarily avoid sanctions by terminating a pregnancy. Ivy told us about a friend who left her conservative rural state to get an abortion: "I think she went to stay with her cousin and get it done." This may have been a strategy to ensure the secrecy of the pregnancy. "Anyways, she got an abortion, and she told two of her friends. And everyone found out. And people are just not accepting of that [abortion]. It is a very, very much 'pro-life' area. So a lot of people felt like she had done something immoral and terrible, and her reputation never recovered from that." Especially if close friends don't uphold the conspiracy of silence, there is often no socially redeeming action for pregnant girls to take. Both staying pregnant and being known to have had an abortion are socially damning in many places.

The teen parent interviewees have been on the receiving end of negative sanctions from peers. Close friends' reactions are important. Patton's speculation above that his friends wouldn't openly sanction him, but instead would not "truly understand" and would drift away from him, accurately reflects many teen parents' experiences. Like many teen parent interviewees, Crystal attributes her friends' distancing themselves from her to being in a different life stage from her school friends. She said, "I had dropped a lot of my friends through my pregnancy. But our other ones that we have, they were very supportive about it, helping us with anything we needed." When asked why she had lost some friends, Crystal said, "They were supportive about it, but . . . we just didn't see eye to eye anymore. I changed so quick, I had to mature so fast, from partying all the time. We just—all my friends are big-time party-goers. . . . And they just didn't understand. I was pregnant. 'Come over, come party!' I was like, 'No, I can't.' I can't be with someone who's going to be calling me to party." Although Crystal chose to distance herself from her friends when they did not accommodate her pregnancy, another interviewee—James—did not. His friends' immediate negative reaction was also tied to his new life phase that they did not share. James said, "I told my friends a day after [he found out about his girlfriend's pregnancy]. They were all different than what I thought. I forget how they said it, but they said, 'You're broke for 18 years.' . . . And they were like, 'That was a stupid move. We ain't going to see you that much no more, huh?' . . . People at school, they called me a stupid idiot. They were like, 'I don't see the point to having a kid this young,' this and that." Even though he is male, James faced a uniformly negative reaction from both close friends and peers, all of whom distanced themselves from him. In Caroline's case, peer social exclusion was severe enough to contribute to her decision to transfer to a school with a teen parent program:

> I'm still going to high school, and I was pregnant. So that kind of—there was conflicts with my friends and that stuff. . . . I guess they weren't my friends after all. [Laughter] Some of them stopped talking to me, and stuff like that. That was hard. And then I had to switch schools. . . . That changed the type of friends that I hang out with now. Because I only have one friend that actually I had when I was in high school, and that actually stayed my friend after that.

Although most teen parent interviewees had experienced negative sanctions from peers, many were not as susceptible to social exclusion as the interviewees in the college-bound sample. This is because even before becoming parents, many of them were socially isolated with few close friends and sporadic school attendance.[31] Social scientists would expect that with less time spent in the "fishbowl" of school-based peer groups and less attachment to close friendships, these teenagers would be less influenced by peers' norms.[32] Anabele told us, "I'm the shy kind, so I didn't go out very much. I didn't have very many friends except for in school." She only told one friend about her pregnancy before transferring to a school for teen mothers. That friend "didn't believe it. She said, 'No, you couldn't be pregnant, not you.'" Adriana was even less attached to peers because of her weak ties to school. She said, "Before I was a mom, I didn't really go to school. I didn't like school. I would just stay at home and clean the house, because I was living with my mom. And I would just clean, and that way she wouldn't get mad if I didn't go to school. . . . I really don't have lots of friends. I only have a few friends, because I don't really like girls. They're too dramatic. . . . I'm a family person." After an embarrassing incident when she threw up in class during her pregnancy, Adriana transferred out of her school to a teen parenting program and attends it consistently.

The vacuum left by a lack of friendship in many of our teen parent interviewees' lives was often filled by a romantic partner, who strongly influenced the teen and sometimes lobbied for a pregnancy (unlike everyone else in the teen's life). Returning to Adriana's experiences, she met her boyfriend one summer and after that "wouldn't really go to school." Spending time with her boyfriend "was all I would do. . . . We were inseparable. We were together all the time." After they were together six months, Adriana got pregnant. She didn't say whether her boyfriend wanted her to get pregnant, but he was "happy" and "over-excited" when it happened. He moved in with her family, then "he got me my own place." After they started fighting, Adriana decided to end the relationship and move back in with her family.

Rose's boyfriend had a more direct influence on her pregnancy, in a story that was typical of many teen mothers. She said of getting pregnant, "I never thought it would happen to me." Rose said of her baby's father, "He planned it [the pregnancy]. I didn't. He was my best friend for four years, and I would never be with him. And then one night we were drinking, and then we ended up having sex. He did it on purpose. . . . He got me pregnant on purpose. So then five months later, I found out I was pregnant, and I told him. And he was all happy about it, and then he told me he planned it. I wasn't ready for a kid." Her baby's father is "still in the picture," but they are not a couple.

Whether reactions come from close friends, the wider peer group, or a sexual partner, young parents are starkly affected by negative and positive sanctions from similarly aged peers. In many cases, the social exclusion they face drives them out of their schools to environments in which their norm violation doesn't make them a target. Social isolation sends many into the arms of partners, some of whom desire a pregnancy in contrast to everyone else around them. This is particularly problematic for young mothers because in many cases, the relationship does not last and the responsibility for raising the child falls mostly or entirely on them.

CONCLUSION

Because most teens' lives are structured by school, their social worlds are shaped by the near-constant presence of similarly aged peers. Peers' norms about sex are often different from those of parents, intensifying the mixed messages teens hear. The fishbowl of school constrains teens' social interactions and forces them to face the same people day after day, creating a potent recipe for social exclusion by peers to have a strong effect. Yet sexual activity doesn't usually happen in public, which means that teens can do one thing sexually and act like they're doing another. Rumors about other people's sexual behavior often can't be convincingly confirmed or denied—short of visible pregnancy, what proof can a teen provide? Yet the stakes are high because adults are watching and judging teens. Girls tend to face a lot more social control of their sexuality than boys, including gossip and reputational threats, and the sexuality norms being enforced differ a lot from place to place. All this means that, for boys but especially for girls, interactions with close friends and peers are potentially dangerous and need to be handled carefully.

To my interviewees, close friends' and peers' influences on young people's sexuality is more complicated than that of parents. Parents typically don't want teens to have sex, even if the rationale underlying that norm may differ. They would rather not know what teens are up to because if they did, they might feel forced to sanction the teen in ways that could damage her future. So the conspiracy of silence is often easy to maintain, and even though teens' behaviors may not be in line with parents' preferences, everyone tends to have the teen's long-term best interests at heart. This is not necessarily true of peers. There's a lot more variation among peers in the acceptability of sex and in the ways that acceptability differs by gender and relationship context. But in general, teenage peers aren't putting a lot of pressure on each other to have sex. Instead, close friends may be quietly helping each other get away with sexual activity while hiding it from the larger peer group. This wider group does not usually have a young person's best interests at heart—instead, social exclusion is a way teens can publicly perform their own sexual conformity and avoid exclusion themselves. Sanctioning someone else may be the surest way to sidestep being sanctioned,[33] and reputational aggression is a good way to gain social status.[34]

Parents and peers represent two different arenas of powerful social pressure around teen sexuality. Given the risk of social sanctions from both family and friends for having sex or having risky kinds of sex, it may be surprising that teens engage in these behaviors at all during high school, let alone the majority of teens. This social control often isn't effective at curtailing sexual behaviors, but it does have problematic unintended consequences in terms of stigma and social exclusion. When adults in positions of authority at the school are added into this mix, as they are in the next chapter, the norms and social control around teen sexuality become even more complicated and interesting.

5

"SCARE IT INTO US"

School Norms and Social Control

SCHOOLS ARE VERY important for communicating and enforcing social norms about teen sexual behavior. They are a social space in which peers who might not otherwise know each other are brought together for several hours each day. But schools are also formal institutions bound by law, supported financially by the community, and required to provide students with information about sexuality and health. Reflecting the schools' exclusive focus as described by interviewees, this chapter describes dynamics around heterosexual sexuality norms.

Alana attended a racially and socioeconomically diverse public high school in an equally diverse Western city. This diversity seemed to have pros and cons. She said:

> I loved it. I hung out with all different groups and races and stuff. And I mean, yeah, there were like the people, you know, you wouldn't hang out with, and when you walk into the cafeteria there would be all the Black kids sitting in the cafeteria in one section, all the Hispanics in one.
>
> *And what about the White kids? Did they hang out together, or did they scatter out?*
>
> They kind of scattered out, but I kind of noticed that the White kids were the ones who would go to their cars and wait for off-campus lunch. And there would be a certain Black group, Hispanic group who would hang outside the

[convenience store], and that's where a lot of the trouble happened, like the fights and stuff, 'cause you'd always see the cops there circling the area.

Racial tensions among the students apparently led to institutions monitoring students closely, which may have further fed those tensions. Alana also thinks the school's academic tracking contributed to the racial splintering of the students' social networks. "I wasn't really aware of that stuff, but I would definitely say that in the advanced classes, a lot of my friends were in AP [Advanced Placement] classes, and it was mainly White." She says her close friends came from this group, even though she wasn't in the most advanced classes herself.

Alana says, "There were quite a few girls who were pregnant that were in school at least for a while. . . . I don't think the teachers liked it." These girls, she says, were not in college prep classes and were "definitely more Hispanic girls." She's not sure if the girls then dropped out or transferred to another school that "the bad kids, the troublemakers, would go to." Alana's community was "religious," and an Evangelical Christian youth group was active within the school.[1] Yet she says, "I definitely don't think there was the abstinence thing in high school at all," and among her sexually active group of friends, an abortion would have been an appropriate response to an unintended pregnancy. Sex education was an elective option, and the class she took was comprehensive rather than abstinence-only. She said, "That's where I learned about contraception and all the types of birth control and stuff and STDs." Having sex was socially acceptable for boys, and within a serious relationship for girls, but "not thinking straight with contraception" was judged harshly. Teens who had violated this norm tried to hide pregnancies for as long as possible or quietly get an abortion.

Like Alana articulates, schools loom large in teenagers' lives as sites for the communication and enforcement of social norms.[2] Schools are important contexts for informal interactions with peers and adults, as well as formal social institutions authorized by society to exercise considerable physical and social control over teenagers. Not surprisingly, then, high school was a main character in most teens' stories about sex and pregnancy norms and behaviors.

SCHOOLS AS ARENAS OF PEER INTERACTION

School came up almost immediately when my research team started asking interviewees about their friends and communities. Many of teenagers' close friends and romantic or sexual partners come from within the school.[3] A school can be visualized as a bounded social network that can be mapped out by asking who is friends with whom. Some schools have one cohesive, homogenous social network, while others are a patchwork of more isolated friendship groups. Teenagers are often aware of how social characteristics are related to friendship patterns within their school. For example, Larena told us about her urban public school:

> My group of friends in high school, we were very athletic, at the top of our class, and everything like that. . . . We were involved in high school. We were at the top. We were educated [she may be referring to a more rigorous academic track]. Most of my friends were part of that middle-class group, and then the rest of the high school was the lower income.
> *So would people in the more educated middle-class group that you're describing, did they interact with the lower-class people?*
> They would, but not as much. Because I figure when you're more educated, it's hard to have a conversation with someone who's not on your intellectual level.

Larena articulated a fundamental socioeconomic divide in her school, but she "missed" social class in explaining why the school's friendship networks were fragmented.[4] Instead, she credited that divide to differences in educational achievement, participation in extracurricular activities, and perhaps more advanced tracking into a college preparatory program. Sociologist Annette Lareau has shown that these factors are indeed important ways in which parents' higher SES is translated into socioeconomic advantage for children.[5] Interestingly, although Larena recognized some of these structural reasons, she settled on the questionable narrative of her friends' intellectual superiority to explain why there was a divide in the school social network.

Many of our interviewees described a social environment in which groups of close friends, or groups of peers who participated in the same extracurricular activity, were loosely arrayed within academic "tracks" and kept largely separate from peer networks in other academic programs. School social networks are often clearly divided by demographic characteristics like race or SES.[6] These characteristics tend to map onto academic tracks, but there can be socioeconomic or racial divides within academic tracks. Interviewees also said splits existed because of religious or political differences among teens, such as the rift between Mormons (LDS) and non-Mormons in one high school or the divide between a politically liberal minority and the conservative mainstream in another. When a school has a social divide across which fewer people are friends with each other, the lack of communication across that gap has implications for the social norms within the school. Chapter 4 showed that close friends are an important influence on teenagers' sexual behavior. When friendship groups are segregated, the norms about sexuality that are communicated within those groups have an opportunity to diverge. For example, Finn belonged to a "deviant" group of friends in his highly religious city, who "hated the community" and encouraged sex out of "spite" and to have fun. These close friends developed sexuality norms that differed starkly from the more conservative norms typical of the school and community. Yet gossip about peers and metanorms about how to treat peers who have violated norms can be more crosscutting across social groups than the norms themselves.

Social divisions within a school shape how norms are perceived and how students respond to them. Several of our interviewees described "split" schools that were starkly divided along racial, socioeconomic, religious, or ideological lines.[7] They perceived these groups as having very different norms about sexual behavior. These divisions sometimes seemed to be exacerbated by the separation of students from different racial and socioeconomic backgrounds into different academic programs, such as college preparatory and vocational tracks. Rochelle's sharply divided school in a low-income Rust Belt community was split along ethnic lines, with a dominant White group and a more impoverished Latino group. Rochelle grew up the White daughter of a shop owner and a college-educated manager. She said that teens didn't date or make friends across the ethnic divide: "They stuck to their own groups." Rochelle characterized White teens in her public high school as subscribing to a moral rationale that considered teen sex and pregnancy to be wrong on religious grounds. She said of teen pregnancy, "It would be the worst thing in the world." In contrast, she said Latino teens did not communicate these moral concerns; Rochelle claims they "were encouraging it [teen pregnancy]." Rochelle's disapproval of the Latinas who ended up pregnant was very strong because she felt they didn't adhere to the "right" (i.e., her own group's) norms. She identified the teen moms in her school as Puerto Rican, though when asked she acknowledged teen pregnancy was somewhat common among Whites as well.

It seems that the ethnic divide in her school strongly influenced Rochelle's perceptions of both Whites' and Puerto Ricans' norms and behaviors.[8] She said that the Latina moms in her school "were proud of it [pregnancy]. . . . They'd have parties [baby showers] in the hallways with balloons. . . . They would carry around their balloons all day." Rochelle said, "Now they have their babies, they're just like, 'That's the best thing that ever happened!' And you're like the last person that should reproduce on this planet. Not to sound totally awful, but it's the truth!" Rochelle's vitriolic reaction stems from her perception that pregnant girls on the other side of the ethnic divide aren't ashamed about having violated the dominant White group's norms. It's very important to note that neither among the predominantly White college student interviewees, nor in interviews with the predominantly Black and Latina sample of teen mothers, did anyone say their *own* peer group or school actually encouraged teen pregnancy. So Rochelle's perceptions of norms among Latinas likely had more to do with racism or her lack of familiarity with the Latina group's norms than with an actual positive pregnancy norm in that group.

As in Rochelle's case, people from split schools often talked more openly and negatively about people who violated sexuality norms. It seems that the constant presence of an "othered" group with different norms helps strengthen cohesion and norm consensus with each of the groups. By exaggerating differences in their sexuality norms and behaviors and condemning the Latinas, Rochelle was performing symbolic boundary work between the two groups in her school, which is a form of social control.[9] Teenagers from outside her group who violated her group's norms against teen pregnancy faced extremely negative reactions from Rochelle, but she looked the other way when teens in her own group engaged in the same behavior.

This kind of symbolic boundary work doesn't only happen in the dominant group. People in the subordinate group are sometimes acutely aware that because more girls in their group portray themselves as sexually active or get pregnant, their group may be viewed as encouraging this behavior. Lillian, who came from this kind of group in a lower-income urban area, had a reaction nearly as strong as Rochelle's but against people like Rochelle:

> I, honestly, I'm sure that kids have sex at different times. But when I hear stories from these girls from [wealthy White suburb] about when they started having sex, or when they started doing sexual things when they were like fourteen and fifteen, there's nothing wrong with that. But I think about that, and I think, you know, I bet you sit at your [wealthy White suburb] house and you talk about these people who are in [names two low-income urban neighborhoods, including her own] or in whatever, and you talk all this shit about how you think they're having sex and doing all this shit when they're young. But look at you. It's not even like that. Look at you. You are way nastier.

Lillian is stung by what she perceives as the dominant group's reaction, so she does boundary work of her own, even though in this case the dominant group isn't located within her own school. She uses this group from another part of the city, which may be more hypothetical than real, to judge both the girls' assumed sexual behavior and their condemnation of people like her.[10]

Many other interviewees described having had a school friendship network that was free of major divides. This tended to be the case in smaller public schools, schools in smaller communities, and above all private schools (whether or not they were affiliated with a religion)—in other words, in schools with more homogenous student populations. These school environments were socially cohesive and usually had one strong set of norms about sexual behavior. Bryce described his private

Catholic school in a wealthy suburb in the Rocky Mountains: "I grew up in a Catholic environment where we were taught that premarital sex and pregnancy outside of wedlock is against God, and therefore wrong. . . . We went to a private high school where it was actually stated in the rulebook that if you did get pregnant, you had to leave school." Even so, a pregnant girl at his school received what he called "special treatment" and was allowed to stay. This was not well received by many in the school community. "I know my mom was disappointed to hear of such a thing at our school, thinking that this sort of stuff might be avoided in a private school environment." Bryce's mother's attitude about "this sort of stuff" has two interesting implications. First, she seemed to expect that norms against teen sex and pregnancy would be more strongly enforced in this small private school. Second, Bryce implied that she and other parents and students may have chosen the school because they agreed with the sexuality norms there. Although this was not the case in small communities with just one high school, it may have played a large role for families selecting private schools and small schools in communities that had many options. In Bryce's school and many others like it, sexuality norms were quite cohesive, and teens often felt like people monitored their behavior closely, resulting in high levels of social control.

In sum, schools are a crucial space for peer interaction. Teenage students form social networks within the school and relay norms, gossip, and social control through those networks. These social relationship structures matter, as Chapter 2 showed. But the networks themselves are strongly shaped by school structures like academic tracking and by existing social divides in the surrounding community. These influences create patterns of norm communication and enforcement that look different in different schools. Teen peers aren't the only people in a school, though, and its primary purpose isn't informal socializing. As a key institution in the lives of teenagers, schools are run by adults who have their own agendas and who are held accountable to other institutions.

SCHOOLS AS INSTITUTIONS

Schools are both an important setting for peer interaction and a physical place that structures that interaction. But they are also formal institutions administered by adults representing the community; bound by local, state, and national laws and regulations; and often charged with teaching students about sexuality. This means that schools have their own agendas for shaping teenagers' sexual behavior, and they have the instructional means to communicate norms to teens. This makes them an important institutional norm enforcer. Interviewees were acutely aware of the power school administrators and teachers held over them. Many made it clear that they knew the adults in the school were trying to control their sexual behavior. What was less obvious to interviewees is that (particularly public) schools work within structural constraints created by the school district, state laws, and national regulations.[11] For example, in the past few years (but in the period after most of the interviewees from that state were in high school) Colorado's state legislature passed a sequence of bills defining the required content of sex education instruction in its school districts.[12] Schools must follow these changing legal guidelines. The rest of this chapter details the ways in which school administrators and teachers operate within such constraints to communicate sexuality norms, strategize to ensure that teens conform to these norms, and sanction teens who violate norms.

WHAT NORMS ARE COMMUNICATED

Some teachers and school administrators have influence over their teen students' sexual behaviors. The interviews suggest that these adults' attitudes about teen pregnancy often conform to the norms of the local community. Lilly, whose community in a diverse large city adopted a practical rather than a moral rationale about teen sexuality, said, "I think at my school the teachers are mostly accepting. They're like, 'You know what, kids have sex and sometimes crap happens.'" This negative but resigned attitude toward teen sexuality as "crap" that happens is typical of adults who espouse a practical rationale. Although many teachers and administrators were more negative about teen sex and pregnancy than those in Lilly's school, none encouraged these behaviors. In this way, they were similar to parents.

Sometimes teachers' and school administrators' relatively higher SES puts them at odds with community norms. Larena, who went to a lower-income school in a large city, said of school administrators and teachers, "They weren't accepting of [teen pregnancy] at all. You know, if you're pregnant and a teacher walks by you, they'll definitely give you that look of almost disgrace. And most of the teachers there were middle class, and they just looked at the girls like they didn't have any respect for their body and they weren't educated on teen pregnancy." This normative stance was more strongly negative than what the families of most of the students in the school may have expressed, but it was in line with the norms among Larena's elite peer group of higher-SES, academically high-achieving teens (described in the previous section). This is typical of a normatively split school—the teachers and administrators share the sexuality norms of the more privileged group of students. In this way, cultural heterogeneity in peer norms about sexuality is not mirrored among the adults in the school. Students tend to perceive consistent, negative norms against teen sexuality emanating from school staff.

These norms seem to emphasize a perceived link between sexual restraint and socioeconomic success—the two related norm sets described in Chapter 2. The practical rationale discourages sex, inconsistent use of contraception, and pregnancy because they can ruin a teenager's future. In a diverse urban area, Joel articulated his father's view of sex as a competing activity that takes energy away from schoolwork: "This isn't what you should be spending your time on. You need to get good grades." Claudia talked about people in her wealthy, White, liberal town who said of teen mothers, "How is she going to get her own education and take care of a family?" Larena told us that although students in her low-income urban school were "more accepting" of teen pregnancy than teachers, "they were still the same as the teachers—you have your whole life to live, and it's like you've lost it all in a heartbeat." This practical rationale is strongly espoused by many school administrators and teachers, who may be seen by the community as the most appropriate enforcers of these particular norms about sex and pregnancy.[13] For example, Liam said of teen pregnancy in his wealthy Western suburban school:

> Health teachers always seemed to be very, very biased against it.
> *What kinds of things did they say?*
> Just that basically, you're ruining not only your life but the child's life. We got a lot of that propaganda thrown at us.[14]

Isabella similarly referenced the practical rationale when asked how teachers would have reacted if she had gotten pregnant in her mostly White, middle-income small town: "There are some teachers that would probably be really disappointed and probably not treat me the same, thinking I wouldn't have the same potential or something now. That I wouldn't be able to go as far if I had to have a baby. Obviously, I mean, it's really hard to try and go to college and have a child."

The perception that teen parents are bound to be educational failures makes it possible for a school's reputation to be tarnished by having students who are parents. The link between visible violations of sexuality norms and school reputation was clear to several of our interviewees. Jessica explained of her politically moderate, middle-income suburban school: "I don't think that the [school] administration would be necessarily for teen parenting, because it would put a bad rep[utation] on our school. Because we have very good and very high expectations of the students, for not having teen moms and things like that. So I think that the lower teen parenting they have, the better for them [the school]." Dylan linked these reputational concerns to his school's reaction to teens' behavior in a large conservative city. He said that if he had gotten a girl pregnant, "I myself was really involved [in school], so I definitely would get a talking-to from the administration, I feel like. . . . 'You're representing the school. You're representing organizations outside of the school. This type of behavior [getting a girl pregnant] is unacceptable.'" When asked what the school administration would be worried about, he replied, "It's probably the consequences, like the image of the school is at stake, or the images of the organizations are at stake." Dylan is implying that his heavy involvement with the school would have given his hypothetical misbehavior particularly strong bearing on the school's reputation as a place where male students get girls pregnant.

When having pregnant or parenting students enrolled damages a school's reputation, it can give schools even more motivation to discourage teen pregnancy. Liam's wealthy suburban public school did this by encouraging "careful" sex. Liam said his school communicated information about sex and contraception so that students were "very, very well informed":

> It probably has to do with the stress that our district put on education about sex.
> *Why do you think they stressed it so much?*
> Because they saw it [teen pregnancy] as something that the poor people did. They wanted to separate themselves from it the same way they wanted to be blue ribbon schools and have the best football team and have, you know, the most diversity without the problems of normally diverse schools.

As the discussion below shows, other schools worked to discourage teen pregnancy, and thereby maintain their good reputation (which Liam linked explicitly to social class), by promoting abstinence from sex instead.

HOW NORMS ARE COMMUNICATED

EXPLICIT TALK THROUGH SEX EDUCATION: "SCARE IT INTO US"

In many states, high schools have a legally mandated responsibility to explicitly communicate information to students about sex, contraception, and pregnancy through sex education.[15] Some states also mandate the content of that curriculum. In many contexts, parents can opt their teens out, but the default option is for students to receive sex education.[16] This gives schools the opportunity to implicitly or explicitly communicate social norms together with factual content. Sex education is the only direct communication of sexual information some teenagers receive from adults. Helena said, "I don't think they [her parents] ever even had the sex talk with me. So they just trusted the school system to do that." Sex education fills the vacuum created by many parents' silence around sex, making schools an important conduit for formal socialization about sex, contraception, and pregnancy.

Communities and states have picked up on the importance of this educational role, leading to bitter struggles over control of the normative messages conveyed in sex education classes.[17] Across the United States today, there is a struggle for dominance between proponents of "abstinence-only" (e.g., teaching teens to remain sexually abstinent until marriage) and "comprehensive" or "abstinence-plus" (e.g., promoting abstinence but also teaching teens about contraception) sex education. Much of this struggle is at the state and district levels rather than the school level. Interviewees' schools fell on both sides of this ideological divide, with stark differences in both the norms and concrete information that were communicated. Some teens learned about types of contraception and how to use them in "comprehensive" sex education programs. Alana tells a typical story of this type of curriculum in her urban public school: "I think it was my freshman year. It was an elective, so you weren't required to take it. And that's where I learned about contraception and all the types of birth control and stuff and STDs more. . . . Our teacher definitely showed us pictures of all the different STDs and even brought in, I think it was an IUD [intrauterine device, a long-acting contraceptive] and showed us how it worked."

In contrast, "abstinence-only" programs do not provide information about how to use birth control, but rather tend to focus on potential negative consequences of sex (including failure rates of contraceptives) and the benefits of sexual abstinence. Madelyn's highly religious suburban public school is an example:

I think a lot of kids, especially the LDS [Mormon] faith, is very against teen-age pregnancy. And even in middle school when we do that safe sex week, our whole safe sex week, we didn't learn about condoms. We didn't learn about birth control. We didn't learn about any of that. We learned about abstinence. That was the only thing we learned about. . . . They were like, "Don't have sex until you get married. That's the way to do everything." And so we just, that's just how we learned about it in school.

The contrast between these two typical descriptions of sex education curricula is striking and illustrates how implicit or explicit support of a behavior can be communicated by including it in sex education. The first teacher's demonstration of an IUD could seem like an implicit endorsement of contraception, while the second example includes explicit normative support for abstaining from sex.

The crux of the debate between proponents of the two types of curricula is this: By presenting information about contraception, are teachers and schools implicitly endorsing teen sex? Some schools, like those in Finn's conservative community and

Haylie's low-income small city in a rural area, cover both bases by offering an "alternative" sex education class. Haylie explained how this worked: "You could either choose if you wanted to do sex-based [comprehensive] or abstinence-based. . . . Basically your parents had to decide for you and fill out a consent form. So almost everyone did the sex ed [comprehensive] version, but there were two people in my class whose parents for whatever reason said they should do the abstinence one instead. So for that portion of the semester, we were divided into separate groups." Although the school was in charge of the sex education curriculum, it let parents make the ultimate decision about which content their teenagers would learn. Schools in lower-income communities may have had fewer resources to provide these different curricular options, and their choice of curriculum often tracked with the salience of conservative religion in the community.

Sex education classes clearly teach more than abstinence or correct contraceptive use. Even in Madelyn's more liberal sex education class described above, teachers used what I call *scare tactics* to communicate norms against teen sexuality. Scare tactics were quite typical in interviewees' descriptions of sex education. As in Madelyn's case in a highly religious suburb, the most common scare tactic was for teachers to show images of people with STDs. This tactic made a strong impression on our interviewees, many of whom described their fearful reaction to the "STD slideshow." Finn told us that in his sex education curriculum in a conservative city, "There was an STD slideshow that was really gross. Everybody had to see it." He later went on to say, "Everyone was kind of afraid of STDs. Even though nobody had sex, they were so afraid of STDs, and I was, too. And that was pretty thoroughly ingrained in our brains. . . . I think it's the slideshow." Makayla articulated the normative message beyond the slideshow in her wealthy suburban school:

It was the scary "look at these diseases," and—
Like the slides?
Exactly, like the "Don't do this [have sex], look how awful."

Even with the frightening slideshow, though, Makayla said her sexually active friends were more concerned about pregnancy than about STIs. This lack of apprehension about STIs relative to pregnancy, even when they received so much attention in sex education, is perhaps surprising and certainly calls into question the effectiveness of scare tactics.

The other school-based scare tactics the interviewees discussed focused on teen pregnancy. They included assignments calculating the cost of parenting a child, bringing in teen parents as motivational speakers to talk about how hard their life is, having teens care for a "fake baby" doll for some period of time, and viewing graphic images of childbirth. Julie talked about the full spectrum of scare tactics and the norms they communicated at her high school in a very conservative middle-income suburb:

> *Did you have any kind of sex ed in your high school?*
>
> We did. It was called "personal survival," and we had different segments. So we did CPR [cardiopulmonary resuscitation], and we did alcohol and drugs, and then we spent time on sex. And we learned the form of sex education where we looked at slides of STDs, we watched a birth, we watched a documentary called *Teenage Father* and it was made in the 80s. And it was about a girl who got pregnant, and it was about the girl and the boy that were going through this, the parents. And it was really sad because the guy really didn't want anything to do with the girl, and there was a lot of animosity between the parents. And then also it talked about the community as well, so that's kind of interesting. But we had that kind of sex education to, like, scare abstinence or scare safe sex into us [laughs].

The sex education Julie describes does not educate teenagers about sex or contraception, but rather about their potential negative consequences. Her curriculum ran the gamut from showing frightening visual images to communicating the idea that parenthood ruins relationships. In the end, Julie knew they were supposed to be scared but wasn't sure what they were supposed to be scared of. This suggests that the norms in the class, while heavily emphasized, were still implicit.

Sex education content tends to reflect the community's norms about teen sexual behavior. When communities advocate a moral rationale saying that teen sex is wrong, schools often reflect that message, as does sex education. The curriculum in those cases tends to be abstinence-only, communicating that refraining from sex is the only "safe" way to avoid the negative consequences of sex.[18] Communities with a practical rationale underlying norms about teen sexuality tend to provide comprehensive sex education in their schools, which emphasizes ways of using contraception to make sex as "safe" as possible. Schools can also sidestep both of these strategies by relying only on scare tactics rather than promoting either abstinence or contraceptive use, as in Julie's case above. However it is communicated, the normative message is what I call the *hidden agenda* of the sex education class, while the content being formally taught is the *explicit agenda*.[19] Unlike those of parents and peers, schools' explicit agendas are often constrained by laws and institutional practices. This makes it more likely that their explicit agenda differs from the hidden agenda.

The hidden agenda can come through strongly in moments that are not formally scripted by the sex education curriculum. Two stories interviewees told us about the instruction they received in sex education classes illustrate the way in which some teachers depart from a standard curriculum in order to forcefully communicate norms about teen pregnancy or sex. Makayla, who came from a fairly conservative suburban school with wealthy students, described her teacher's communication strategy that reinforced the community's focus on discouraging teen sex: "In health class, our health teacher, . . . he said, 'Do you guys know that you can use aspirin as birth control?' and we're like, 'Oh, and how does that work?' 'Oh well, girls, you just put it between your knees and you hold it there.' [laughs] . . . It was a joke, of course, but [trails off]." The male teacher communicated an explicit norm about avoiding teen sex while implicitly minimizing the importance of effective contraception. He also encouraged girls (but not boys) to take responsibility for conforming to the community's norm. This instructional interaction imparted no useful information that would have helped meet the course's sex education goal.

This kind of normatively motivated but pedagogically dubious communication also took place in a lower-income urban school, but with a very different normative message. Sociologist Lorena García has detailed the ways in which gender, race, social class, and heteronormativity play into sex education messages for minority youth.[20] In Lillian's story from a low-income urban school, the teacher communicated the community's norm encouraging the use of contraception, but not by providing instruction on the use or effectiveness of contraception:

> I saw that we were a lot, because people had stereotypes about us [many students were lower-income racial minorities], they would talk to us a lot more about sex. And I don't know if people in middle school had these experiences, but I vividly remember that teachers would really have a much lighter way of teaching. And I remember once I had a health teacher, which, she was a bitch, in other respects. . . . She was like, . . . "Tyrone, come up here," and Tyrone went up there . . . and Tyrone was Black, and she was like, "Ladies, don't let anyone ever tell you they are too big for a condom." And she put this condom all over Tyrone's arms, and I just remember that and think back on it, and I think that would never happen in any other school. I really don't think it would, I really don't think that the talk about sex would be that open. So that's some of the views that I've picked up about sex.

The teacher communicated not only the community's norm encouraging contraception in this interaction, but also assumptions about the roles of gender and race in teens' sexual encounters. She explicitly communicated norms that girls should be responsible for contraception during sex and articulated assumptions that (especially Black) boys will try to avoid contraception. The teacher's handling of Tyrone's body in this encounter, which evoked racial stereotypes, also demonstrates the tendency in lower-income urban and minority communities for teachers and administrators to regard teens' bodies as appropriate targets of physical intervention in order to prevent pregnancy.[21]

SILENCE AND INVISIBILITY: "WE DON'T NEED TO TALK ABOUT IT"

While talk about others (particularly girls who have violated norms against sex and pregnancy) looms large as a way that parents and peers communicate norms about sexual behavior, interviewees didn't see it as a common tactic for teachers and school administrators. Outside of sex education, in many communities teachers were expected to at least make a show of being willing to support pregnant teens and not gossip about norm violators. Ella told us that if she had gotten pregnant in her wealthy, liberal small city, "I think that individually everyone [teachers and school administrators] would have had their own opinions, but in general they would have been supportive, not like kicked me out of school or anything." This school "support" isn't overwhelming, especially since kicking pregnant girls out of school is illegal, but many interviewees felt teachers had an obligation to at least appear somewhat neutral.

Instead of engaging in informal gossip about—and thereby social exclusion of—norm violators, adults working in schools tended to minimize opportunities for such gossip to occur by making teen sex and pregnancy as silent and invisible as possible. In interviews, silencing and hiding sexuality were very common strategies used by adults in schools. As the discussion of parents showed in Chapter 3, silence can communicate norms. Veronica said misinformation about sex was prevalent among students in her private Catholic school. Some teens thought you couldn't get pregnant during your menstrual period or if withdrawal was used, but others thought giving oral sex could make a girl pregnant. After an embarrassed laugh, she explained, "We didn't have sex education." Earlier in the interview she said, "It was always understood, especially in religion class, that we don't need to talk about it [teen pregnancy] because Catholic girls and boys don't have sex until they're married." In this school, it appears that silence around sexuality was meant to communicate that sex was expected to be nonexistent among students. This is similar to the ways in which many parents use silence to communicate sexuality norms, and it may stem from emotion norms prescribing feelings of shame around teen sex.

Unfortunately, in Veronica's account the school's silence about sexuality seemed to be exposing some teenagers to unnecessary risks through their ignorance about sex. Other interviewees said similar things. Annika told us her high school in a low-income mining town taught "abstinence-only" sex education. She said that sex was prevalent among students, but she didn't think most people used condoms. This was despite the fact that STIs were "one of the big messages of our abstinence-only education." Annika said that she didn't think people connected condom use to STI prevention because their sex education classes didn't give them that information:

> I feel like it's pretty obvious that you would know a condom would prevent contracting an STD, but nobody actually said that. . . . It was very, very strictly, just "don't have sex before marriage," and they had all those reasons not to do that. But I don't think we ever actually had somebody come in and say, "This is how you prevent getting these STDs." It was kind of like assumed that once you're married then there were no STDs or something.

Outside of sex education classes, many schools strive to maintain public silence on the issues of teen sex, contraception, abortion, and pregnancy. Makayla told us that in her "fairly religious," wealthy suburb, "our school really didn't like to talk about issues like pregnancy or contraception." She went on to say that despite strong norms against teen pregnancy in her community, "I don't feel like the administration at school would even allow a campaign like that [against teen pregnancy] because they didn't want to touch on that issue." This illustrates how strongly committed to silence schools can be—they may not even be willing to permit student campaigns that articulate the norms they want to communicate.

A problem with silence as a strategy for communicating norms is that although school staff members may intend their silence to express disapproval and instill a sense of shame, students and others may interpret it as tacit support of the school's status quo. When this status quo entails nearly nonexistent teen pregnancies and a normative climate discouraging pregnancy, as in Makayla's case, the school's silence may be interpreted as disapproval, as it was by Makayla. But when the school's status quo involves quite a few teenage mothers and visible teenage pregnancies, the school's silence may instead be interpreted as approval of teen pregnancy. This was the case for Rochelle, whose lower-income Rust Belt community, discussed above, was divided along ethnic lines with different pregnancy norms. Rochelle repeatedly brought up "parties in the [school] hallways with balloons" for female students who were having babies. When asked how the school felt about this, she implied that some teachers may not have approved but school administrators wanted them to stay silent: "I don't think teachers could say anything about it because they didn't want to get in trouble, so I don't think you can really say anything, you know." The school's tolerance of baby showers in its halls communicated tolerance of teen pregnancy to Rochelle. I return to strategies of silence and invisibility later because they are also strategies schools use to enforce norms.

HOW SCHOOLS TRY TO ENSURE CONFORMITY

Schools are often normative environments in which teen pregnancy is uniformly discouraged and teen sex is either proscribed or seen as an unfortunate inevitability. Schools of the former type tend to stay silent about contraception in order to avoid suggesting implicit approval of sex, while the latter tend to provide contraceptive information to students. The norms schools communicate and the ways in which they communicate them often differ. But across the board, schools try to ensure that students conform to their norms about sexual behavior. For all schools, this means trying to discourage teen pregnancy. Some also try to discourage sex, while others encourage contraception. Like parents, schools have legal authority over their students, giving them more opportunities for physical control over teenagers.

CONTRACEPTION IN SCHOOLS: "THEY WERE OPEN ABOUT IT"

The question of whether to provide contraception in schools is hotly debated in the United States. As with comprehensive sex education, the crux of the issue is whether making contraception available implicitly condones teen sex, or simply makes sex that was going to happen anyway have fewer negative consequences for teenagers. As expected, schools with a moral rationale specifying that teen sex is wrong tended not to make contraception available, choosing to keep sex and contraception invisible in the school context and thus express disapproval. Schools without a moral rationale varied in their approaches, but some distributed contraceptives. In Drake's high school in a small, "liberal" community, he said, "For the most part, I think everyone practiced safe sex methods." He told us, "We had this program through the nurse's office where it was confidential from your parents. But you could go in there, and the ladies could get birth control [pills], day after pill [emergency contraception], stuff like that. And they had drawers of condoms. I think a lot of people utilized that." In Spencer's posh private school, he estimated that nearly every student had sex by the end of high school and nobody became visibly pregnant. Spencer said, "You could go into the advisor's office at any time and go get condoms, and it would not be a problem. They were open about it, so we were open about it, and we were safe about it." Spencer believed free access to contraception worked for preventing teen pregnancy in his school.

The low-stigma environment for getting contraception these two male interviewees described wasn't available at every school that offered these kinds of services. For example, in Larena's urban public high school, "Our school nurse, it was part of the hospital, so they were able to distribute birth control pills. . . . As long as you had to have a certain form that the nurse was sort of your doctor, then they'd be able to prescribe it to you." Parental consent was needed if you were under "16 or 17." But although this resource sounds fairly accessible, Larena says most people didn't use it. "I think a lot of people were embarrassed. But they just weren't educated on the fact that it's okay to take birth control, or go see the nurse about different things, or talk about sex." Larena claims that "a lot of the people couldn't afford" birth control if they went somewhere other than the school nurse. But instead of facing the stigma of seeing the nurse, "they would steal condoms" or "have sex and use the pull-out [withdrawal] method." This illustrates how important social norms can be—it has to be socially acceptable to access contraceptives, or some people won't use them even when they are readily available.

Few of our interviewees said there were contraceptives available at their schools. When there weren't, sometimes the adults at the school served an important purpose through shaping teenagers' access to contraception outside the school. Certain teachers or school counselors were known to be willing to help students find contraceptive alternatives, especially in communities where such options might not otherwise have been widely known or available. Annika told us that in her small conservative town, "My home ec[onomics] teacher would always try to get girls to go get birth control or whatever, or go get the morning after pill. . . . She's the kind of person who if something happened, you would go talk to her. And she would say, 'Okay, you can leave class, leave school, ditch home ec[onomics] and go take care of that.'" Several interviewees brought up these adults as important resources for sexually active teens who didn't know where else to turn in their community. In this way, when schools tried to maintain the invisibility of sex and contraception, adults who disagreed could work around the school's intent by making use of clinics and other resources outside the school. They served as "beacons" of contraceptive information.

INVISIBILITY TO PROMOTE CONFORMITY: "YOU WOULDN'T KNOW ANYONE EVER GOT PREGNANT"

Beyond communication, silence and invisibility are also effective forms of social control to get people to conform to norms. Many schools and school districts (particularly ones serving families with higher SES) use a variety of strategies to make violators of sexuality norms invisible in the school context. Although being expelled is illegal in public schools because of Title IX, some schools' strategies result in students voluntarily leaving the school or being shifted into a low-visibility program for young parents.[22] Private schools have more leeway and can legally "state in the rulebook that if you did get pregnant, you had to leave school," in Bryce's words (though his private school later made an exception for a pregnant student). Regardless of its legal basis, expulsion from the school peer group can be seen as a kind of "social death," one of the most extreme sanctions a norm violator can face. In this way, some schools formalize the sanction of social exclusion that peers enforce at the interpersonal level when teens (especially girls) violate sexuality norms.

Students who have not publicly broken the social rules observe the negative sanctions faced by peers who have violated these norms as an implicit threat. Watching norm violators being sanctioned is an effective norm enforcer strategy that tends to make people more likely to conform to a norm.[23] This certainly seemed to be the case for interviewees, who often had a clear understanding and fear of their schools' treatment of pregnant girls. As discussed above, becoming visibly pregnant is an obvious sign that sexuality norms have been violated, whether those norms pertain to sex, contraception, or childbearing. This makes girls, not boys, the main targets of school sanctions.

Many interviewees told us their high schools encouraged pregnant girls to leave the school or transfer into a segregated, alternative program for young parents. Dylan described a typical situation (except for the adoption, which was rare):

> In my high school, at least, there was an alternative center, so if a female got pregnant and when she started to show, they would pull her out of the main high school and put her in the alternative center. So I mean, in high school, if you weren't directly related to the situation or by a friend or something, you wouldn't know that anyone in our school ever got pregnant unless you kind of knew the person or through the grapevine, so I guess it definitely wasn't a norm to be pregnant and it definitely wasn't accepted. One of my friends actually got pregnant, and her parents took her out of school completely immediately until she was done with the whole pregnancy. And they gave the baby up for adoption. When she came back, I mean, she looked the same, like nothing ever happened.

Several aspects of Dylan's story, which took place in a conservative large city, are worth pointing out. First, a girl would be convinced to move to the alternative center "when she started to show" signs of pregnancy. This is long before the typical services at a parenting center, such as childcare, are actually needed, so it suggests that the school is taking action to keep the pregnancy invisible from the school community. It also sounds like students in the alternative center are being kept separate from the "main high school." Because of that, as Dylan acknowledges, "you wouldn't know that anyone in our school ever got pregnant." None of these actions are illegal since the school isn't expelling the girls. But it is also common for families to remove pregnant girls from school voluntarily, as in the case of Dylan's friend. In this way families and schools often cooperate to keep teen pregnancy invisible. This kind of collaboration between norm enforcers is common.

Some interviewees told us that they thought their public schools had official "no-pregnancy policies" in which girls "were pushed out" (in Makayla's words referring to a high-performing public school in a wealthy suburb). Such instances still occur but are decreasing because of Title IX legal protections of pregnant girls' right to attend public schools.[24] Makayla's perception is striking, though, because it implies that pregnant girls rarely defied the school's unofficial recommendation to leave. Even when interviewees did not think their school had an official no-pregnancy policy, pregnant girls seemed to comply with the school's wishes. Sometimes there was no clear educational motivation for girls to move, but they did anyway, which interviewees tended to attribute to a school policy. Madelyn said in her wealthy, conservative suburban school district:

> What they do in our school is you have a choice to go to our high school, and then we also have another school in our district called Clearview.[25] And a lot of the girls, when they get pregnant and it starts to show and stuff, that's where they would end up going to school to finish.
>
> *So why would they switch?*
>
> Just because they didn't like to be around the other students, and so—
>
> *Why would they not want to be around the other students?*
>
> I don't know why they didn't want to be around them, because I didn't care really. Growing up, I heard of kids getting pregnant, and they just disappeared suddenly from our high school. And I later found out that they went to Clearview or something until they had the child. And then they would come back to our high school because we have a daycare at our school. So then they could go to our school with the daycare, or they just wouldn't come back to our high school.

Madelyn attributed this situation to school policy, although it would not have been legally enforceable. She later identified Clearview as "where all the druggies go and then all the pregnant people." This (likely voluntary) segregation of pregnant girls had no obvious motivation beyond social exclusion, since the daycare center was located in Madelyn's own school.

Especially in larger, more densely populated districts, schools are able to offer pregnant girls "carrots" instead of "sticks" when encouraging them to leave. The "carrot" is often an alternative program offering valued services such as a childcare center, an evening course schedule, or parenting classes.[26] Adrian talked about this dynamic in his large suburban school district:

> I didn't see anybody carry the pregnancy [at school]. I mean, there were rumors that if somebody got pregnant, they would go to Mountain High School, and for the whole district it seems like that's where you went if you got pregnant, but I didn't know anybody who did that.
>
> *So no one would stay at your school?*
>
> No, definitely not.
>
> *Was there a policy about that?*
>
> I don't know if there was actually a, I mean it wasn't something I signed in the handbook, 'I will not get somebody pregnant.' But it seemed like there was a reputation to uphold [for the school] ... Like, our students don't get pregnant, and we don't have any pregnant women here. And maybe they would argue, we don't have the ability to deal with pregnant women. I don't know really why someone pregnant would make a difference, but maybe they would. I mean, having a child would make a difference, and that's why you went to Mountain, I guess, 'cause they have a daycare program, so I heard.

Here, Adrian articulated the synergy between the school's explicit and hidden agendas. The school's explicit agenda is to offer better support in an alternative program because "we don't have the ability to deal with pregnant women." The hidden agenda is to communicate that "our students don't get pregnant," thereby upholding the school's reputation. Both of these agendas are served by using the "carrot" of an alternative program to render pregnancy invisible.

Julie felt her school in a very conservative middle-income suburb had a different hidden agenda: "I think administration in schools doesn't want, they do not want, pregnant girls around. I think that it's viewed really negative, and I think that they think that if girls see other girls getting pregnant, they'll want to get pregnant, too, or something ridiculous of that nature." Julie scoffed at this hidden agenda, but fears of teen pregnancy being socially contagious have been widely publicized and discussed in media, such as the alleged but disputed "pregnancy pact" among a group of friends in Massachusetts.[27] Sophie detailed how the interaction offering a "carrot" might look in her predominantly White, middle-income suburb:

> I guess my impression too is overall, my school would have wanted to put the student in the best situation for being pregnant. Maybe the counselor would

have sat them down and talked to them. "You know, you can stay here, but is there another school where maybe other girls are going through the same thing that might be a better environment for you?" So not necessarily pushing them away, but letting them know their options so they maybe don't feel quite so, I don't know what the word is, discriminated against.

Sophie sees this "carrot" as a benign offer preventing discrimination, but if the student faces disapproval for choosing to stay in the mainstream school, it actually creates discrimination.

Even though alternative programs were seen as "carrots" to support pregnant girls, their dual purpose of social exclusion was clear to some of our interviewees. Ella said of her school's program for teen mothers in a wealthy, liberal small city:

It wasn't meant to be a program for them to be chastised. It was designed so they can continue their education, graduate, get a good job, support their kid, as well as teaching them basic parenting and life skills. But I think in the process, maybe since they're segregated from the rest of the school, it may kind of feel like a sanction, because they're not exposed to anyone else, and they're clearly different than everyone, being pregnant.

Even with this segregation, the stigma of having teen parents enrolled caused contention: The affluent families served by this high school lobbied to have the parenting program moved, and it is now housed in a lower-SES school in the same city.

Not all schools choose to make teen pregnancy invisible, but a decision to acknowledge its presence can sometimes result in clashes with students and community members who feel the school isn't doing enough to sanction teen mothers and discourage pregnancy among other students. Rochelle's example above of the school that allowed baby showers in its halls resulted in substantial hostility among students and families who advocated a stronger stance against teen pregnancy. Bethany talked about a different situation that resulted in similar sentiments:

Well, I remember actually that at my high school graduation, a girl got an award. And she had gotten pregnant while she was in high school. But I don't really remember who she was. But I remember they gave her an award for being responsible and being able to finish high school with a good GPA [grade point average] afterwards. And I remember we thought that it was stupid because why did she get an award above everyone else for making what we considered a mistake?

So do you think that they created that award for her? Or was it there in the past and she met the expectations for that award, or they created it once she finished school?

I would think they just created it for her and were trying to prove they were proud of her for being so—taking responsibility for what happened.

And so your friends had a chuckle about it because you deemed it as being irresponsible from the get go?

Yeah, because I mean, she finished high school, and she did have a baby, which is commendable in some respect. But none of us got awards for *not* getting pregnant and finishing high school. [Laughs]

These two situations elicited similar reactions because in different ways, the teachers and school administrators permitted celebrations of girls who combined school and teen pregnancy—thus making it more visible. This violates a metanorm prescribing that schools should work to discourage teen pregnancy.

Do schools' control strategies—providing or withholding contraception and making teen pregnancy invisible—actually succeed in discouraging additional pregnancies? I can't fully answer this question with my interview data, but birth certificate records certainly show that U.S. teen birth rates spike sharply at age 18 and 19 (when teens are finishing or have finished high school) compared to younger ages.[28] Interviewees tell us that norms about sex and pregnancy are much stronger in high school than afterwards, and many of them feel that becoming sexually active shortly after high school graduation at the latest is the only "normal" thing to do. Several interviewees said that teen pregnancy after high school was much more common than during high school. Alana told us that in her urban community, "I just kept hearing . . . right after high school everybody started getting pregnant." All of this suggests there is something about high school that tends to reduce teen pregnancies compared to immediately afterwards. It may be that the normative environments and social and physical controls schools use reduce teen pregnancy, even as they create negative consequences for teens who do end up pregnant.

MANAGING NORM VIOLATIONS

The previous section showed that many schools segregate pregnant and parenting girls or push them out of the school. Some students interpret these actions as being intended to socially exclude such girls and make pregnancy invisible in the school. Offering alternative programs that provide needed services to young mothers gives school districts the opportunity to simultaneously pursue an explicit agenda (supporting pregnant and parenting teens' unique needs) and a hidden agenda (discouraging teen pregnancy by making it invisible). I could imagine an educationally beneficial alternative to this state of affairs: In-school childcare centers could be an opportunity for all students to learn about parenting skills and child development. But nobody reported this happening in their schools. This suggests that the hidden agenda is at least as important to schools as the explicit agenda.

From a different perspective, though, school-based programs for teen parents can be very beneficial for the students they enroll.[29] Because so many schools strive to make teen pregnancy invisible, it is highly stigmatized in many mainstream academic programs. Chapter 4 detailed the interpersonal social exclusion faced by pregnant and parenting girls within their schools. In interviews with teen mothers and fathers, it was clear that negative experiences in mainstream schools are widespread among and damaging for pregnant teens. In a fairly typical story, Nicole attended a mainstream high school when she got pregnant. Teen pregnancy was not entirely invisible there because "there were a few pregnant girls." But students "always stared at me," and girls who had competed with her to date her boyfriend reacted to her pregnancy by saying, "Oh, now we don't like her even more!" Teachers' reactions were also problematic:

> There was one teacher, it was a guy, he was kind of nice about it. He used to tease me a lot, in a funny way. And then a lot of other teachers were really mean to me. Like, I had a lot of morning sickness, so they told me to eat crackers and stuff. So when I would eat a cracker, they said, "You can't eat that in here." I even had a doctor's note, and they were like, "We don't care. You can't do it. Nobody told you to get pregnant." They were really rude. And I missed a lot of days also because I always had to go to the doctor a lot because of my sickness. I was losing weight. And they used to get mad at that, too, that I missed a lot of days.
>   *Even though you had doctors' notes?*
>   Yes.[30]

The teachers and school administrators did not expel Nicole, but they still made it nearly impossible for her to keep attending school while pregnant. Six months into her pregnancy, Nicole dropped out of school because "my mom just thought it was too dangerous with girls running into you and stuff like that." She is eager to return to high school.

Dropping out of school as Nicole did is one common response to negative experiences with students, teachers, and administrators. To avoid social exclusion and access important resources like childcare, many other teen mothers voluntarily transfer to alternative programs (these programs' counterparts for teen fathers tend to be support groups or specific services, but not separate educational programs). Casey is one such teen mother. At her mainstream public school, people "were always talking about me because I was pregnant. I missed a lot of school because I was pregnant, and during class I'd have to ask the teacher because I would need to throw up. And girls just looked at me like, 'Gross! Little slut!' or whatever. 'How gross! How could she be pregnant?'" Casey knew about her city's charter school for teen mothers because her sister and cousin had attended. "I said, if I can take my kid to school [to the childcare center], of course I'll want to go there." It seems that a mixture of social exclusion, unforgiving attendance policies despite her medical excuse, positive recommendations from family members, and the resources offered by the alternative program led Casey to switch schools.

Teen mother interviewees' experiences with alternative programs were overwhelmingly positive and often described as life changing. Some alternative programs simply offer more flexible class scheduling, but others include free childcare, parenting classes, diapers and baby clothing, access to medical care and social worker support, and more. Beyond this considerable material support, the young mothers talked about the emotional support and empathy they received from teachers and other students. This lack of stigma and the social cohesion in the student body (because all the students are combining school and motherhood) are a marked departure from their experiences in mainstream schools. Like many others, Casey highlights both the resources and the interpersonal cohesion when talking about what makes it possible for her to keep attending her new school:

> Having daycare here. Just having the people care about you. This school's very small, and it's just like, everybody knows everybody. So it's just like, there's people that care about you, people that look up to you, too. It's good to come. I like coming here, because when I have a bad day, there's always somebody that's gonna cheer me up. If it's not my kids, it's here at school. Feeling loved, too. . . . I love this school. It's good.

Casey is "excited" because she is about to become one of the first high school graduates in her family. Her career plans have been informed by her experiences at the new school:

> I want to become a [preschool] teacher. After I graduate, I already have a job set up for me to work at a learning center where my daughter goes to preschool

[job placement is a benefit the program offers]. So I'm going to go do that, and to school to get higher [education] than just being a helper in the learning center, just working with the kids. I want to [get to] the point where I can have my own learning center.

Many of the teen parent interviewees who were enrolled in alternative programs were formulating concrete career plans like Casey's.

The paradox of school-based programs for young mothers is that although they help stigmatize teen pregnancy in mainstream schools by contributing to its invisibility, they are often tremendously beneficial for the students who attend them. This makes mainstream schools' negative sanctioning of pregnant teens particularly interesting. The powerful combination of sanctions from students, teachers, and administrators usually pushes mothers-to-be out of schools (at least among the teen mother interviewees, almost none of whom stayed enrolled in mainstream programs throughout their pregnancy). For the many young women who drop out, these negative sanctions can be permanently damaging, even if some later go back to finish a high school degree or GED.[31] But those who find their way into an alternative program often seem to be better off educationally than they were before the pregnancy.

School administrators and teachers appear to be navigating potentially treacherous terrain when they react to teen pregnancies. On one hand, they are legally and ethically bound to adhere to the school's explicit agenda of supporting its students' education. On the other hand, they often face pressure from the community, district, students, and families to pursue a hidden agenda of discouraging teen pregnancy and making it invisible, in order to protect the school's reputation and keep students from violating sexuality norms. The hidden agenda stems from adults in schools being regulated by a metanorm encouraging negative sanctions against pregnant teens. Metanorms are social norms about the appropriate ways to positively or negatively sanction people who have conformed to or violated a norm.[32] People who violate metanorms face sanctions themselves. This is evident in the strongly negative reactions to school administrators and teachers in Rochelle's school—which allowed baby showers—and Bethany's school—which gave an award to an academically successful teen mother. By choosing not to negatively sanction these girls, the adults in the school did not violate a norm against teen pregnancy themselves, but rather violated a metanorm regulating people's reactions to pregnant teens.

In contrast to these two schools, most of the schools our interviewees talked about conformed to this metanorm rather than violating it. Schools' formal negative sanctions against teen mothers are constrained by Title IX law, but teachers and administrators can still sanction girls informally. These sanctions ranged from the interpersonal—such as public shaming and teasing of girls—to the potentially illegal—such as giving girls trouble for missing school because of pregnancy-related complications and refusing to accommodate their medical needs in the classroom. When sanctions from adults in schools are combined with the severe social exclusion typically meted out by peers, they form a negative school climate that is effective at driving pregnant girls out of mainstream programs, despite legal protections.

Even alternative programs have to operate within the constraints of the meta-norm encouraging schools to negatively sanction teen parents. Between the college student and the teen parent interviews, I have heard about several ways alternative programs have navigated this metanorm while still supporting pregnant and parenting teens. These included kicking students out of the school or the childcare program if they had a repeat pregnancy, denying services if students' attendance slipped, and requiring that incoming students sign a contract promising to avoid specific problem behaviors. As Logan (from the primary interviews) told us about the teen parenting program at an alternative school in his middle-income Western suburb, "I think you either had to sign a contract going in, or there was some kind of code of conduct. Because if you were there, you were there to continue your education, not to get an easier diploma type deal. So it was a pretty well-run school, from what I've heard." Logan implies that the program's tight restrictions on teen mothers' behavior garnered social approval and the judgment of being "well run"—these are social rewards the program received for adhering to the metanorm. His account also emphasizes the important relationship between a school and its broader community.

As formal institutions, schools are legally accountable for what they teach students and how they treat them. I have also shown that they are held morally accountable for the norms they communicate and the ways in which they enforce community norms. This can create tensions between the explicit agenda and the hidden agenda a school communicates with regard to teen sexuality. Schools' formal sex education curricula are a political battleground, as other social actors seek control over the norms about sexuality that are communicated to teens. But schools can also face criticism for how they treat pregnancies among their students, and even for what they are implying if they impose silence around teen sexuality.

CONCLUSION

School plays a complicated part in regulating teenagers' sexuality. School is the fishbowl that contains peer interactions and social exclusion. It's also the key pathway to the future socioeconomic success that parents emphasize in the practical rationale that sometimes underlies teen sexuality norms. But school administrators and staff are powerful social actors in their own right, within constraints placed by the district, state, and nation. They communicate teen pregnancy norms to teens, act as agents of formal socialization through sex education, and often exercise physical control over pregnant girls' bodies by transferring them out of the school. In many cases, these actions facilitate a climate of silence and invisibility around teen pregnancy in the school. In communicating and enforcing teen sexuality norms, schools often act as a mouthpiece of the broader community, which is the focus of the next chapter.

As each new layer of social contexts unfolds, from families, to friends and peers, to schools, the norms about sexuality teenagers hear get more complicated. So do people's efforts to control teens' sexual behaviors. Many people, such as parents, close friends, and teachers, really do try to have a teenager's best interests in mind when they encourage her or him to behave in certain ways. Others, like some peers and school administrators, aren't necessarily out to hurt the teen deliberately, but they have their own agendas to pursue. Both peers and school administrators are interested in protecting their own reputations from the courtesy stigma faced by those who associate with teens who "misbehave" sexually (such as teen mothers). Peers avoid this stigma by socially excluding teens who have broken sexual rules. Many schools take steps that amount to the same thing, working to make pregnancy and parenting as invisible as possible in the school. This can improve a school's reputation. Because of the rampant stigma and social exclusion of teen mothers in many places, ironically school is also the most important safe haven many young mothers experience. The special programs for pregnant and parenting teens that some girls choose—or are pushed into, depending on the situation—give them a respite from the social sanctions they face in many other areas of their lives. This alternative vision of schools' messaging and enforcement around teen sexuality shows how important a school's normative climate is for teens' lives.

6

"CARRYING A STIGMA"

Communities and Teen Sexuality

TEENS HEAR MIXED messages about sexuality from their families, peers, and schools. Yet all these norms stem from within the same community—a community that also includes other people and institutions.[1] This creates a complicated context for the communication and enforcement of norms. Interviewees tended to clearly differentiate between norms in their broader community and those in their family. Sometimes the norms communicated privately by families and the public messages from the community came into conflict, and sometimes they reinforced each other.[2]

To many interviewees, communities are an important source of normative communication and social control of teen sexuality. Many different social actors are working, sometimes collaboratively and sometimes in conflict, to transfer their cultural values to a new generation of young people. Compared to families, peers, and schools, people and organizations in the rest of the community often have less direct lines of communication to teens and fewer opportunities to enforce norms. But communities are crucial as settings in which families, peers, and schools are situated, and they hold each of these social actors accountable for their interactions with teens in complicated ways. In other words, communities are a major source of metanorms— norms about how to appropriately enforce norms. They are also settings for formal institutions, like religious and healthcare organizations, that have their own agendas for influencing teens' sexuality. This chapter addresses communities both in terms of their direct communication of norms and social control and in terms of their influence on teens via other social actors.

Isaac stressed the importance of his community for understanding teens' sexuality. He grew up in a large but isolated mountain town surrounded by rural areas. He said, "It's a small enough community where everybody knows everybody, and everybody knows where everybody comes from, and everybody knows everybody's family, so your place is sort of made for you." Isaac's community is described in more detail later in the chapter, but for now I'll lay out the complicated norms communicated by his community. Isaac said:

> It was considered that a person in their teens was not ready to have a child. That's definitely a general conception. However, at the same time, terminating pregnancies [abortion] was also not generally accepted by the majority of the population of my community. . . . I knew those expectations of me. I knew how my community thought and my family thought about those issues, so the goal was certainly not to get [a girl] pregnant.

Isaac is describing conflicting norms in his community—don't have a baby, but don't have an abortion either. Assumptions were made about the sexual behavior of pregnant girls in Isaac's community: "If you got pregnant, that means you had not had sex once and happened to get pregnant. You had a lot [of sex] and with lots of different partners. However, I don't know where that perception comes from because the majority of the teen parents I knew were pregnant by their steady boyfriends."[3] Accompanying the strong norm of avoiding pregnancy was a striking silence around how to avoid pregnancy beyond avoiding sex:

> Abstinence was certainly promoted. . . . It's not that people, the community, didn't want students to get pregnant, so therefore promoted contraception. . . . It was considered a lot of times, "You don't want to get pregnant, so you figure out how to not get pregnant." . . . "Don't get pregnant. I don't care how you do it. I'm not going to give you condoms. You're not supposed to get pregnant when you're seventeen."

These strictures against sex and pregnancy without much accompanying information or practical support are typical of the norm set of a particular type of community in the sample—usually lower-income, highly religious towns in rural areas. They are strikingly different from the norm sets described by other interviewees in wealthier, less religious urban or suburban communities. These different sets of norms show that the United States is starkly polarized about teen sexuality. This polarization tends to overlap with the political divide between conservative "red states" and liberal "blue states."[4] Interestingly, statistical analyses have shown that it is the conservatively religious "red states"—the ones that have traditionally held the strongest norms against teen sex and pregnancy—that tend to have the highest teen pregnancy rates.[5] In this chapter I describe this stark variation in norms across different U.S. communities.

COMMUNITY NORMS ABOUT TEENS' SEXUAL BEHAVIORS

Interviewees were asked to talk about the norms communicated by their communities when they were attending high school, leaving it up to them to define that community.[6] Letting interviewees decide which broader reference group was the most relevant for communication about teen sexuality norms permitted a better understanding of their social worlds as they perceive them. Outside of urban areas, interviewees like Isaac often considered their community to be their whole town. A community tended to be a neighborhood or school for interviewees from larger cities, and those in smaller or religiously based schools frequently considered the people involved in the school to be their community. Across the board, though, interviewees tended to stress the norms communicated by *adults* when discussing community norms.[7]

Studying norms in communities that encompass families, teens, schools, and other people and institutions is fascinating because it takes a "big picture" perspective on norms about teen sexual behavior. But it's also messy and difficult because of the many people and organizations involved and the variation in what interviewees consider their community. Perhaps surprisingly, like many other interviewees, Isaac had little trouble articulating the seemingly complicated tangle of teen sexuality norms in his community. The co-occurring norms I identify in his account are a strong norm against teen sex, a stronger norm against frequent or promiscuous teen sex, a weak norm against contraception for teenagers, a very strong norm against abortion, and a very strong norm against teen parenthood. I call this a *set of norms* (see Chapter 2). The five norms Isaac identified above are part of a norm set that is communicated as a whole, despite being internally conflicting. These multilayered normative messages about teen sexual behavior have appeared in the chapters on families, peers, and schools. But in communities, sets of norms tend to become especially complicated because there are so many social actors involved.

Sets of norms simultaneously target the *chain of interrelated behaviors* that lead to teen parenthood: sex, contraception, pregnancy, and abortion. Teens who avoid the first link in the chain by staying abstinent can conform to the whole norm set.

But as soon as they have sex, as Isaac estimated 85 percent of the teenagers in his community did during high school, the normative prescriptions in the set become inherently contradictory.[8] In Isaac's community, teens are told not to get pregnant but are simultaneously discouraged from accessing contraception (or from planning to have more sex in the future, which makes it hard to use contraception in future sexual encounters). They are supposed to avoid having a child at all costs, but definitely not have an abortion.

Norm sets in a community also include metanorms about how to sanction people who violate sexuality norms. Isaac identified conflicting metanorms regulating community members' reactions to teen parents. People were expected to show disapproval "of the lifestyles of teen parents," but at the same time, "they weren't outspoken against them being pregnant or carrying the pregnancy to term, because it would sort of be hypocritical to also be not supportive of terminating pregnancies." In other words, community members could face criticism for not being anti-abortion enough if they were too disapproving of teens who had decided not to abort an unintended pregnancy—yet they were simultaneously supposed to disapprove of teen parenthood. This linking of the social "problem" of teen pregnancy to anti-abortion rhetoric in many communities is a recent development, detailed below.

Even though the norms and metanorms within a set conflict, community members can still enforce the conflicting prescriptions by sanctioning teens no matter what they choose. For example, Lucy talked about negative sanctions against both pregnant teens and teens who had abortions in her wealthy resort town. Her cousin from Texas:

> ended up having to borrow money from a friend to go through with the abortion because she couldn't tell her parents why she needed it. Because she felt like if she told her parents, they would completely disown her. So she went through with the abortion. Her friend that she told ended up telling someone else, who told the whole school. My cousin would walk down the halls, and people would yell, "Baby killer!" to her. And it was a really, really hard time for her.

Her parents ended up being supportive when they found out, but walking the halls at school would have been a shameful experience whether she had an abortion or a pregnancy. Oftentimes people are aware of the conflicting norms communicated to teens. Henry said in his community (which he defined as revolving around his Catholic school in a conservative Southern city), "it was a very hot issue to talk about abortion. People really had different opinions about whether these girls should even have their children, whether or not it was right for them to go through with the pregnancy." Community members recognized the conflicting norms against teen parenthood and abortion. This meant there was no acceptable way for teens to behave other than abstinence, which many didn't see as a realistic option, and interpersonal sanctions could be severe.

Many communities described in the interviews don't have the anti-abortion sentiment articulated by Lucy and Henry. Instead, a different set of conflicting norms, part of the practical rationale, is more salient: Don't have sex, but make sure to use contraception. A competing pair of metanorms is also important in many of these typically more liberal communities: Disapprove of teen parents because they behaved irresponsibly, but don't disapprove of them because our community should support young people who need help. This pair of conflicting metanorms arises from a practical rationale rather than the moral one that was present in Isaac's, Lucy's, and Henry's communities, but the behavioral prescriptions are still the same: Disapprove of teen parents, but also support them. This is why it is important to consider both the behavioral prescriptions and the underlying rationale being communicated to teens.

In interviewees' communities, teenagers faced competing norms about sexual behavior, just as community members experienced conflicting pressures about how to treat pregnant and parenting teens. As Henry described above, sometimes people were aware of and uncomfortable about these inconsistencies. So why do competing norms persist? I argue that norm sets are shaped by an overarching *rationale*, or an acceptable reason why a behavior should be encouraged or discouraged. As Chapter 3 showed for families, there are two rationales in the communities our interviewees described: a *moral rationale* and a *practical rationale*. Previous chapters have discussed the moral rationale against teen sex, pregnancy, and abortion—almost without exception in these interviews, the moral rationale arises from conservative Christian values. In the practical rationale, a threatened future and immaturity are pragmatic reasons why teens should not have sex, should use contraception carefully, and should not have children.

Each of these overarching rationales gives rise to an internally contradictory norm set. The *moral rationale* says that teen premarital sex and abortion are wrong. Using this logic, teen contraception is also wrong because it helps teens avoid sanctions while committing the sin of sex. Teen pregnancy and parenthood are both wrong because they mean that a teen has had sex. But teen parenthood is also good because it means that a teen has not had an abortion. In terms of metanorms, people should disapprove of teen parents because they had sex, but approve of them because they did not have an abortion. This messy set of competing norms and metanorms thus arises from a consistent moral rationale.

A very different but still consistent logic motivates norm sets when a *practical rationale* is used. Here, teen sex is discouraged because it exposes teens to practical risks to their futures—STIs, pregnancy, and assuming the responsibilities of parenthood. Contraception is encouraged because it can greatly reduce many of these risks. Pregnancy is strongly discouraged because it means a teen made the wrong decisions about sex and contraception. Abortion is less problematic than parenthood because it helps teens avoid the heavy responsibilities of parenting. Teen parenthood is the most discouraged behavior of all because so many negative consequences are expected to occur. The practical rationale also results in conflicting metanorms: Community members should disapprove of teen parents because they made irresponsible decisions, but they should support them because they will need lots of practical help to avoid even more negative consequences in their lives. Like the moral rationale for norms regulating teens' sexual behaviors, the practical rationale provides a coherent logic underlying an internally conflicting set of norms and metanorms.

COMMUNITY TYPES

Interviewees seemed to consider it obvious that their normative environments regulating teen sexuality were complicated and contradictory. In many cases, they explicitly described their communities' norm sets.[9] The behaviors interviewees described among teens in their community didn't follow directly from the norms in the set, but rather were driven in part by other factors. There are four predominant types of communities in the data, summarized in Table 6.1.[10] Because all the interviewees were college students, their educational aspirations and family backgrounds may have shaped their perceptions of their communities. The sample did not include sizable groups of communities that were dominated by a non-White minority or a non-Christian religion. But racial/ethnic and socioeconomic divisions *within* communities were often important for understanding sets of norms about teen pregnancy.

Table 6.1 displays the four predominant community types in the center. Community-level religious influence and SES are the characteristics that typically combine to divide the communities into types. Community religious influence tends to shape the set of publicly communicated norms and teens' public portrayals of sexual behaviors. Community SES instead has a greater influence on families' privately communicated norms and teens' actual sexual behaviors. The relationship I found between lower community SES and higher teen birth rates is supported by others' statistical analyses.[11] Combining the information in the relevant row and column for a particular community type shows the features of that type of community's typical norm set and norm outcomes.

TABLE 6.1

Typology of perceived community-level norm sets and norm outcomes, with percentage of cases

Norms for all groups: Teen sex and pregnancy are discouraged	**Lower** community SES	**Higher** community SES	*Publicly communicated norms*	*Teens' portrayals of sexual behaviors*
Less religious influence in community	**"It Could Be You" Communities** (18%)	**"Be Careful" Communities** (35%)	Practical community rationale and norm set	Less careful about hiding sexual behaviors
More religious influence in community	**"It's Wrong, But…" Communities** (12%)	**"It's Wrong" Communities** (30%)	Moral community rationale and norm set	More careful about hiding sexual behaviors
Privately communicated norms	Heterogeneous/ **weak** family rationale/norm set	Practical family rationale/norm set		
Teen sexual behaviors	**High-risk** sexual behaviors	**Low-risk** sexual behaviors		

I emphasize a final, important point in Table 6.1 before describing the predominant community types: *None of the interviewees said their communities encouraged teen sex or pregnancy.*[12] Many interviewees assumed that *other* communities believe teen pregnancy is a good thing, but none said this was true in their own group. Some interviewees thought their communities tolerated teen parenthood as a life choice that some people unfortunately make, while others perceived their communities as encouraging parenthood for girls who regrettably were already pregnant because it was morally preferable to the alternative of abortion. But I consistently heard that nobody thought it was a good idea for a teenager to get pregnant in the first place. Despite considerable community variation in the content of teen pregnancy norms, then, interviewees described an overarching *societal* norm against teen pregnancy in the United States and a less consistently strong overarching one against teen sex.

Table 6.2 summarizes the norms, metanorms, and norm outcomes in each of the four community types described next.[13] Each of the four community types of norm sets and prevalent behaviors is named after a unique message communicated to teens by community members. The first community type, found in 18 percent of my cases, is dubbed "it could be you" because of the community members' sense that their teen-agers run the risk of ending up pregnant. These communities are mostly urban with lower or mixed SES, are less religious or religiously heterogeneous, and have greater racial/ethnic diversity than most other communities in our sample.[14] According to interviewees, these communities also tend to have relatively high numbers of teen parents. Societal stereotypes about teen parents often identify teens from these communities as the main "problem" demographic because of the overrepresentation of lower-income teens and those from some racial/ethnic minority groups among teen parents,[15] though these stereotypes are biased because rural White teens are also at high risk for teen pregnancy.[16] Because teens in these communities are identified as "problems," adults in the communities seem to have greater license to openly exercise control over teens' sexuality.[17] Sex education in this community type tends to be comprehensive with explicit instruction about contraceptive use, and reproductive health clinics (sometimes working within or near high schools) actively distribute and encourage contraception. The communities' rationale for attempting to control teens' contraceptive behaviors and reproduction is practical rather moral, focusing on the expected catastrophic consequences of teen parenthood for teens' futures and for U.S. society.[18]

In a community like this, Joel described a set of community norms that was quite complex, with some norms conflicting and some working together to influence teens' sexual behaviors. Joel is an Asian American first-generation college student, the child of a government worker and a food service employee who went to a Western big-city high school located next to a reproductive health clinic. Another interviewee said the school had the nickname "Ghetto Womb," which is telling not just because of its racist, classist, and sexist overtones, but also because it shows that teen pregnancy was salient to the school's reputation. He described his friends' families as "low middle income" and his community as politically liberal. Joel's large school included a wide range of academic programs, from an academically rigorous program with a high college placement rate to less academically oriented programs that he described as having high dropout rates, "gang problems," and "known drug

TABLE 6.2

Contents of community norm sets and perceived norm outcomes

Norms, Metanorms, Behaviors, and Public Portrayals	"It Could Be You"	"Be Careful"	"It's Wrong, But"	"It's Wrong"
	Low religion	Low religion	High religion	High religion
	Low SES	High SES	Low SES	High SES
	Practical rationale		Moral rationale	
PUBLIC NORMS REGULATING TEENS' BEHAVIORS				
Against teen sex				
• Because it can have negative consequences	Moderate norm		Weak norm	
• Because it's morally wrong	No norm		Strong norm	
For teen contraception if having sex				
• Because it can alleviate negative consequences	Strong norm		No norm	
Against teen contraception if having sex				
• Because it could encourage teen sex	No norm		Weak norm	
For abortion if pregnant				
• Because it can alleviate negative consequences	Strong norm		No norm	
Against abortion if pregnant				
• Because it's morally wrong	No norm		Strong norm	
Against teen parenthood				
• Because of its negative consequences	Strong norm		Weak norm	
• Because it's morally wrong	No norm		Strong norm	
For teen parenthood				
• Because it means fewer abortions	No norm		Emerging contested norm	

METANORMS REGULATING SANCTIONS

	Practical rationale	Moral rationale
For support of teen parents		
• To alleviate negative consequences	Weak norm	No norm
• Because it could happen to anyone	Weak, only with lower SES	No norm
• Because they didn't have an abortion	No norm	Emerging contested norm
For negative sanctioning of teen parents		
• Because they're irresponsible/immature	Strong norm	Weak, with higher SES
• Because they behaved immorally	No norm	Strong norm

PUBLIC PORTRAYALS OF BEHAVIORS

	Less careful	More careful
Hiding sexual activity	Frequently	Very frequently
Hiding/giving innocent reasons for contraceptive use	Frequently	Very frequently
Hiding abortion	Frequently	Very frequently

TEENS' ACTUAL SEXUAL BEHAVIORS

	Riskier	Less risky	Riskier	Less Risky
Heterosexual intercourse	More frequent	Less frequent	More frequent	Less frequent
Consistent contraceptive use	Less frequent	More frequent	Less frequent	More frequent
Pregnancy	More frequent	Less frequent	More frequent	Less frequent
Abortion if pregnant	Less frequent	More frequent	Less frequent	More frequent
Parenthood	More frequent	Less frequent	More frequent	Less frequent

problems." Students were "pretty sexually active," and there were multiple girls each year who carried pregnancies to term. Most of them, but not all, eventually left the school. When a friend of his got pregnant, she received "a lot of support," and students threw a baby shower for her.

In describing the community's norms about teen pregnancy, Joel said, "The sex part of it wasn't really that big of a deal because everybody was doing it." Yet at the same time, "I don't think any of them really would have told their parents" that they were having sex, suggesting that parents disapproved. Norms about abortion were heterogeneous within the community: "It seems like everyone who did get pregnant did have their child. The people that wanted to have an abortion, I think, there would be some support [he later clarified the basis for that support as, 'You should have that abortion because you're still young'], and others would say no" for religious or other moral reasons. Discussing teen pregnancy norms, Joel said adults felt that "if it happens, then that's fine, even though we don't like it. It's, let's be there to support them if it does happen." School programs available to pregnant teens tried to provide this kind of practical support, but teens had to transfer elsewhere in the district to access most of them.

Joel described a normative context in which adults attempted to control teens' contraceptive behaviors: "We knew [were taught] a lot about STDs because that has always come up. It's been a really big problem. The people I hung around with were just, 'Make sure you have a condom. Be safe. Don't be stupid about it.'" He said that teens themselves were more worried about pregnancy than about STIs. The normative language framing sexual behavior as "safe" or "stupid" is a hallmark of the practical rationale for norms about teen sexuality, typically found in less religious communities.

Coming from another "it could be you" community, Lillian is the Latina daughter of a food worker and a warehouse manager. She went to an urban high school with "a lot of different cultures" that "treat sex . . . and talk about contraceptives . . . differently, or you don't talk about it at all." She said that although she talked about sex with her friends "all the time," in her family, "culturally, we just don't talk about sex." In Lillian's school, although most kids were having sex, some parents knew about it and some did not. The number of teen pregnancies in her school was "more than I could probably count," and even though pregnancy "carried a stigma" for girls that was attached to a perception that their future socioeconomic chances would be ruined, she perceived that abortion was rare. This was interesting given the lower salience of religion in the community. At the same time, norms about teen pregnancy were not brutally negative. Lillian described families' attitudes when talking about teen pregnancy to children as, "You could be in that situation, and thank God you're not, but you need to be nice to her." This perception that teen pregnancy could happen to anyone was common in "it could be you" communities, unlike many others in the sample. In all of these ways, Lillian's and Joel's descriptions of their communities' sets of norms and prevalent behaviors were similar. And although both Lillian and Joel identified as racial/ethnic minorities, the White interviewees from "it could be you" communities described a comparable norm set and teen behaviors.

Lillian told a story that illustrates how motivated her friends and family were to prevent teen pregnancy. Importantly and similarly to Joel's story about STIs above, the behavior targeted by the relevant norms in this story was contraception rather than sex. When asked how her friends would have reacted if she had gotten pregnant, Lillian said, "Once I had to go to [a reproductive health clinic—she later clarified that she went to get Plan B medication after unprotected sex], and there were like five of us in the car. In fact, I wasn't gonna go to [a reproductive health clinic] because I thought I was fine. My parents, my friends were like, 'We need to go. We need to go right now. We need to go today.' And so we did, and so they were very supportive of it." Lillian was apparently willing to violate her family's norm of avoiding talk about sex in order to enlist both family members' and friends' support to avoid a potential teen pregnancy, highlighting her community members' practical approach towards controlling teens' bodies to prevent unintended childbearing.

Some interviewees in "it could be you" communities were aware that their communities were stereotyped as encouraging teen pregnancy. Lillian reacted strongly against these stereotypes when talking to her peer interviewer, who came from the same community. Lillian emphasized that even when sexual behaviors look similar in communities that differ along socioeconomic and racial/ethnic lines, norms and stereotypes frame these behaviors as a bigger problem when they are done by lower-SES, minority teens. This mapping of supposed tolerance of teen pregnancy onto racial and class disadvantage was widespread, justifying direct control of "it could be you" teens' reproduction.[19]

"BE CAREFUL" COMMUNITY TYPE

The remaining three community types tended to be predominantly White. Like "it could be you" communities, "be careful" communities (35 percent of the sample) are similarly less religious, but they typically have higher SES. It's important to note that community-level, not family-level, religion and SES drive the community norm set. Interviewees believed teen pregnancy was infrequent because sexually active teens usually used contraception consistently. Some interviewees told us that people in the community thought of teen pregnancy as more rare than it actually was because most teen pregnancies ended in a secret abortion. Sets of norms for this community type typically include norms prescribing public tolerance and even material support of teen parents, as well as conflicting norms that strongly and privately encourage teens to use contraception and avoid pregnancy. As with the "it could be you" community type, a practical rationale underlies the set of norms. Unlike the strong community-wide efforts to control teens' behaviors in the lower SES "it could be you" type, in "be careful" communities the communication and enforcement of norms about teens' sexual decision making seems to be primarily considered the private domain of families. Parents ignore their teens' sexual activity while strongly encouraging contraception and, if necessary, abortion. One interesting and surprisingly prevalent strategy parents in these communities use in managing these conflicting normative pressures to remain silent about sex while ensuring that a teenage girl uses contraception consistently is to put her on birth control pills for stated reasons other than sexual activity, such as acne or menstrual cramps.

Patton is the White son of two nurses from a medium-sized, predominantly White, higher-income city he described as "very liberal." He felt that in his community, pregnant "girls were shunned" (or as another interviewee from the same community put it, "a pregnancy is just like a physical marker that you are a slut"), yet using politically correct language, he also acknowledged that "there's often a lack of support for individuals who become pregnant when they're in their teenage years." As in Joel's example above, then, the community's norm against teen pregnancy is paired with a competing metanorm encouraging the support of young parents. Patton's high-achieving school reflected this tension between social distancing and providing support:

> That wasn't the case [pregnancy was not accepted] in my high school, even though they did have a teen parent program within our high school, but . . . if you weren't in that program you knew nothing about it. While it was in the same building and the students had the same access to everything, we didn't really see those students, know what was going on. They weren't a part of the whole community of the high school, because I knew that there was a teen parenting program, but I never saw anyone that was in the program. I never saw their kids. I didn't see what their life was like.

After contention about the teen parenting program among the school community, it was later moved to a more vocationally oriented high school.

Teen parenthood, then, was carefully tolerated in public, but also actively silenced so that the topic would not come up too frequently. Patton said it "was kind of pushed into the dark corner—the taboo topic that we don't want to talk about." Teen sex was somewhat different because "there was a perceived notion that there were a lot of kids that were having sex." Patton estimated that in fact, "about half" or fewer, particularly "cool kids," had sex by the end of high school. Because "for the most part they [teens] were practicing safe sex," few ended up pregnant and parents were able to quietly ignore teen sex. Patton said, "I think that some parents probably turned their head because they didn't want to know what their kid was doing."

Although interviewees in this community type said many adults tacitly tolerated teen pregnancy and ignored teen sex, they were not passive about their teens' sexual socialization within the privacy of the family. Parents made sure to communicate a strong norm encouraging careful contraception, but at an abstract level divorced from any concrete discussion of the teen's current sexual activities. In Patton's case, the discussion about how to have "safe sex" happened "way before the thought of me having sex was in consideration." Patton confirmed that the community norm encouraging contraception was more important than the competing one discouraging sex: "As a whole, it was more kids practicing safe sex rather than being a focus on being abstinent."

Sophie is the White child of an engineer and a consultant from a predominantly White, middle-income suburban community. Her "be careful" community echoes Patton's in many ways, including her description of the tolerant but negative norm about teen pregnancy: "I think if someone was to get pregnant in our school, it would maybe be talked about and they'd get looks, but they wouldn't be so shunned that they couldn't keep going to school, whereas I think some [other] places, you would have to find another school to go to." When asked how people in the community felt about teenagers having babies, Sophie's answer illustrated the community's practical rationale for its norm against teen pregnancy and the focus of other norms in the set on contraception and the stupidity of teens who get pregnant: "You're like, 'How could she let that happen?'—more, maybe even, 'Stupid kids. In this day and age who doesn't use a condom, who doesn't know what they're doing?'" At the same time, Sophie said, community members were "overall pretty understanding, kind of wanting to help."

Sophie perceived teen sex as somewhat more prevalent than in Patton's community, with "most" teens having sex before entering college. As in Patton's case, "a lot of times parents choose to be ignorant because they don't want to think about it," but some parents knew their teens were having sex. Interestingly, although teens who got pregnant in Sophie's community were informally sanctioned as stupid, sexually promiscuous, and academically underachieving, she acknowledged that unprotected sex sometimes happened and placed many teens at risk for pregnancy. She said:

Once you decided to have sex, for the most part I think people used condoms and were pretty smart about it. But the problem is condoms aren't totally reliable, and in high school I don't think birth control [the pill] is very common. I guess it also depends on which situation you're in, a relationship versus you're at a party and you have the random hookup when maybe you're drunk and not making good decisions. So I don't think anybody intentionally doesn't use protection.

Sophie's language throughout the interview absolved "responsible" teens like her of culpability for an "accidental" unintended pregnancy while placing explicit blame on teens who ended up carrying a pregnancy to term. This suggests competing norms, in which *getting* pregnant is much less of a problem than *staying* pregnant. These rapid shifts between blame and pity, condemnation and support, reflected a set of conflicting norms about teen pregnancy and sexual behaviors in these communities.

As in Patton's community, teen pregnancy was kept fairly quiet, often through abortion. Sophie said, "I don't know if I would have told anyone. I mean even now if I got pregnant, I don't know that I would tell anyone unless I was going to keep it." "It could be you" and "be careful" communities tend to regret the necessity of abortion, but because of practical concerns about the girl compromising her future, their norms encourage it over becoming a mother. Other interviewees' narratives help illustrate these normative messages. As Nadia said of her "be careful" social network within a hybrid community type, "If you were to get in that situation, you probably would not have the baby. You would get an abortion." Similarly, Claudia said that her friends, family, and teachers in her "be careful" community "would have told me to have an abortion and really heavily encouraged me in that direction" because "it is the easiest, cleanest, most discreet thing."

Although these types of communities tend to encourage abortion as the least problematic solution to the "problem" of a teen pregnancy, abortion is still stigmatized. In some cases, teens took steps to avoid potential pregnancies without telling their parents because they were afraid to make their norm violation known to their families. For example, Isabella helped her friends in a "be careful" community get Plan B medication after unprotected sex so they would not need to tell their parents: "A couple of times, . . . I got the 'morning after pill' for a girl who didn't have . . . an account with [a reproductive health clinic], I guess. So, I would get it for her. I mean, it's so easy to do that how can you not, really, if you're even worried about it at all?" The many steps teens in "be careful" communities took to hide their sexual activity from their parents underscore that norms against teen sex and pregnancy felt strong to teens, even in these relatively tolerant contexts.

Although both types of communities have higher SES and teen pregnancies are perceived as infrequent, the differences in sets of norms between "be careful" and "it's wrong" communities are stark. A consistent demographic difference between these two community types is community-level religious composition. "It's wrong" communities (30 percent of my sample) are dominated by conservative Christian religious organizations such as the Roman Catholic Church, various Evangelical Protestant churches, or LDS (Mormons), while "be careful" communities are less openly religious. This difference is tied to the moral rationale for norms and meta-norms about teen sexuality.[20]

In "it's wrong" communities, even religious families often privately communicate a practical rationale and related norm set like those in the community types above, but communities and most families also communicate a strong moral rationale. Teen pregnancy is talked about as "wrong" more than "stupid." Community norms focus on discouraging sex rather than encouraging contraception. As I discuss below, there is a publicly communicated norm dictating that teen pregnancies should not end in abortion because the strong anti-abortion discourse in most of these religious communities holds that abortion is morally wrong. In private, though, families' norms and rationales are split. Some are more likely to pressure teens to have a secret abortion on practical grounds, while others encourage the teen to continue the pregnancy on moral grounds.

Brooke is the White daughter of a shopkeeper and a salesman from a predominantly White, higher-income "it's wrong" suburb. Her interviewer remarked that she seemed uncomfortable talking about teen sex and pregnancy. She perceived that although most teens had sex during high school, teen pregnancies were rare. Her description of her friends' reaction to the one pregnant girl she knew was, "I can't believe she's having sex. . . . We wouldn't have gotten into that situation." As was typical for "it's wrong" communities, Brooke's and her friends' reactions revealed both a focus on the community norm proscribing premarital teen sex and a sense of moral superiority among those not having sex (like Brooke and her friends).

As was true to some extent for both "be careful" and "it's wrong" communities, teen pregnancy was a "taboo subject" in Brooke's community and "obviously not a desirable situation." She reflected, "You know, I think my knowledge on how many people were having babies wasn't reflective of the actual number. It was reflective of how 'hush hush' it was." In particular, many religious groups in her community were explicitly "against" teen sex and "promoted abstinence." She summed up the set of norms communicated to teens as, "If you're going to do it, be safe and don't tell me about it." Brooke's description of her community's norms revealed the conflicting rationales and related norm sets that are unique to "it's wrong" communities: a moral rationale communicated publicly in the community and privately by many families, accompanied by a practical rationale communicated privately in some families.

These norms against sex and pregnancy loom large in teens' lives and regulate their behaviors, especially their public portrayals of their behaviors. When asked why teens might have chosen not to have sex, Brooke explained, "There was definitely like an element of fear involved. Of what your parents would do. . . . A fear of being judged if you did get pregnant." She felt that community norms against teen parenthood "definitely" affected teens' sexual behaviors and public portrayals. Despite often being sexually active, teens in her community could easily avoid pregnancy and were motivated to do so in Brooke's view: "I feel like contraception was very accessible to us. We were rich White kids."

Finn is the White son of a nurse and an engineer in an "it's wrong" community he defined as "pro-religion" and "upper middle class" in a racially diverse, middle-income, midsized city. Christian religion "totally" dominated social life at his high school, with the most popular teens heavily involved in an Evangelical youth group. This Christian youth group's pro-abstinence norm successfully influenced teen culture, curtailing sexual behaviors and leading to the perception in the community that teens (particularly girls) who had sex were "sluts, whores." Finn became sexually active in his sophomore year of high school while flouting other community norms together with his close friends, but "most kids were not having sex." Among those who were, "everybody was really careful about it because they were so afraid" of being publicly portrayed as sexually active. Their fear, according to Finn, was "all about reputation."

Some parents' norm sets in "it's wrong" communities combine a practically rationalized norm prescribing contraception with a morally rationalized norm proscribing sex. Finn identified this contradiction when telling us that his parents "would've said, 'It's really irresponsible. You should use a condom. You're not supposed to be having sex with girls anyway.'" Finn also described a stringent community norm against teen pregnancy, even though the issue was not talked about frequently:

It was strongly looked down on. I mean, we were nice to those people [teen parents], because we're all nice Christians who were like, "Oh, we'll help you," but at the same time those people are never really accepted into the social realm again. It's like the silent treatment almost. It makes it so uncomfortable that they just have to leave. They got so uncomfortable they had to get out of there.

When asked whether people in the community felt that a pregnant teen should get an abortion, Finn replied that although norms publicly prohibited abortion, for families privately considering how to resolve a potential pregnancy, "it was on the fence." He perceived that norms about aborting teen pregnancies were shifting in his community, which is discussed further below.

Teens in "it's wrong" communities are often torn between competing abortion norms: a strong, publicly communicated community norm against abortion, and a privately communicated but often equally strong family norm that pregnancy should be "dealt with" quietly through an abortion based on the rationale that parenthood would ruin a teen's life. Other interviewees supported this point. Charles described this tension in his "it's wrong" community, saying that abortion is "a bigger taboo [than parenthood] where I'm from." Then he corrected himself to separate actual behaviors from public portrayals of behaviors: "I wouldn't say *having* one [an abortion]. But *speaking* about it, *being open* about it, that stuff. . . . You're shunned. . . . Many people that would do the same thing [have an abortion], but just keep it hidden" [emphasis added]. Describing his "it's wrong" community, Adrian echoed, "I think the people who were judging about the abortion would have done it themselves also if they were in that situation." And as Logan told us about his "it's wrong" middle-income Western suburb, "Well, obviously in the church community and my family, abortion is kind of like, just compounding the mistake. . . . So if you get pregnant, you're pregnant. You already made your choice by having sex." This public message is repeated over and over in "it's wrong" and "it's wrong, but" communities (described below) in our data, as is the rhetoric of referring to having sex and getting pregnant as a "mistake."[21] In this community type's rhetoric, a contrast is drawn between the "mistake" of sex and pregnancy, for which a teen has less moral responsibility, and the "choice" to abort or not, for which a teen's moral responsibility is greater.

Although it protects teens from publicly portraying themselves as sexually active and pregnant, having an abortion either with or without a disapproving parent's knowledge entails substantial risks. Perhaps the most severe is the threat of being removed from the community in order to hide a norm violation. This happened to Henry's friend, whose "very ashamed" father "made her live with her mother in Florida" after she had an abortion. Even when parents didn't find out about an abortion, their lack of support can create negative psychological consequences, as it did for Veronica, who said, "I guess the lack of information I had about abortion . . . really led to me making a bad decision" in having the abortion.

"IT'S WRONG, BUT . . ." COMMUNITY TYPE

The final community type is similar to "it's wrong" communities in terms of the influence of community-level religion and the moral rationale for the community's set of norms. However, "it's wrong, but" communities (12 percent of the sample) typically have lower SES. In this sense, they are more similar to the "it could be you" communities. As in that community type, community members consider it appropriate to strictly control teens' sexual behavior rather than leaving that work to families, but the control that communities work to impose has a moral rather than a practical rationale. Both communities and families seem to consistently communicate a morally rationalized set of norms about teen sexual behavior. Despite this community type's normative pressures against having sex, interviewees think teen sex and pregnancy are fairly common. Teens who are already pregnant are encouraged not to have an abortion—marriage and adoption are often held up as ideal moral solutions for avoiding stigma when experiencing a teen pregnancy.[22] But as interviewees said and statistics for such communities show, most pregnant teens do not actually marry or give up their children for adoption.[23]

Annika's "it's wrong, but" community was a "very conservative" small, rural, lower-income mining town with "a lot of meth [the illegal drug methamphetamine]." Christianity, particularly Baptist and Mormon churches, was "big." Few teens went on to college, and "there were a lot of people that were pregnant in high school." A college-bound, sexually active liberal, Annika felt like an "anomaly" in her community despite her White, working-class background as the child of a miner. In Annika's town, the norm "was very, very strictly . . . don't have sex before marriage." Yet she described a situation in which most teens were having sex but hiding it from their families and adults in the community: "I don't think it was very surprising that people were having sex . . . it was more that they were, I don't know, that they were pregnant." In other words, teens frequently violated the norm against sex but worked to hide their norm violation from adults. Annika believed that because most teens were partnered with the person they expected to marry sooner or later, they did not feel as concerned about delaying sex or using contraception consistently as they otherwise would have. The socially approved path for a pregnant teen was clear: "People were very anti-abortion, so that was kind of a given. . . . Everybody I know kept their baby." Anti-abortion norms were strong and explicit in the community, with teens frequently coming to school in "abortion is homicide" sweatshirts. Teens were by no means encouraged to get pregnant, but the sanctions they faced were not as severe as in many other communities. Annika said, "I think the teachers may not have been very excited about it [teen pregnancy], but everybody was very supportive." For example, "our senior class president was actually, like, eight months pregnant at graduation," and rather than working to push her out of the school as some communities did with their pregnant teens, school administrators allowed her to give the graduation speech.

Teens from "it's wrong, but" communities often conform to the norm against abortion if they get pregnant (which interviewees said they more often do because sexual activity and inconsistent contraceptive use are more common). Annika described her community as being a bit more tolerant of teen pregnancy than most others, but with similar reasoning behind adults' reactions:

> The older people, they were always very excited [about teen pregnancies], which I thought was kind of weird. But I think it's a part of the whole religious thing where . . . everybody thought, I don't know, that it was a gift from God, and they were very excited about it. And then, within the high school, I don't know. I don't think anybody was ever made fun of. . . . It wasn't like a good thing or a bad thing. . . . It's kind of like they [older adults] took the religious aspect of, like, children are very welcome. . . . That was more important than the fact that people weren't married and [had engaged in] premarital sex.[24]

The less attractive socioeconomic opportunities for young people in communities with lower SES like this one,[25] their lower average ages of first marriage and birth,[26] and the large proportion of rural U.S. counties without access to abortion providers[27] may help explain why pregnant girls in this community type more often adhere to norms discouraging abortion than in higher-SES "it's wrong" communities.

Isaac, whose norm set was described above, grew up the White son of a doctor in a lower-income, overwhelmingly White town located in a rural area. He estimated that 85 percent of teens in his tightly knit, highly religious "it's wrong, but" community were "sexually active to some degree" during high school. He thought that if asked, the adults in the community would have guessed that the figure was 20 percent. Isaac said, "Every girl was on the pill, it seemed like," and "they took care of it [getting the pills] in secret almost . . . without their parents knowing." Pregnancy was fairly prevalent in Isaac's view, with about 10 to 12 girls he knew getting pregnant each year. Like Annika, Isaac explicitly linked the issues of teen pregnancy and abortion when asked about the community's norms around teen pregnancy: "In general I would say it [teen pregnancy] wasn't accepted. It was considered that a person in their teens was not ready to have a child, that's definitely a general conception. However at the same time, terminating pregnancies was also not what I would call generally accepted by the majority of the population of my community." As in many other communities, there were stereotypes about the types of teens who ended up as parents. Isaac said of his segment of the community, "People of high socioeconomic status were generally viewed as trying to be understanding or accepting, but it always carried that undertone of, you know, 'I would never let that happen to me, or you know it's not my kids, that's what happens to the poor kids or the Hispanic kids.'" He also identified stereotypes of pregnant girls as "promiscuous." In other words, teen pregnancy was heavily linked to class, race, gender, and sexual morality in Isaac's community, in ways that enabled advantaged groups to do boundary work that enhanced their standing.

In contrast to the silence around teen pregnancy in the higher-SES "be careful" and "it's wrong" community types, Isaac perceived that teens "absolutely" talked with their families and each other about teen pregnancy because many families had been through the experience.[28] Although lines of normative communication were unusually open, practical information about contraception was not forthcoming. As described above, Isaac summarized the set of norms communicated to teens by community members as follows: "Don't get pregnant. I don't care how you do it. I'm not going to give you condoms. You're not supposed to get pregnant when you're 17." Anti-abortion norms were also an important part of this norm set, as I discuss below.

Although "it's wrong, but" communities share a moral rationale against sex with "it's wrong" communities, the anti-pregnancy voices, rather than the voices of people proposing to shun teen parents, are silenced in public discourse. Isaac explained:

> If people didn't accept what was occurring, they usually kept quiet about it. The most outspoken people were usually supportive of the entire event [teen pregnancy]. I never personally heard any really outspoken comments from, maybe those groups that I would have expected. We did have a substantial Mormon community. Also, people in my community in high school were predominantly Christian. I think it was sort of revered as an issue correlated with terminating pregnancies, abortions, so it made it sort of a hot topic for . . . the more religious communities. . . . Even though they sort of disapproved maybe of certain lifestyles, the lifestyles being those of the parents, of teen parents, they weren't outspoken against them being pregnant or them carrying the pregnancy to term, because it would sort of be hypocritical, to also be not supportive of terminating pregnancies.

Isaac saw people working actively to navigate conflicting metanorms about how to treat teen parents—and he perceived that community norms prohibiting abortion explicitly trumped those discouraging premarital sex. Uniquely among the four community types, this latter dynamic was nearly ubiquitous within "it's wrong, but" communities, though it was starting to spread to "it's wrong" communities as discussed below.

"It's wrong, but" communities are not always as lenient about teen pregnancy as those described by Annika and Isaac. Pregnant girls in these communities are often targets of public scorn. Other interviewees' stories support this. Josiah told of the sanctions faced by a pregnant girl at school in his "it's wrong, but" community: "Every time she walked down the hall, people would look at her and then whisper behind her back, like, 'I can't believe she's pregnant—she's only 16.'" Perhaps not surprisingly, Josiah knew of another girl in his community who had been encouraged by her family to get a secret abortion. Even outside of school, the mere sighting of a pregnant or parenting teen provoked anger in many communities, such as Rochelle's description of the reaction of her "it's wrong, but" social network to teen mothers in the "it could be you" segment of her hybrid community (described below): "I mean, if you drive through there, you're going to see they're pushing their kids around, and they're like all doing whatever they want. You know, like, walking around with their kids." This objection to teen mothers being visible at all in public is a sign of strong disapproval.

HYBRID COMMUNITY TYPES

Although most communities fit into one of the four types described above, 5 percent of the sample reported a hybrid of two community types. In each case, the communities were sharply divided along racial or socioeconomic lines into two groups with contrasting community types. In hybrid communities, each group's norms appears to be stronger because of the constant presence of an "othered" group with different norms.[29] Interviewees in hybrid communities performed symbolic boundary work between the two groups, which is a form of social control.[30] The social divisions that foster a split in community norms are often both socioeconomic and racial/ethnic, and these divisions sometimes seem to be exacerbated by the separation of students from different backgrounds into different academic programs. Rochelle's ethnically divided low-SES Rust Belt community is one example, with Whites having an "it's wrong, but" community type and Latinos viewed by Rochelle as having an "it could be you" community type. Rochelle's extreme racist rhetoric about teen pregnancy was among the most vitriolic in a dataset full of derogatory stereotypes about teen parents, perhaps because she portrayed it as only being prevalent among Latinas in her town. When probed, however, she acknowledged that teen pregnancy was somewhat common among Whites as well.

Nadia took a more politically correct approach in describing the socioeconomic and racial/ethnic divides in her large Western city where she attended a large, diverse high school. She said:

> In my high school, it was more like half and half. Like, a lot of people thought it [teen parenthood] was a bad thing, and a lot of people didn't think it was bad at all. But, in my neighborhood and my community, it was looked down upon.

Um, 'cause my school was inner city so, like, there were people from a bunch of different areas. And my neighborhood was more of like, an upper- to middle-class neighborhood, where it usually isn't okay to have a child.

Nadia said that "African American and Hispanic" girls got pregnant, but "Caucasian" girls did not. She attributed this to normative differences between racial groups, saying, "I know that in my high school there were a lot of instances where there was girls that got pregnant and had the babies or whatever, but they, their cultures supported it. Um, and that's how their family has kind of brought them up. So, but for me, I don't really agree with it." More subtly and tentatively than Rochelle, Nadia is doing boundary work by characterizing other racial/ethnic groups in ways that don't match how people from those groups described their own communities, but that bolster her own perception that her own group has a superior culture around teen sexuality.

CHANGING COMMUNITY NORMS

Communities' norms can change over time. In some "it's wrong" communities, interviewees believed that families who recently would have quietly encouraged an abortion for their daughters were in the process of shifting their attitudes to conform to the prevailing public norm against abortion. Finn was unusual in articulating the reasons for this recent shift in his "it's wrong" community:

> I mean, everyone in that . . . area is really on the fence about abortion. It's like, "Oh, my God, I should get an abortion. It's stupid." . . . I mean, back then. It's changed recently, as we got older. . . . We've gotten more inclined to say we should take care of the baby. I remember it was right after [the movie] *Juno* came out [in 2007] . . . stuff started to shift. . . . Everybody started to be, like, "Whoa, she [the character Juno in the movie] went through with it [the pregnancy]. Is that what you're supposed to do?" Because nobody knew. We weren't really educated on it. So we must all, after that, we all started to look for . . . more statistics, looking for more reasons why you shouldn't abort. . . . And now it's like right on the fence. It might even be leaning towards the other way. . . . Every point of view on this that teens have, adults seem to share. Because they talk about this more with their parents than anybody else. I'm more inclined to talk about this with my mom and dad and my friends. Or my teachers. And so their point of view is changing at exactly the same rate that ours is.

Besides the movie *Juno*, another high-profile event around the time of data collection that highlighted the tensions between anti-abortion rhetoric and norms against teen pregnancy was the 2008 pregnancy of unmarried teenager Bristol Palin, politician Sarah Palin's teenage daughter. The Palins and others emphasized Bristol's bravery in adhering to anti-abortion norms by carrying her pregnancy to term.[31] Events like these seem to have fueled discussion in some highly religious Christian communities about how best to resolve teen pregnancies. Logan's description of his church in an "it's wrong" community echoes this. He said that church members openly discussed if they should be approaching teen pregnancy differently by being more welcoming of young parents. He told a story about an unwed mother being "really welcomed" into his church "even though obviously everyone would have preferred if they had gotten married" that suggests these ideas were gaining purchase over time.

HOW COMMUNITIES TRY TO ENSURE CONFORMITY

Depending on their SES and the salience of Christian religion, communities have different norms about teens' sexual behavior—which may or may not conflict with norms being privately communicated within families. But what are communities' norm enforcement strategies to socially control teens and get them to conform to norms? As Chapter 5 showed, schools (including their sex education curricula) are important agents of social control. Boards of education—which can decide school policies and curricula—are often controlled by elected community members, and tax levies that financially support public schools are put to a local vote. Therefore, communities have considerable power over schools and often work actively to control norms about sexuality being communicated there. But here I focus on other formal institutions in the community that work to influence teens' behavior by shaping the normative messages they hear and the opportunities they have for different kinds of sexual behavior.

FORMAL INSTITUTIONS IN COMMUNITIES

Other community institutions work, sometimes in concert with schools, to communicate and enforce teen pregnancy norms and control teens' behaviors. Here I focus on two institutions that interviewees said strategize to regulate the roles of sex, contraception, and pregnancy in teens' lives: reproductive health clinics and religious organizations.[32] The physical location of these institutions varies, but they often try to occupy space in the school or as close to the school as possible. Schools' cooperation in granting access is therefore key for understanding these institutions' influence over teens.

Reproductive health clinics

Not all interviewees told us that there was a reproductive health clinic in their community. They seemed to be more common in communities with a practical rationale. Interviewees brought up clinics as particularly visible in the "it could be you" community model, which encourages the community's direct intervention to control teens' contraception and fertility. In these communities, reproductive health clinics are often located in close proximity to teens' everyday lives. For example, Larena (who came from such a community) said that a nurse was authorized to distribute birth control pills onsite in the high school, "as long as you had a certain form" and parental consent. Joel talked about a reproductive health clinic that occupied a site adjacent to his "it could be you" community's high school. Although these strategies are intended to increase teens' use of contraception, teens' own strategies turn out to be important: Larena told us that in her community, many teens chose not to use the services.

Even if they are not physically located near teens, reproductive health clinics are often successful in making their services known and available to teens, as many interviewees attested. For example, Lillian talked about driving to a reproductive health clinic with her parents and friends to get needed medication.

Religious organizations

Although their typical norm discouraging teen sex is quite different from the clinics' encouragement of contraception, religious organizations' norm enforcer strategies for influencing teens' behavior are quite similar to those of the clinics. These organizations tend to be most influential in communities with a moral rationale. Some schools, like Alana's, had Christian youth groups operating on school grounds.[33] In other cases, religious organizations would occupy a site adjacent to the school and work together with the school to ensure influence over students. Madelyn (who was a non-Mormon student in a predominantly LDS/Mormon community) told us about an LDS "seminary" (youth theological education program) adjacent to the school: "They [the LDS students] had seminary [available] every single class period, and it was right next to our school, so it was off campus because of the separation of church and state. But they had a period of the day that they could go there for an hour. Like, it was called free period, and they went there." In other communities, Christian youth groups were physically separate from the school, but they still became important institutions in the social lives of teens by succeeding in getting popular teens to attend regularly.

Religious organizations sometimes attempt to intervene in teens' decision making about pregnancy. As I describe in greater detail below, a primary goal for many of these institutions is to avoid abortion. Madelyn said:

> The LDS church supports adoption to the point of, they have their own adop-
> tion agency. And we'd see commercials that say, "If you don't want your baby,
> they deserve a good family, so put them up for adoption." So I think that's the
> way of the church getting around . . .
> *So they would match them up with an LDS family for adoption?*
> Yeah. And I think that's like the church's way of kind of helping out some of
> those families who stuff happens to.

Although Madelyn did not say whether the adoption agency was located near the school, it attempted to influence teens through advertisements.

Both reproductive health clinics and religious organizations seem to recognize the importance of schools as gatekeeper institutions into teens' worlds. Schools are sometimes willing to act as partners when the norm set of the community considers the organization's focus to be appropriate (the clinics' encouragement of contraception is appropriate for the practically oriented "it could be you" and "be careful" community types, while the religious groups' message of discouraging sex and abortion is appropriate for the morally oriented "it's wrong" and "it's wrong, but" community types). In many interviewees' communities, then, the norms represented by key social institutions—including both schools and others—align with the community's norm set.

INFORMAL SOCIAL CONTROL IN COMMUNITIES

Like parents, communities use norm enforcer strategies to try to influence teens' sexual behaviors by enabling or restricting access to sex and contraception. Earlier I talked about many parents' rules restricting opportunities for sex at home. The effectiveness of this strategy depends on parents being available for consistent monitoring and on opportunities also being absent outside the home. Finn noted that when parents and community members work together to minimize physical opportunities for having sex, teens aren't "put in very many situations where it [having sex] was possible. . . . You don't have a bed anywhere." Beyond having few opportunities in the home, Finn talked about teens' limited access to cars (a traditional site for sexual activity among American teens)[34] and the possibility that police would identify teens in parked cars and send them away. If outside opportunities for privacy are few, teens become reliant on spending time either in school activities or in each other's houses under the control of their own or friends' parents. In this way, close collaboration among families and with community institutions such as police and schools can lead to stronger monitoring and social control of teens.

Besides teens' homes and in-school activities, two other sites of social interaction for teens came up a lot in the interviews. One is religious organizations and youth groups in the community, which aren't intended to give teens opportunities for sex. In some communities, the other opportunity for teen social interaction outside of school is parties, which many interviewees viewed as events that can facilitate sex. But parties are complicated settings for teen sex. They are fairly public spaces with high levels of peer scrutiny, and having casual sex at parties is discouraged in many peer groups. Even in the communities with a practical rationale in which parties were mentioned more frequently, people (especially girls) who have sex at parties are often judged as deviant. Kaley's account of teens' sexual activity in her wealthy, suburban "be careful" community is pretty typical:

> I think a lot of the people who were in relationships had sex. But there's also the stories that went around about girls at parties hooking up with guys in rooms and stuff. Pretty funny sometimes. You want me to tell a story? . . . There's this girl who just transferred to our school from Texas. And like, she like hung out with the popular crowd, if you will. And apparently at a party she got drunk and [describes an extreme, explicit sexual act "someone" did to her, apparently without her consent, then laughs].
>
> *Was this a common thing at your school, or was this a one-time situation?*
>
> I mean, specifically I think that's the only one I heard of. But I heard of people [having sex] in the kitchen and stuff like that. [laughs]

Even in the relatively permissive normative climate of Kaley's community where teens had opportunities for sex at parties, girls who had this kind of casual sex faced very serious threats to their reputations. It's important to note even though Kaley's supposedly "funny" story may have been describing a violent sexual assault, which is a common threat for teens, the male perpetrator remained blameless and completely anonymous in the story while the female victim faced horrible embarrassment.

Thus, the parents in a community can facilitate sexual activity by hosting parties or curtail it by carefully monitoring teens in their home and reducing opportunities for sex when the parents are not home. Formal institutions in the community— police and religious organizations—can restrict sex through monitoring and providing opportunities for teens to interact socially without sex. Collaboration among adults' and institutions' norm enforcer strategies strengthens their social control, while a family hosting an unmonitored party can undermine it. Similarly, community members and institutions can restrict or enable contraceptive use by teens. I have discussed how school-based nurses and clinics provide contraception in some communities and how in the absence of this on-site availability, specific teachers act as "beacons" of information to connect teenagers with contraception outside of parents' purview. The information provided (or not provided) in school-based sex education also shapes teens' access to contraception by influencing their knowledge of what to ask for and where to get it. And the last section showed that the presence or absence of a reproductive health clinic affects teens' access to contraception. As Madelyn said, in her area (which was conservative but fairly urban), girls who "didn't want their parents to know" could go to the local reproductive health clinic and get birth control pills "on their own."

Even if parental consent is required, a reproductive health clinic can sometimes enable contraceptive use for many teens. Annika said that although there was no clinic in her rural town, "we had a visiting nurses' association." A friend of hers used these medical providers to act as a beacon of contraception, rather than of information: "For some reason she went and got birth control for everybody else because nobody else wanted to go, because you had to have a parent or something. . . . So yeah, my friend Christy would just go and be like, 'Oh, I lost my pack [of birth control pills]. Can you give me another one?' And they'd just give her birth control. And she would distribute it to everybody else." In contrast, in Ivy's small rural town in a neighboring state, "if you did have sex, it was more acceptable to get pregnant and have a kid than to use birth control or some kind of contraceptive." Whether because of that norm or other factors, Ivy told us that contraceptives weren't an option for teens, and they didn't usually use it: "It was impossible to get hold of. . . . If I would have gone to the store to buy condoms, it would have been absolutely ridiculous. To be honest, I don't think I would have even tried. . . . Birth control is not known like it is in other places." Ivy also said a friend had to go "out of state" to have an abortion (and her reputation was subsequently ruined when the news leaked). Although Annika and Ivy described similar norm sets in their communities, the visiting nurse in Annika's town made a big difference for some teens' contraceptive use.

SOCIAL CONTROL WHEN PARENTS AND COMMUNITIES CONFLICT

An important theme in this analysis of communities' strategies to control teens' sexual behavior is that communities can either reinforce or undermine the social and physical control parents exert over teens. Ivy's community's strict limiting of contraceptive options reinforced the norms she said families were communicating to teens.

But the visiting nurse in Annika's town, by collaborating with the teen who asked for many more birth control pills than she actually needed, was able to undermine several families' attempts to refuse their daughters access to contraception. Parents and youth groups that provide nonsexual opportunities for social interaction reinforce many parents' norms, but parents who allow unsupervised parties in their homes undermine other families' limits on teens' access to sex. In this way, communities and parents can sometimes struggle for control over teens' sexual behaviors. This conflict over control of teenagers' sexual decision making is evident in media firestorms like the 2013 controversy around over-the-counter access to Plan B emergency contraception.[35] Medical scientists recommended allowing prescription-free access to all girls and women, but facing pressure from conservatives, the Obama administration proposed restricting access to girls below age 15 by requiring parental consent. The contested issue here is whether parents should decide their young daughters' contraceptive behaviors, or if the decision to make contraception available should instead reside with community pharmacies.

Conflicts between families and communities are most evident in two of the community types, "it could be you" (low religion, low SES) and "it's wrong" (high religion, high SES). "It could be you" communities have a practical community rationale and accompanying norms, but heterogeneous family rationales and norms (see Table 6.1). As is typical for communities with lower SES, the school and community institutions often feel free to apply norm enforcer strategies, regardless of whether these strategies conflict with family norms. They tend to use comprehensive sex education and extensive access to contraception as tools to control teens' bodies and reduce teen pregnancy, rather than leaving that task to families. Alana described her urban community as a diverse mixture of highly religious and nonreligious families. She received sex education in elementary, middle, and high school (ending with a comprehensive curriculum that involved showing contraceptives to students). The normative message she described was, "Use contraception. Use condoms. How could you screw that up?" Most teens had sex in high school, some at parties. They knew how to access birth control and Plan B emergency contraception, and they used both. Alana was somewhat dismissive of parents' ability to support or control teens. She said, "The poor minority kids who were having the babies . . . you know the statistics. Most of their parents were divorced. So it's not like they had their parents to help them." This attitude that parents in the community aren't much help to their teenage children may have been a justification for community intervention from schools and clinics in providing knowledge and contraception, as well as support to teen mothers like school programs and childcare.

Like "it could be you" communities, community institutions in lower-SES "it's wrong, but" communities also tend to more strongly control teens, but because of their moral rationale, those norm enforcer strategies are religiously motivated. Community institutions often work to restrict sexual information and contraceptive/abortion access rather than providing them. Because most families also subscribe to the moral rationale, the strong control over teens exercised by the community doesn't often conflict with family efforts like it sometimes does in the "it's wrong, but" communities. Similarly, there are few conflicts between communities and families in the higher-SES, lower-religion "be careful" communities because communities' control efforts—providing sexual information and contraceptive access—tend to support families' strong norms.

The greatest struggle between parents and communities—even though it is not an open conflict—is in the higher-SES, more-religious "it's wrong" community type. These communities are torn in responding to competing metanorms for appropriate reactions to teen parents—sanctioning them because they had sex versus supporting them because they did not have an abortion. From interviewees' accounts, it sounds like parents are also torn because they tend to subscribe in part to the moral rationale communicated by the community, but often even more strongly to a practical rationale, linked to their higher SES, that focuses on preventing detrimental negative consequences of sexual behavior for their teenage child. Earlier, Finn described the struggles that can arise as families and communities try to decide which norms and social control are appropriate.

Logan defined his higher-SES, conservative community primarily around his church. The main norm discouraged teen sex, which like teen parenthood is a behavior that both the moral and practical rationales agree on proscribing. He said, "Premarital sex wasn't really something that was an option for us." The strong anti-abortion norm he heard is typical of a moral rationale: "Well, obviously in the church community and my family, abortion is just compounding the mistake." Logan thinks teens tended to follow these norms, with most abstaining from sex and abortion being kept "*real* hush-hush, if it happened" [Logan's emphasis]. So far it sounds like the morally based norm set in the community and his family were in alignment.

But Logan's account highlights inconsistencies and questions in community members' reactions to teen pregnancy. In discussing "the abortion thing," Logan told us about attempts to support teen mothers: "At one point we had a church discussion as a youth group over teen pregnancy. If it's something we should be doing—reaching out to the community more, to single teenage mothers more." But Logan's description of how he thinks his community (which he interpreted as his church) would react if he got a girl pregnant suggests a competing metanorm encouraging social sanctioning of teen parents: "Ostracized would be really strong. But I mean, it would just be one of those situations where I wouldn't see them nearly as much. You know, the community in our church really thrived off of quality time spent together, with activities. I just can't imagine me spending time with a lot of the same people anymore." Logan suggests that his social exclusion from the church would become a reality, even though people might ostensibly blame it on a lack of "quality time spent together."[36]

Even though the church community was struggling to come to terms with internal contradictions in its norms about teen sexual behavior, these inconsistencies were all within a moral rationale. In contrast, Logan described the practical rationale communicated by his mother (a never-married single parent): "My mom always stressed education as a big thing. And so I mean, if my sister ever got pregnant, that would be kind of a blowout, because I think she'd just view it as a really big opportunity lost." This focus on avoiding pregnancy because of lost opportunities more than on avoiding sex is typical of a practical, but not a moral, rationale. Yet Logan also introduced the moral rationale his mother increasingly subscribed to: "[Religious] faith was something that me and my mom were kind of just finding when I was in high school. And so under that context, I'm sure it [a teen pregnancy in the family] would have, potentially could have been something that could have torn our family apart." Although Logan did not spell out what the conflict would be, my reading in the context of his interview is that he means his family could have been "torn apart" about whether to abort the pregnancy—which is a clear point of contention between the moral and practical rationales.

As Table 6.1 shows, the moral rationale tends to control teens' public portrayals of their behaviors rather than their actual sexual behaviors. This gives teens (and sometimes their families) in the inherently contradictory normative environments of "it's wrong" communities a chance to adhere behaviorally to the family's practical rationale while publicly portraying their behavior as adhering to the community's moral rationale. Getting an abortion but doing so secretly, which was frequently described by the interviewees in this community type, fits with this complicated dance of conformity. So does putting girls on birth control pills for nonsexual reasons such as acne or menstrual cramps, another common tactic parents and teens used in these communities.

MANAGING NORM VIOLATIONS

COMMUNITY METANORMS FACED BY TEEN PARENTS' FAMILIES: "DID YOU DISOWN HER?"

Both the college student and teen parent interviewees talked about communities' sanctions when norms were violated. The support many parents provide to teens in getting birth control pills for reasons like acne and cramps or in secretly having abortions suggests that parents, and not just teens, are motivated to avoid sanctions from the community. Like friends, families of teen parents experience courtesy stigma and confront metanorms that expect them to enforce the community's norms by sanctioning their teenage child. If they don't enforce the norms, they face negative sanctions.[37] Families of teen parents can reduce their courtesy stigma by adhering to community norms when sanctioning their teenager—this is how they prove to others that they believe in the community's norms even if their child violated those norms.

Faith described the complicated metanormative dynamics facing parents of pregnant teens in her highly religious suburban community. She told us, "I think they [community members] felt probably sad like I do, and maybe a little embarrassed that we're not past the point where girls know more about contraception, or their parents aren't raising them to have better values." The last part of her statement places blame on parents for their teens' childbearing. Faith thought the focus on blaming a pregnant teen's parents may have reduced some of the stigma pregnant teens faced from teachers and school administrators. "I think they [teachers and administrators] look down on you, or they feel bad for you. But I think also they're trying to, they probably feel bad for you because they think you come from a, you know, not very good family, or the way you are, like something happened in your past, so they already feel bad for you. So I don't think they would treat you badly." But Faith believed metanormative sanctions against parents should be tempered in favor of more direct sanctions of the teen: "That's another thing I think about teenage pregnancy. It's like, you can blame the parents, but at the same time they can't always be with their child, and they're going to do what they want to do."

Sophie (from a "be careful" community) told a story that illustrates the interpersonal sanctions parents of pregnant and parenting teens can face: "My mom was telling me about a friend of hers that she knew, that her daughter got pregnant. And we were talking about it one day, and my mom was super surprised that her friend was really excited for her daughter to have the baby. And my mom was almost angry with this woman that she was supporting teen pregnancy." Through anger, Sophie's mother was enforcing a community metanorm by informally sanctioning the pregnant teen's mother. Sophie disagreed with her mother, saying, "Mom, at some point, what good does it do to think of it so negatively anymore?" Sophie didn't see that the negative sanctioning of family members her mother was engaging in—whether directly to the girl's mother, or indirectly when gossiping about it with Sophie or others—is a form of social control that tries to ensure others' future conformity to community norms. Community members are motivated to enforce metanorms because, as Mackenzie put it, "if you got pregnant, it was reflected a little bit on the community—they could look at you with judging eyes."

To avoid these "judging eyes," some parents hide their teenagers' pregnancies by helping them get a secret abortion, sending them away to another location, or pulling them out of school.

The supplementary interviews with teen parents paint a similar picture of meta-norms regulating families of teen parents. Fabian talked about his religious community when they found out he was going to be a teen father: "As a Muslim, the reaction was more on my parents. 'What's going on over there in that family?' You'd see the weird looks, people looking at you strange, shaking their head. I had a person shaking their finger, 'You're not supposed to do that!'" Fabian agreed with metanorms blaming parents: "Kids are impressionable. It boils down to what's in the household." But he also felt that "we all make some type of mistakes." Crystal's church was even more explicit in its enforcement of metanorms sanctioning her grandparents when she got pregnant:

> My grandparents are very involved with the church, so they know a lot of people and they run the Hispanic community at the church, or I should say used to. But they still know a lot of people, and a lot of them were saying, "What did you do to her? Did you kick her out? Did you disown her? What sanction did you give her?" My grandmother just told them, "It's not my choice. She's 19. She's of age. She's not under 18. I can't control her anymore." . . . They thought that she would have done something and that she should have done something.

Standing by their decision to violate the church's metanorms, Crystal's grandparents still provide a lot of material support to her and her child. Despite their negative reaction, people from the church community attended her baby shower, but then their involvement tapered off.

COMMUNITY SANCTIONS FACED BY TEEN PARENTS:
"WHAT WAS SHE THINKING?"

Many of the community sanctions teen parents face are similar to the social exclusion meted out by peers (such as gossip) and schools (such as invisibility). Girls who do not choose abortion usually keep their babies. Despite explicit encouragement from some communities, it's rare to hear of a girl giving her baby up for adoption. Except in unusual cases of highly religious, lower-SES "it's wrong, but" communities that encourage marriage at early ages, girls whose pregnancy becomes publicly known are almost always destined to become targets of public scorn. Because teenagers spend almost their entire daily existence in their communities, their sanctions are even more far-reaching than those of peers and schools.

Even in her large urban "it could be you" community that might be expected to have weaker social control, Abby illustrates how widespread community sanctions of teen parents can be. She said people in her area were "really gossipy" about teen pregnancy. "All the parents were gossiping about it. I mean, even though it's a public high school, a huge school. . . . My neighborhood is one of those things where all the moms get together, like book clubs and stuff like that, and they gossip." Abby talked about how people reacted to her childhood friend who got pregnant: "I found out about it at work, because I worked at a restaurant that a bunch of my high school friends worked at, too. So it was really bad. People would gossip about it in the kitchen. . . . I am sure there was gossip going around the school with the faculty." This sanctioning reflects peer dynamics of gossip as a form of social exclusion, but it's more pervasive.

Besides negative interpersonal sanctions like gossip, another strategy is to sanction teen parents for being visible in the community. This echoes the invisibility of teen pregnancy and parenting that adults often try to achieve in schools. Although some teens choose to reduce their public visibility themselves, in many cases families play a part. In Sydney's urban neighborhood, "my neighbor, when she was 16, got pregnant. I didn't find out until after she had the baby, because they kept her indoors. And nobody really found out about it. Because the neighborhood was so critical." Keeping a girl under effective house arrest for the duration of a pregnancy is a severe sanction indeed, as is sending a girl away. Ivy's childhood friend who "got pregnant at 17 . . . went and stayed with nuns." In Jessica's community, pregnancy was usually "covered up." She said, "Almost every girl that got pregnant at our school stopped attending school. They would either finish schooling online, be home schooled, or transfer to a different school until they had the baby. Rarely did we ever see pregnant girls walking around. And by rarely, I mean never." Often it's less clear what happens to girls who disappear from the community. Camryn said of pregnant girls in her school, "We would hear about it [the pregnancy] after they disappeared from school. We never really knew what happened to them."

From interviewees' accounts it's clear that being invisible is often considered the only appropriate choice for a pregnant or parenting girl (but not usually for a boy). Lots of interviewees from all types of communities detailed community members' negative sanctions of girls who chose to remain visible. An expecting couple in Bryce's private school "were so secretive about it [the pregnancy] in the beginning," but after their child was born, "they used to bring him to sports games and after-school activities. Every conceivable place where a baby could be shown off, they brought him. I thought this was strange." It's interesting that Bryce considers teen parents simply appearing in public with a baby to be "showing off." Although people in Bryce's community simply seemed irritated, in other places the reaction was stronger. For example, Rochelle became angry when talking about the visibility of teen mothers on a particular street where people from the Puerto Rican community lived: "Most people were like, 'Don't go there. It's awful.' . . . You would see, like, 16-year-old girls pushing their baby strollers and all. It was like, 'Oh, God, I'm not driving down that road.'" There was clear pressure for teen parents to quarantine themselves within Rochelle's community, or for their families to do it for them.

In the supplementary interviews, many teen mothers felt this pressure acutely (the teen fathers faced interpersonal sanctions from strangers much less frequently). Public spaces are where most of this negative sanctioning of visibility plays out, especially places like city buses and doctors' waiting rooms where teen parents are a "captive audience" and can't easily leave the interaction. Adriana described how pervasive these negative sanctions were in her everyday life:

> Sometimes I would be on the bus, and people would just stare at me. Or, like, when I went to . . . prenatal appointments, people were like, "How old are you? What are you going to do with a kid this young?" Stuff like that. I'm like, "Obviously you see that I'm going to have a baby, so I might as well try to find positive things." It was kind of awkward, because I know that people looking from the outside to the inside. It looks kind of bad to see a really young girl pregnant, but also, they don't know me, what I do. Now when I look at people, I'm like, "Whatever. You don't even know me." They see me in the store with my daughter, or anything that I do, if I take her to her doctor's appointments, some people just start talking to me. "Oh, you're young to have a kid." Like, for example, I got to get my nails done and I have my daughter. They're like, "Is that your daughter?" I'm like, "Yeah." "You look really young to have a kid," kind of ridiculing me. I'm like, "I still go to school." I can throw that in their face, because I still do what a lot of girls who don't have babies do. And I have a baby, and that makes me stronger than they are, because I have something that would possibly hold me back, and I still do it.

Adriana was cowed by these negative reactions at first, but now she uses her success in school—an unexpected outcome for a teen mother in many strangers' eyes—to try to shield herself from negative sanctions. It's unclear how well this norm target strategy works. Teen mothers almost always paired their accounts of strangers' negative sanctions with a discussion of the strategies they deployed to face this criticism, such as reminding themselves to be proud, thinking of the support their family gives them, or telling strangers they don't know the whole story.

Casey also talked about her traumatic experiences on public buses:

> When I found out I was pregnant, I came to enroll myself in this school [the charter school for pregnant and parenting teen girls], and I had to take the bus in the morning, and you get criticized by older people.
>
> *They'd say stuff?*
>
> Yeah, like, "Oh, my God, look at that little girl. She's pregnant! What was she thinking?" Or, "Look at that." Laughing, you know. It was bad.

The school for young mothers was able to supply free bus passes for its pregnant and parenting students, which enabled many of them to keep attending. Some girls spent hours each day commuting by bus. Yet serious problems with bus travel were widely acknowledged among students. Strangers on the bus harassed young mothers, and some bus drivers refused to stop at all for the mothers. Some students' fear of facing these reactions was so strong that it jeopardized their continued attendance in school. In this way, despite the extensive material support provided by the school, a negative normative climate in the surrounding community can have very real consequences for teens.

CONCLUSION

Communities are the outer circle of the social worlds interviewees described when talking about norms and social control around teens' sexuality. Families, peers, and schools are embedded in communities. These and other people and institutions in the community exert norm enforcer strategies, trying to control teens' access to opportunities for sex, contraception, and abortion. They can strengthen these strategies by collaborating with each other, or weaken them by conflicting with each other. The threat of social exclusion from the community affects teens' behaviors and their public portrayals of their behaviors, as well as other people's enforcement of teen sexuality norms. Although the set of norms and metanorms in a community is usually confusing and contradictory, an underlying moral or practical rationale provides a cohesive logic. These rationales, which tend to track with the importance of religion in the community, combine with its available socioeconomic opportunities to shape teens' behaviors and their public portrayals and justifications of these behaviors.

Clearly communities are important for understanding teen sexuality norms. But why don't interviewees talk more about broader *societal* norms around teen sex?[38]

One likely possibility is that these influences are harder for people to see, like a fish not seeing the water in which it is swimming. The interviewees had left their home communities to attend college—even for the few who grew up in the same town where the university was located, the campus community is very different than the surrounding town in terms of its norms and enforcement of young people's sexuality. Because they had arrived in this new community, interviewees could probably see their old one more clearly, but they were still in the same U.S. society.

It's also likely that the norms and social control around teen sexuality coming from our society aren't as visible in everyday life. The media sends a lot of messages but doesn't have control over young people. Without the opportunity to sanction teens who violate them, media messages aren't social norms. Societal messages and enforcement are both important, but teens' everyday social worlds are smaller than that. If a teen breaks a social rule about sexuality, a sanction is usually going to come from someone the teen knows or from a local institution the teen relies on. This makes norms and social control feel very local.

Societal norms often reinforce the norms teens are hearing in their communities, but they also complicate them. In U.S. society, I argue, nearly every teen has come into contact with both the moral and the practical rationale—the competing rationales that underlie complex sets of norms regulating teen sexuality. This means that no matter how strongly the community's rationale is communicated, the teen knows there is more than one way to approach the issue of teen sexuality in our society. As with competing norms within a set, these widely known competing rationales within a society may give teenagers more behavioral leeway because they understand that, at least in the long run, they can find a community whose rationale better supports the ways they'd like to behave.[39] The norm target strategies teens adopt in response to their normative contexts are the focus of the next chapter.

7

"SAY ONE THING AND DO ANOTHER"

Teens React to Norms and Social Control

PARENTS, PEERS, SCHOOLS, and communities use norm enforcer strategies to pressure teens to internalize their norms about sexuality and behave accordingly. Young people talk about feeling very afraid of flouting those expectations, and many believe in the severe consequences norm enforcers say they will face if they do. But somehow, most end up having sex sometime during high school. It's clear that teens typically do follow norms throughout much of high school, but at some point most take what they see as a major risk and break the rules. Why does this happen if they believe the consequences can be so dire? This puzzle can't be answered simply by looking at other people's communication and enforcement of norms, as earlier chapters have. This chapter focuses on the norm target strategies of teens to understand how many of them first follow, then violate, other people's norms about teen sexuality.

Teenagers are the targets of the norms, rationales, and norm enforcer strategies described in earlier chapters. Teens are navigating complex normative environments with regard to sexual behaviors. How do teens respond to normative pressures in their social contexts? High school students are in a unique phase of the life course because they are still very much under their parents' legal and physical control, yet they have a lot of leeway in deciding their own behaviors. This makes them a particularly fascinating group for studying the interplay between cultural and structural pressures and individuals' responses. Of course, these responses—also known as agency—aren't distinct from cultural and structural constraints. A teen may have internalized norms from her family and community that shape her behavior but that *feel to her* like her own independent choices. Sexual decision making is interesting to study because of its private nature. With the exception of later-term pregnancy, people's actual behaviors and their public portrayals of those behaviors can be quite different. This gives people more behavioral options than a more public type of behavior would, and it keeps teens' sexual behaviors beyond the full reach of norm enforcers' control.

This chapter starts by talking about how teens negotiate their own sexual behaviors and their dependence on people who discourage those behaviors. I then describe specific strategies teens use to navigate their normative climates in an attempt to maintain what sociologist Lorena García calls "sexual respectability."[1] Some of these strategies involve teens behaving as they want and justifying those behavioral decisions to themselves. Other focus on minimizing negative consequences when violating teen sexuality norms, through hiding norm violations and managing public norm violations.

NEGOTIATION AND DEPENDENCE

Interviewees viewed themselves as agentically negotiating their sexual behaviors and public portrayals. A pregnant teen in a higher-SES, highly religious "it's wrong" community has a variety of choices open to her that all entail violating one norm in the norm set while conforming to another. But each of these choices entails risks. Teens subjected to the same normative pressures in these communities make different choices, such as Veronica who got an abortion without telling her parents, Henry's friend who got an abortion and told her parents, and several teens discussed by our interviewees who chose to become mothers—some of whom stayed in school and some of whom dropped out or transferred. In each of these cases, the teenage girl faced negative consequences for having violated one or more norms: Veronica regretted her abortion, Henry's friend was sent away to a different state by her father, and the teen mothers regularly faced negative interpersonal sanctions from community members and schoolmates. Although no choice was beneficial for the girls, the community's internally conflicting norms did result in decisions they needed to make personally. Pregnant girls could choose to violate a norm against abortion in order to conform to the community's competing norm against teen motherhood, or they could do the opposite.

But even more than many interviewees could see, these choices are constrained by teens' dependence on other people and institutions. Although teens usually decide their own sexual behaviors, adults—parents, school administrators and teachers, and other community members—who are trying to control their sexual behavior still have a lot of leverage over them.[2] Most high school students are dependent on their parents for housing, food, living expenses, and emotional support. They also rely on adults in their schools for the curricular placements, grades, and personal references that undergird their future educational credentials, which are increasingly critical for employment and earnings throughout life.[3] Social scientists have long known that being dependent on someone for a resource that you need gives that person power over you.[4] Parents and school administrators explicitly or implicitly threaten teens with the removal of these resources if they violate norms regulating sexual behaviors. Because the adults control these resources, the threats feel real to many teens. Peers and community organizations such as churches also hold power over teenagers, but their resources are more social than material, and their threats involve social exclusion rather than resource withholding. Still, teens take these threats seriously as well, suggesting that they feel reliant on their friends and organizations for social interaction.

High school students' strong dependence on the various norm enforcers in their communities has an important consequence: Very few teens "go public" with a violation of sexuality norms.[5] About 40 percent of my college student interviewees remained virgins throughout high school, thus conforming to their communities' sexuality norms (although a couple said they were "technical virgins" who had engaged in heterosexual sex other than penile–vaginal intercourse as a conformity strategy). Importantly, in every community type, fewer than half of the interviewees were sexually abstinent throughout high school, revealing that anti-sex norms had a fairly weak hold on teens' private behavior.

Another 40 percent of the interviewees had heterosexual intercourse during high school and said they or their partners used contraception every single time. At least in less religious communities, protected sex is viewed as less normatively encouraged than abstinence but still conforms to the set's arguably most important norm—the norm prescribing consistent use of contraception. The vast majority of these teens did not make their sexual activity public, with the common exception of one or more close friends who were supposed to keep quiet about it.

Finally, 20 percent of the interviewees had sex during high school and used contraception inconsistently. Most of these interviewees said they almost always used contraception but made an occasional "mistake." They also tended to work hard to keep their sexual activity and their occasional violations of contraception norms private. The two interviewees in the sample who ended up pregnant both got secret abortions, one telling her family (and subsequently conforming to their pro-abortion norm) and the other not. Not one interviewee in this college-bound sample said they had publicly violated anti-pregnancy or anti-abortion norms.[6]

These behaviors, in combination with interviewees' accounts, tell us that most teens are too dependent on the people around them to risk an open violation of norms regulating their sexual behavior. They see two viable options: conforming to prevailing sexuality norms by refraining from penile–vaginal intercourse, or *appearing* to conform while privately violating norms in a way that usually minimizes the risk of exposure. As I discuss below, which of these options teens choose seems to depend on which norms and rationales they have internalized. Claudia talked about these options in her "be careful" community. She said that "behavior really changes" depending on whether it's public. She points out that because sex is private, "you could do what you wanted," including not having sex. But public violations of sexuality norms, like pregnancy, have to be "dealt with" publicly, so "you would probably do what your community would want." Charles talked about the power hierarchy underlying this public conformity in his "it's wrong" community: "There's a very, how do I want to put this, a very patriarchal way, but also there's a hierarchy set up. . . . So they [teens] are expected to do exactly what their parents tell them, or what other parents tell them. So there's an authoritarian, authoritative thing they [parents] teach about it." He went on to say that he thought lots of teens covered up pregnancies by getting "a fair amount of abortions that were just never heard about."

In contrast, people who are teen parents have publicly violated norms against teen sex, contraceptive use, pregnancy, parenthood, and—depending on the community type—abortion. The fact that the vast majority of teen pregnancies are unintended suggests that these young people didn't set out to flout norms openly.[7] Even so, they pay a price for their norm violation because after the birth, they are often increasingly dependent on norm enforcers who are inclined to sanction them. The sanctions teen parents experience, from being encouraged to leave their schools to receiving limited material support from family and community members, show how teenagers' dependence really does matter.[8] These negative sanctions are often problematic for the futures of young parents and their children, constraining their options after the pregnancy even though they made their own choices before it.[9]

HOW TEENS NEGOTIATE THEIR NORMATIVE CLIMATES

Because most of them have sex during their high school years, it's clear that teens find ways to negotiate the constraints adults place on their behavior.[10] But why do they do it when the potential negative consequences are so severe? Biological forces are part of the answer. Across time and place, people in their late teenage years have often been sexually active, and in recent decades average ages of the onset of puberty, or biological sexual maturation, have dropped in the United States.[11] Sex is often pleasurable. It sometimes happens as part of forming new emotionally intimate relationships, a part of the process of establishing independence from one's family of origin.[12] Sex is also an activity associated with adulthood—a status many teens aspire to. As I describe below, being sexually active when most peers are doing the same can make a teenager feel normal. If close friends have started having sex, teens may even feel social pressure to conform to that behavior. Teens may have sex to please a romantic partner or (especially for some boys) to impress friends whose group norm encourages it.[13] Finally, many teens begin experimenting with alcohol or other substances at about the same age, and those substances can serve to enhance the in-the-moment upsides of sex while minimizing in-the-moment perceptions of the longer-term risks it entails.[14] For all these reasons, teens may decide they'd like to have sex even though many people in their social contexts are discouraging them.

VIOLATING SOCIAL NORMS: "JUST DOING IT"

During high school, interviewees usually chose one of two sexual behaviors. The most common choice by far early in high school but the less common one by graduation was abstinence from penile–vaginal intercourse (which is what "sex" refers to in this chapter). The second choice was sex with consistent use of contraception (contraception is strongly encouraged by less religious communities and by many families in higher-SES communities). Abstinence conforms most closely to adults' and institutions' norms, but as I discuss in a later section, with a bit of luck, sex with consistent use of contraception can be kept secret. So although one of these behaviors involves risk, both offer teenagers a reasonable opportunity to appear to conform to adults' norms and avoid negative sanctions.

Teens who decide they want to have heterosexual intercourse face problems negotiating normative contexts that are unwelcoming of that behavior. Either they must make an unusual decision to violate the norm publicly and disregard the negative consequences, or they have to strategize to minimize the risk of sanctions. I talk about the second, much more common, decision here. There are two main strategies available to people who want to violate a norm without facing the full negative consequences: finding ways to change the normative pressure itself, or finding ways to violate a norm without being sanctioned too much. Here, I talk about several specific tactics teens use to negotiate normative constraints and achieve their own goals. The first three seek to change the normative expectations teens conform to. The last two seek to violate norms while minimizing or avoiding negative sanctions.

First, teens can choose which of their existing reference groups' norms to conform to. Although school and community norms about teen sexual behavior tend to be similar, family and community norms sometimes differ. This is especially true in "it's wrong" communities, where the importance of religion drives a moral rationale for community norms, but high SES drives a practical rationale for family norms (which is often combined with the moral rationale in families). The largest disjoint in norms is usually between peer norms and those of the other (adult) norm enforcers. Although teens are often expected to keep their sexual behavior quiet, peer norms often tacitly or openly support sex with consistent use of contraception. The decision to conform to peers' versus adults' sexuality norms allows teens some choice in their behaviors while still conforming to their chosen reference group's norms.

Second, teenagers can change the reference groups that are available to them— which also changes the norms they're expected to conform to. Disowning one's parents or switching communities usually isn't feasible, but researchers have found that teens commonly change their close friendships during high school.[15] Shifts in friendship groups often happen because a teenager's friends either are or aren't engaging in behaviors the teen wants to engage in or avoid, such as studying hard or smoking.[16] Changing friendship groups because of those groups' sexual behaviors— or their norms regulating those behaviors—is a very real option for the many teens whose social contexts include a variety of norms and behaviors. But I can only speculate that teens do this because not enough interviewees talked about it. In contrast, I do know that interviewees (especially the pregnant and parenting teens) moved into and out of religious organizations and schools, sometimes explicitly because of the norms they were communicating about teen sexuality and sometimes for other stated reasons. For example, teen mother Olivia told us:

> Two years before I was pregnant, I started going to Catholic [church], and I was involved in the youth group and the church choir and everything. In August of last year I stopped going.
>
> *Was this when you found out you were pregnant?*
>
> Well, it was when I was pregnant, but I stopped going because in the church it was too hot, and I fainted once. It was so hot, so I just took off, and when I was pregnant, I didn't go back.

Going to church didn't stop Olivia from having sex when she wanted to, but once church members were about to be able to see she had violated their anti-sex norm, she exited that reference group. Although a too-hot church might have prevented Olivia from attending in August, it does not explain why she stopped going in the longer term. A triggering event like Olivia's fainting spell is often the catalyst for a teen's decision to leave an organization or school that disapproves of him. Leaving the church presumably diminished the anti-sex/pregnancy norms in Olivia's social context, making her feel less deviant.

A third way teens can negotiate normative pressures is by choosing which norm to conform to in a reference group's norm set. This is particularly useful when the norm set is internally contradictory, as the teen sexuality norm sets for all predominant community types are. For example, communities with a practical rationale for their norm set (the less religious "it could be you" and "be careful" communities) hold both a norm discouraging teen sex and a stronger norm encouraging consistent use of contraception. A teen who remains a virgin is conforming to the first norm without violating the second. A teen who has sex but uses contraception consistently is violating the first, weaker norm but conforming to the second, stronger one. As long as the teen does not publicly flaunt her sexual activity, in many communities either of these strategies is tacitly tolerated. This leaves teens in these community types with some limited choice of behaviors. In contrast, a third behavioral option of being sexually active without using contraception consistently would be very deviant at least in wealthier communities and is not considered an acceptable option by many teenagers.

Two additional strategies described below have to do with violating norms while avoiding sanctions. First, teens can violate norms while working to hide their violation from norm enforcers. Many teenagers collaborate in their efforts to do this. Second, teens who have been caught violating a norm can work to justify to themselves and others how this behavior is less problematic than it seems. This can involve excusing the behavior as a "mistake" and thus reinforcing that they have internalized the rationale for the norm that they accidentally violated, demonstrating that they don't belong in the category of deviant people because of other redeeming qualities, or arguing that the deviant behavior isn't a problem after all.

JUSTIFYING BEHAVIORAL CHOICES: "THE NATURAL PROGRESSION OF THINGS"

Norms do appear to shape teenagers' motivations for their sexual behavior,[17] but they use the sets of norms and rationales for norms that exist in their social contexts as a flexible toolkit or repertoire.[18] Young people pick which norm in the set to conform to (for example, an anti-sex norm versus a pro-contraception one), and they also make use of different aspects of the rationales for these norms to *justify* different behavioral choices. Both of these strategies involve choices within the constraints of the norms and rationales available in a teen's social context. This view of teens' negotiation of normative pressure weds older and newer views of norms and culture. Norms constrain the choices for behaviors and justifications of behaviors, but people actively make decisions among those choices and strategize to "spin" those decisions in a socially acceptable way. Although justifications of behavior are just talk, they are important. Sexual behavior is private, so people's talk about their own behavior is an important way that others judge whether they're following norms.

What's not yet clear is whether teenagers have *internalized* the norms and rationales that shape their behavior and justifications for their own behavior. When a norm has been internalized, a teenager personally agrees that its rules for behavior are appropriate. Rationales (agreed-upon reasons why a norm is appropriate) also relate to internalization—people internalize not just a norm, but the shared reasons why that norm is appropriate. Teens may have internalized the norms and rationales they use to explain their behavior. Alternatively, they may simply be "talking the talk" of superficial conformity by doing and saying what's socially acceptable without themselves believing those are the right choices. I argue that in most cases, interviewees had internalized the norms and rationales they drew upon as teens, but they actively chose which norms and which reference groups to conform to.[19]

Justifying abstinence: being moral, being smart, not being ready

Because they didn't violate any sexuality norms in their social contexts (except for peer norms in some schools), interviewees who remained sexually abstinent throughout high school could easily draw on available rationales to justify their behavior. But because the moral and practical rationales each rely on unique reasoning, teens in different communities had different cultural tools available to help them explain their actions. Sociologist Christie Sennott and I identify three justifications sexually abstinent teens use: being moral, being smart, and not being ready.[20]

"Being moral" is a straightforward justification for behavior, most available to teenagers whose families or communities have a moral rationale for norms regulating teen sexuality. In this rationale, avoiding sex outside of marriage is the only morally acceptable choice. Logan made use of this justification when explaining why he remained a virgin throughout high school in an "it's wrong" community (his emphasis): "My *personal* opinion is that sex should occur inside of marriage. And right now I believe that contraception is not really the way to go. I don't really agree with it . . . it's basically an entirely religious conviction. My line of reasoning is that birth is a miracle that God is solely responsible for. Every child is a miracle. Every child is a blessing, and I don't see us having a legitimate role in preventing that." Logan weaves together anti-sex, anti-contraception, and anti-abortion norms using a classic moral rationale. He tracked the development over time of his internalization of the moral rationale and its related norm set, saying that social control by family and community became largely unnecessary:

> *Do you think your friends' decisions to not have sex were affected by either what family members thought, or what the community thought?*
> Up to a certain point. I would definitely say by senior year, . . . maybe even junior year [of high school], our convictions were starting to become much more personal, and much more potent, to the degree that I don't think that was so much of an issue, or our family members or community. I mean obviously that would always be in the back of our minds, but by then it was much more of a personal conviction.
> *And so what do you mean by personal conviction? What was that based on?*
> Our religious beliefs.

Another sign that Logan had fully internalized the moral rationale and norm set is that he was willing to enforce these norms if peers deviated from them. He was "part of the leadership team" of a Christian athlete organization in high school. If someone else in the leadership had gotten pregnant, Logan said, "I mean, yeah, don't ostracize the person, but at the same time I wouldn't feel comfortable allowing them to be a part of the leadership team, you know."

Like many interviewees, though, Logan didn't draw on only one justification for his behavior. He also made use of the "being smart" justification for remaining abstinent. Presumably reflecting his never-married mother's communication of a practical rationale for curtailing sex alongside the moral rationale, Logan spoke disparagingly of the intelligence of teenagers who have sex: "It just kind of seemed a stupid thing to do at that time, you know? To risk premarital sex. Of course if it ends in a pregnancy . . . Premarital sex wasn't really something that was an option for us. . . . It was always looked down on in the sense that it just wasn't a place you should have gone. Not that you were a lesser person for doing it, but it was kind of a stupid mistake to make." It's interesting to note that Logan made this use of the "being smart" justification—which is more widely accepted in his current college environment than a moral justification—early in the interview before switching to a strong "being moral" justification later on. At that point he contradicted his earlier statement that you weren't a "lesser person" for having had premarital sex.

In the "being smart" justification for abstinence, teenagers who have sex are "looked down on" because they're making a stupid, irresponsible decision. In contrast, teens who wait to have sex are smart. Being smart and responsible is part of the practical rationale underlying norms about teen sex. Many teens who use the "being smart" justification also reference another aspect of the practical rationale: that negative consequences of sex can jeopardize a teen's future. Both are evident in Camryn's account. Although she says she doesn't "really agree with value judgments," Camryn seems to have quietly internalized the norm from her "it's wrong, but" community, friends, and "very future-oriented" family that "any type of sex before marriage was very looked down upon." Teen pregnancy was viewed as "the ultimate sign of irresponsibility. . . . Their future is ruined. How could they do that? Why weren't they smarter?" Despite the practical rationale that was unusually prominent in her religious community, "there was no other option than abstinence, and if you deviated from that, then you were considered a deviant." Camryn had not internalized her community's moral rationale like Logan had, but she conformed to the anti-sex norm and had internalized a practical rationale.[21]

Implicit in Camryn's account is the third justification for sexual abstinence, not being "ready." Like "being smart," this justification often references the practical rationale, but it highlights another important concept that cuts across all community types: *age norms*.[22] Age norms determine the appropriateness of a behavior depending on how old people are or what life stage they're in (such as being married, being financially independent, having completed one's education, and so on). Sexually inexperienced teens use age norms when talking about not being ready for sex because they're too young, or not married, or not finished with high school. Claiming "not being ready" as an individual decision that is free from family influence may also help abstinent teens feel that they are being adult without the adult marker of sexual activity.

"Not being ready" is compatible not only with being smart, but also with being moral. In Noelle's "it's wrong" community, "most people had that view, like you should be married. Everyone goes to college. That's not the time to be having a baby." What started out as a moral rationale morphed into an age norm rationale that transcends the moral and practical rationales, about not being ready because it's "not the time." Proponents of this justification, like Chloe who grew up in an "it could be you" community, can be passionate about it. Chloe said she was "damn proud" of her virginity through high school. She told us of teen parenthood, "I think it's sort of a tragic thing. I don't think people in high school are ready to have that type of commitment. I mean, you're still trying to take care of yourself." As is typical, Chloe's condemnation of teen parents (a condemnation that came through much more strongly in the peer interviews than in those with older interviewers) is the clearest articulation of her internalized norms about teen sexual behavior.

Haylie talked more explicitly about not being ready and being too young for sex in her internal decision-making process: "My decision to not have sex was more based around myself not being ready, and not being in serious relationships in high school, and then my friends also not having sex." She said that the idea of sex in high school was "still really new to me, and strange, I guess. So there's that aspect of just being something different, and perceived as older than what I was doing. It wasn't really a moral thing." Unlike the communities of many of the others quoted above, Haylie's "it could be you" community was not highly religious. Her "not being ready" justification was not shaped by moral rationales as Chloe's and Noelle's were (Chloe's by her family and Noelle's by her community). In fact, Haylie pointedly rejected a moral rationale. This shows that like the "being smart" justification, "not being ready" is flexible and can be used in a variety of ways as part of different kinds of cultural toolkits. It's also interesting that even though adults' norms supported their decisions to remain abstinent because they weren't ready, Haylie and several others referenced close friends as important influences on their behaviors.

Justifying sexual activity: being normal and being smart

Interviewees who didn't have sex during high school justified their behavior using aspects of the rationales that adults in their social contexts subscribed to, even though they sometimes said their close friends also influenced their behavior.[23] In contrast, many of those who did have sex shifted the focus of their justifications to the wider circle of peers.[24] In this way, they negotiated their normative climates by changing the reference group whose norms they conformed to. Sexually experienced interviewees identified a norm among peers that tolerated (or sometimes even encouraged) sex and that was justified by an idea that teen sex is "normal." Jillian articulated this justification:

> *What were common beliefs most teenagers had in your community about sex?*
> That it was pretty widely accepted. That it was the norm. It was what people did . . .
> *Why do you think teenagers like you behaved the way you did in terms of having sex and getting pregnant or avoiding pregnancy?*
> It was the norm. We all were just doing it. It was sort of a peer group thing, and everyone just validated it and made it okay. It was the natural progression of things. It is what everyone before us did. It's what the older kids did. Like, once you got a certain age, you partied, and when you were with someone, you were having sex with them. It just wasn't even a question. It was just something you did. It was expected behavior in high school.

When Jillian says sex was "expected behavior in high school," she certainly wasn't talking about adults' norms in her highly religious "it's wrong, but" community with an "attitude of abstinence." Jillian was talking about her peers. Kaitlyn was more explicit about how peers came to be the main reference group influencing teens' sexual activity in her "be careful" community: "Once their friends have sex and start experimenting, it starts to be okay. I mean, once everyone is doing it, you think it is okay. You start to think, 'Everyone is doing it, so why am I not doing it?'" Kaitlyn is demonstrating how this peer norm directly influenced her subsequent sexual activity in asking, "Why am I not doing it?"

In Jillian's and Kaitlyn's descriptions of peer norms, teens' sexual activity is "okay," but it's not necessarily a social norm in the strictest sense because there is very little evidence that teens who didn't have sex faced negative sanctions. Instead, both women are describing a statistical, or descriptive, norm (a prevalent behavior in a particular reference group) that is based on perceptions of what behavior is "normal," but not on social sanctions attached to violation of the norm.[25] Julie talked about how the "being normal" justification was only available to teens later in high school because that's when sex became the statistical norm in her "it's wrong, but" community, as is true in most places:

It changed through high school. When we started, freshman, sophomore year it was, . . . it was less accepted. And I remember when I lost my virginity when I was 16, there were a lot of girls that looked down on me because I was not a virgin anymore. But by the time we were seniors in high school and we were 18, they were all having sex and they were having sex with way more guys, way more partners than I was ever, and their views on it had completely changed.

Julie is describing how a social norm against teen sex early in high school turned into a statistical norm later in high school that didn't have positive or negative sanctions attached. At that point, "being normal" became a feasible justification for having sex.

Besides emphasizing how normal sex was among peers, interviewees who had sex during high school also used the "being smart" justification described in the previous section. But there is an important difference: Abstinent teens usually equated "being smart" with not having sex, while sexually active teens tended to think "being smart" means using contraception carefully and avoiding pregnancy. They used the same justification of being smart as abstinent teens do, but they applied it to different behaviors. In using this justification, sexually experienced interviewees often talked like abstinence wasn't a realistic option. Henry told us, "For me, I was scared to have a child. I knew I wasn't ready for a child and was against abortions. So being safe about what I did was the best option for me. And it was easy to be safe about it." The beginning of

Henry's justification sounds like something a sexually abstinent interviewee would say, but then Henry said "it was easy to be safe" (by which he presumably means use contraception, which he did consistently) and become sexually active in his "it's wrong" community. Not everyone agreed with Henry's sentiment. Carter said of his "be careful" community, "I think most people who were in sexually active relationships in high school knew it [pregnancy] was a possibility and felt more like they dodged a bullet if they didn't get pregnant." Even so, among peers, "no one judged you if you did or did not" have sex, and teens started having sex at "the appropriate time for me" (this is a rare use of the "being ready" narrative to justify sexual activity). Personally, Carter had internalized a "being normal" justification as well as "being careful": "Our bodies are programmed to have sex, and then to just ask it not to is not the right way to take it. It's going to happen." Carter's view of teen sex as biologically inevitable but involving the dodging of bullets reflects known cultural frames about teenagers being driven by out-of-control hormones.[26] Carter's perspective is more risk-filled than Henry's, but Carter felt strongly that the community norm promoting contraception was "very helpful" by enabling teens to be smart when having sex.

Justifying inconsistent use of contraception: secret behavioral "mistakes"

One fifth of the college student interviewees had heterosexual intercourse without contraception at least once (for most of them, it happened rarely). This means that one in three sexually active interviewees had unprotected heterosexual sex at some point during high school. For most of them, this behavior violated a strong community, family, and/or peer norm encouraging consistent contraception. But other than a sexual partner knowing, this norm violation is private unless a teenager chooses to make it publicly known. Interviewees who used contraception inconsistently worked to keep their norm violations secret.

But if you have internalized a norm, then even if nobody knows you violated it, you're probably going to have to justify your norm violation to yourself. This happens because people who have internalized a norm feel shame or guilt unless they can explain the violation away or deny that it happened.[27] Most of the interviewees who inconsistently used contraception chose to deny the norm violation or excuse it as a "mistake" rather than labeling themselves as having done something wrong. Ivy explained why it was okay that she didn't use contraception by refusing to claim a sexually active identity: "I only had sex a couple of times and wasn't experienced or anything like that." She also said that in her isolated, "it's wrong, but" farming town, people disapproved of contraception on religious grounds and "it was impossible to get ahold of." Ivy minimized her norm violation, claimed that she couldn't have used contraception if she had wanted to, and implied that she didn't really need contraception.

Bryce used two other common justifications—denying that his behavior violated the norm and demonstrating that he personally agreed with the norm—to explain why he used contraception only "most of the time." He told us of teens in his "it's wrong" community:

> We would use condoms most of the time, but there would be some times, especially when dating someone exclusively, that contraception was not used. The pull-out [withdrawal, not a very effective method of contraception] was popular among boys, and the "morning after pill" was at almost every girl's disposal. . . . It was equally important for each partner to make sure they did their part to avoid pregnancy and use contraceptives.

Although Bryce acknowledged that he did not use contraception consistently, he suggested that he "did his part" in terms of contraceptive use. He also explicitly demonstrated his internalization of a pro-contraception norm without acknowledging his own norm violation: "I think that everyone who is involved in sexual acts should be responsible for practicing safe sex and using the necessary tools to avoid any unwanted consequences. Women and men alike should have whatever form of contraception they feel works best when they engage in sexual activities."

A related strategy some interviewees used to excuse their behavior is to disassociate themselves—whom they present as innocent people who made an understandable mistake—from those they consider to be the "real," culpable norm violators—pregnant and parenting teens. Some of the most vicious condemnations of young parents came from interviewees who had not used contraception consistently. Lilly first denied her behavior by following her statement that she didn't always use contraception with, "we were always careful, that's for sure." She then set to work "othering" people in her "it could be you" community who had not used contraception consistently.[28] Lilly used a variety of severe racial and class-based insults, including "White trash," to describe the teen mothers in her high school. She condemned teens in her school who didn't always use contraception: "I'm sure they were using condoms and were on the pill, but I guess most of the time they forgot or were like, [spoken mockingly] 'too much in the moment' or something."

Like Lilly, Carsen (from a "be careful" community) adopted a combination of justification strategies. He established himself as someone who is usually careful about contraception, said it's normal to have "a scare now and then," and condemned teen parents even more strongly than Lilly did. But then he justified his inconsistent use of contraception by judging girls who have contraceptives available:

> I just always bought them [condoms]. I mean, you should never go into a situation going, "I bet she has some," because she's not going to. And if she does, then you gotta rethink yourself.
>   *So if she has condoms like in her bed stand then she's probably, maybe slutty?*[29]
>   I wouldn't just label her slutty right off the bat. I would probably think, "Her last boyfriend probably bought those."

Blaming or putting responsibility on the girl was common among the male interviewees who didn't use contraception consistently, but the women didn't blame the men.[30] Spencer was unusual in retrospectively accepting the responsibility for both violating a pro-contraception norm in his "be careful" community and putting too much burden on the girl:

> I mean, in high school we would all joke around about how—or just be like, "Dude! Just pull out!" Like [pretending] that it's not even an issue. But I mean, in reality, we all knew through our various sex ed[ucation] classes at our different schools that that was not effective and that you could very easily get a girl pregnant. But there was also some sort of understanding in our community, I guess, and in our group of friends—not our group of friends, but in our high school circuit, really—that if the girl were to get pregnant, she would almost 100 percent get an abortion. So I guess you could say that for the guys, we weren't really worried about it. I'm sure the girls were, but like . . . It was kind of a douchebag mentality when I think back on it, but at the same time, we were in high school and pretty immature.

Although Spencer didn't dodge responsibility for his norm violation, he excused himself as having been "in high school and pretty immature." This justification is available to him now that he's older and has some distance from the situation.

HIDING NORM VIOLATIONS: "SAY ONE THING AND DO ANOTHER"

Although many teenagers who have sex during high school justify their behavior as being "normal" among peers, they all have to deal with adults in their social contexts who do not consider teen sex acceptable. Because many of these adults (such as parents, teachers, and school administrators) have considerable power over them, young people are motivated to make it seem like they're conforming to the adults' norms. So almost all of them strategize to make it appear to adults that they're not having sex. With a more public behavior, such as reckless driving or dropping out of school, falsely portraying conformity would be less of an option. But with sexual behavior, if you avoid visible pregnancy and convince your sex partner(s) to stay quiet, you can keep your norm violation secret.

Henry talked about how widespread this strategy was in his "it's wrong" community:

> A lot of people would have sex in high school, and a lot of people would say one thing and do another. They'd say how it's a bad thing and that their religion is against it, but at the same time they'd be out sleeping with their partner or random people sometimes, in different cases. And people would be saying one thing, and saying they couldn't engage in a relationship like that, but at the same time they'd be doing it. So it was sort of odd.
>
> *So would you say—well, let me just ask, was there sort of an underlying belief [among peers] that everyone is doing it?*
>
> Yeah. That was how it was acceptable for people to have sex, and when they got pregnant it became unacceptable. And now this result is there. It either has to be dealt with by having a baby or by having an abortion, and most people didn't want to address [that]. . . .
>
> *Do you think teenagers' behavior was affected by what kids in school thought about teenage parenthood, or the community thought about teenage parenthood?*
>
> Like I said, people really said one thing and did another. It was more an issue of people finding out about it and people talking about it, rather than people actually doing it. A lot of it was, if you don't hear it then you don't see it, and it's fine. However, when people find out about it, this girl is labeled as a slut. People start to talk about it and it really changes from their own actions to what others do. If it is them, it is acceptable. But if it is others, it is not.

Henry said many teens were vocal about having internalized the community's religious norm against premarital sex while getting away with having sex. But when teens—especially girls—got pregnant or when people found out they were sexually active, "it became unacceptable." When teens publicly violate an anti-sex norm, adults, teens, and institutions are compelled to stop participating in a conspiracy of silence and sanction their behavior.

Like many other interviewees, Noelle emphasized that parents were the main targets of many teenagers' attempts to cover up their behavior. She said that in her "it's wrong" community, "definitely a lot of parents were left in the dark." But she underscored parents' active role in allowing teens to hide their sexual activity: "It wasn't a subject that came up a lot. . . . It was just kind of one of those things where you just didn't really talk about it. I think that a lot of parents knew what was going on, but they didn't want to directly know about it." Teens would go to great lengths to have sex without parents or other adults finding out. Instead of going to their parents, they would acquire contraception secretly through a free clinic or from a friend. Others, like Nadia in a hybrid community, went through parents to secure contraception without acknowledging their own sexual activity: "When I wanted to get on birth control or something, I told my parents it wasn't for that reason, for sex. It was just to get more regular on my period or whatever. And it wasn't really something that I would directly talk to my parents about." If teens got pregnant, many would abort without telling their parents. Sadly, some tried to induce secret miscarriages in dangerous ways. Julie said her pregnant friend in an "it's wrong, but" community "threw herself down the stairs" and binge drank to the point of blacking out until she eventually did miscarry.

Covering up nonconforming behavior: "keep that behind closed doors"

Interviewees told us about four common strategies teenagers use so they can have sex while appearing to conform to adults' norms: engaging in heterosexual activity other than penile–vaginal intercourse, reserving sex for committed romantic relationships, using contraception carefully, and avoiding public talk about their sexual behavior.

As other researchers have found, when teens perceive there to be strong negative consequences to sex, some choose "technical virginity"—avoiding penile–vaginal intercourse but having oral or anal sex.[31] Technical virginity is a concern because although they rule out pregnancy, oral and anal sex still put teens at risk for STIs. Like many of her friends in their "be careful" community, Makayla remained a technical virgin by having oral sex with her boyfriend. She also talked about others:

> *Were a lot of people having sex?*
> Um, yeah, I think so. Maybe not intercourse, but maybe just oral sex.
> *So oral sex?*
> Yes.
> *And anal sex was. . .?*
> Nah, I didn't hear about it.
> *But oral sex you think was more common?*
> Oh, yeah. Definitely.
> *Do you kind of feel that your friends didn't consider oral sex to be sex?*
> Yeah, I would say that.
> *So intercourse was sex, and . . .?*

Yeah, exactly.
So you could have oral sex and still be a virgin, type of thing.
Yeah, exactly.

Technical virginity through anal sex was rarely discussed in the interviews, but Veronica talked about girls in her "it's wrong" community whose "families were really religious, and they really tried to be technically virgins, so they would have anal sex." Veronica didn't know if they used protection.

Teens who had penile–vaginal intercourse often engaged in the strategy of having sex in the context of a committed relationship. I was surprised to see how little emotional attachment most interviewees described when talking about their high school relationships retrospectively—especially when compared to the strong attachments (whether current or past) the teen mothers and fathers said they had in their high school relationships.[32] As strategic behavior, having sex within a committed relationship achieves several goals simultaneously. In many communities, sex in a relationship is a much less serious norm violation than casual sex.[33] Because the relationship is publicly known, it ensures that a teen's partner is also motivated to keep the sexual behavior private: If one partner is condemned for having sex or getting pregnant, the other will be condemned as well. For this reason, male partners were often seen as interested in supporting the girl through any negative consequences of sex. Lilly implied that she and her friends in an "it could be you" community strategically waited to have sex with their boyfriends until they felt the boys could be trusted. She went on:

> In the [academically high-achieving] program, the girls expected that if something bad happens to them in that area [pregnancy], the guy would take care of it . . . I'd think he'd support me in whatever decision *I* make.
>   *Yeah, and do you think that's because you feel like you waited until you were in a relationship instead of more casual sex?*
>   Yeah, definitely.

This relationship strategy doesn't work as well for girls if there is a strong double standard for sexual behavior that excuses boys from serious sanctions, like some interviewees said their social contexts had. Charles talked about how the stakes of being known as sexually active were higher for girls in his "it's wrong" community:

> "Oh, keep that [teen sex] behind closed doors," you know? Only in certain contexts, and it needs to be something you share with somebody special. It's

also kind of viewed as dirty. . . . Nobody [among his peers] expects a girl to be a virgin. Nobody that I knew in high school. But if you did have sex and it was known, you were seen through a different lens, you know? It wasn't always negative, but most of the time it was.

Besides illustrating a gendered double standard, his account also articulates a norm that sex with "somebody special" is more acceptable than sex outside a relationship and another norm that sex should be kept secret, "behind closed doors."

A strategy that two thirds of sexually active interviewees engaged in is using contraception very consistently. Other than becoming the target of gossip or being caught in the act of having sex by a parent or other adult, getting pregnant is the most common way a teen's secret sexual activity becomes known. This strategy is easier in many of the less religious "it could be you" and "be careful" communities, which teach about contraception in sex education and sometimes make it widely available to teens. In Dylan's "it's wrong" community, when teens had received abstinence-only education they often "didn't know how to use it [contraception] the first time," but they eventually learned.[34] Research has found that teenagers aren't less careful about using contraception than young adults,[35] and many interviewees exercised extreme caution, using multiple contraceptive methods.[36] Like many others, Spencer said lots of teens in his "be careful" community used multiple methods, such as birth control pills with condoms, or birth control pills with withdrawal.[37] In an "it could be you" community, Lillian had sex once during high school. She said, "We used contraceptives, and afterwards, because I was so worried about it, I went and got Plan B at [a reproductive health clinic]." These multiple methods of contraception should be quite effective at preventing pregnancy, thus helping cover up teens' norm violations.[38]

Finally, many teens work hard to avoid becoming targets of public talk about their behavior. Perhaps surprisingly, teens are often motivated to curtail gossip about their behavior even in social contexts where teen sex is a "normal" behavior and is only weakly discouraged. As Helena, from a "be careful" community with pervasive casual sex, said, "I think because it was such a small school, they just didn't want to talk about it [sex] all with people, as things go around really quickly. So, yeah, they would just keep their mouths shut about everything." In other words, even if it's okay for peers to know you're having sex, "things go around really quickly" if teens start talking, so adults can find out and sanction you. The safest strategy is not to tell anyone. Alternatively, a teen might tell his secret to reliable close friends, as Dylan experienced in an "it's wrong" community: "People only talk about that stuff with their best friend, people who you really trusted not to tell." Close friends often collude in keeping each other's sexual behaviors quiet. Interviewees also identify reserving sex for a committed relationship as a strategy for minimizing negative talk. Through some combination of these four strategies, then, most teens work hard to keep their sexual behaviors private in an attempt to avoid negative sanctions from their parents, peers, school, and community.

Collaborating to cover up nonconforming behavior: "Her friends helped her out"

As people who participate in labor unions and social protests know, one way for less powerful people to gain power is by banding together to work toward a common goal.[39] This strategy is trickier when the goal is sexual behavior, which most people engage in with only one partner at a time, but teens do often collaborate to create opportunities for sexual behavior, as well as opportunities to keep their sexual behavior private and portray themselves as conforming to adults' norms.

It's important to understand *why* teenagers are often willing to go to the trouble of helping each other have sex while avoiding negative sanctions for their behavior. Interviewees talked about one important reason: that the stigma of non-normative sexual behavior (such as sex or pregnancy) isn't isolated to the offending teen, but instead "courtesy stigma" spreads to her close friends. Helena said that teens in her "be careful" community who knew a friend was pregnant were aware that the stigma of not being "responsible enough" would spread to them: "And so I think it was just like, 'I don't want to be identified with you, because, you know, you're clearly not responsible enough, so I don't want to be seen as your friend.'" Similarly, Rochelle made it clear that the stigma of teen pregnancy in her school extended to the friends of pregnant girls, who threw the mothers-to-be "parties in the hallways with balloons" (in Rochelle's hybrid community, the friends were allegedly not violating their own ethnic group's norms by doing this, but they were violating the dominant ethnic group's norms).

If friends' reputations rely on each other's outward conformity to adults' norms against sex and pregnancy, then they're motivated to help each other. Two important and very common ways of helping close friends are to engage in a "conspiracy of silence" to avoid finding out about friends' sexual behavior, and to actively curtail the spreading of gossip in the peer group or wider community. Dylan's comments illustrate these strategies in his "it's wrong" community:

Well, the group of friends would know [something about their friends' sexual activity], but most of us, I think, if you were close enough to the person, were pretty good about respecting their privacy. So we wouldn't ask too many questions, and we wouldn't spread stuff. So in the case of that girl [a pregnant girl who was keeping her pregnancy secret], when people were like, "Oh, where is she?" We'd say, "Oh, I don't know, maybe she's sick or has a health issue." It's what she asked us to say.

Besides managing public talk about teens' sexual activity and pregnancy, in many cases friends facilitate each other's sexual activity and contraception. In his "it's wrong" community, Finn told of friends helping each other find safe, attractive places to have sex away from the eyes of their parents or other adults: "There were a lot of situations [with male friends] where I remember it was like, 'You two should have sex.' You know, 'We're going to put you in a situation where you can have sex.'"[40] Friends also help each other obtain contraception (both condoms and birth control pills) or Plan B medication, or get a secret abortion if they end up pregnant. For example, Alexis talked about what happened when her older sister started having sex in a "be careful" community:

When Liz [her sister] became sexually active and stuff with Scott, then when she had to go get birth control pills and buy condoms and stuff on her own because she was 17 and didn't want to go to our parents, obviously—because who wants to go talk to their parents about, "yeah, I'm having sex?" So her friends helped her out with that, and they knew that you could get free birth control at [name of clinic], and how to go about getting all of that.

Alexis was then able to use information gathered from her sister's experiences to inform her own sexual health.

Sometimes teens are forced to go to friends for resources they need, even when the risk of disclosure is high. Parker's friend in an "it's wrong" community is an example:

And my sister, one of our mutual friends, she's in my sister's grade two years younger than me, she also had an abortion in high school from her high school boyfriend of like three years.

They never told their parents?

No. She had to go to one of my sister's friends for the money—still never paid her back.

When teens have their own resources like money and information, they can choose a safer strategy and not tell anyone, like another of Parker's friends did: "One of my best friends, she ended up having an abortion without telling any of us. She told us months later that she had one." For many teens, close friends are trusted collaborators who can help them manage their sexual behavior safely and privately while "flying under the radar" of their parents' and communities' sexual norms. But telling anyone about sexual activity—even a close friend—entails risks.[41] Dylan talked about how in his highly religious community, many teens saw even friends' knowledge of their behavior as a threat to public conformity: "Even if you had a girlfriend and you were having sex, even within the guys, it wasn't talked about. And I know we joked about it with a friend—she was a girl—and she got so pissed off at us just hinting at her and her boyfriend having sex. So it's definitely something that was probably not talked about, even with your close friends, I would say." Given the social exclusion peers in many communities use to sanction girls known to be sexually active, it takes a lot of trust to tell a friend you've violated a sex norm. Lucy's newly pregnant cousin experienced what happens if you misplace that trust, when a friend told "the whole school" about the cousin's secret abortion and she faced widespread interpersonal sanctions. So even though friends can be a source of support for having sex while portraying conformity, this support is full of risk because it increases the chances of a norm violation becoming public. Even when collaborating, teens are clearly constrained by their lack of resources and dependence on adults.

MANAGING PUBLIC NORM VIOLATIONS: "DAMAGE CONTROL"

Although teenagers strategize to appear as if they're conforming to sexuality norms, if they are actually violating those norms, people may find out. If that happens, a teen's only option is "damage control"—working to minimize negative sanctions. Scholars of deviance and social control have a long tradition of studying people's attempts to avoid sanctions by justifying or "neutralizing" their deviant behavior.[42] These justifications are sometimes different from the ones discussed above because the person has been caught violating a norm, so isn't simply justifying the behavior to herself or to an interviewer. Several of the justifications college student and teen parent interviewees used when they were caught violating sexuality norms are similar to those people have used in explaining other kinds of behavior, such as theft.

Teenagers use three main strategies to try to minimize negative sanctions for their behavior: calling the behavior a "mistake" and thus demonstrating that they have internalized the norm they violated, explaining that they shouldn't be sanctioned because they are "better" than people who violate the norms, or rejecting the idea that their norm violation is a problem. The success of these strategies depends a lot on the social position of the teen who tries to use them. Socially privileged teens have more success avoiding sanctions for missteps than do marginalized teens, such as minorities or those with low SES.[43] I draw both on the college student interviews and on the interviews with teen mothers and fathers—who have all publicly violated multiple sexuality norms—to talk about how these strategies are used and how they're received by others.[44]

First, teens who violate norms can try to sidestep violations by calling their behavior a "mistake" that is not in character with their own typical behavior or their internalized norms.[45] The last section showed that a lot of teens who used contraception inconsistently but suffered no negative consequences (like a pregnancy or STI) used this kind of strategy to justify their behavior to interviewers. It's less convincing the more serious or repetitive the mistake is perceived to be. But many teen parents used the language of mistakes in interviews. Teen mother Crystal told us that unprotected sex between her and her partner "just kind of happened on accident one or two times, and I never got pregnant, so we were just like, 'I guess not.'" If Crystal had received sex education reporting the actual (quite low) odds of getting pregnant from any single unprotected sex act, she might well have reached a different conclusion and continued using contraception. Instead, she and her boyfriend stopped using contraception because they thought she was infertile. She emphasized that "we weren't trying" to have a baby; "It just happened." Fabian had an even stronger "mistake" justification for how he became a teen father: "We were using protection, and the condom had broke. . . . We were using protection, and it snapped, and one thing led to the next, and she ended up being pregnant."

But teen parents who talk about accidents and mistakes still face substantial sanctions from the people around them. Even if they accept that the pregnancy was accidental, many people still believe that negative sanctions are appropriate because of the severity of the "mistake." Lilly said with "conservative people" in her "it could be you" community, "there would be an encouragement not to keep the baby. 'We don't want this on our name. This is really embarrassing to have our daughter make such a mistake.'" Lilly thinks family members would have accepted that the pregnancy was a "mistake," but that wouldn't have stopped their negative sanctions. To avoid violating metanorms that expect family members to sanction pregnant daughters, Lilly believes parents would have demanded a secret abortion.

Especially with less severe norm violations than teen parenthood, the strategy of calling behavior a mistake can sometimes be effective because it implies that the teen agrees with the rationale underlying the norm and is willing to comply in the future. Carter had a negative opinion of teen parenthood in his "be careful" community, calling it "unfortunate." But when asked if there were any special issues or exceptions to consider, he replied, "Yeah, when there was an obvious step taken, but just a mistake was made. And I don't think that makes a person a bad person." I interpret his condition of "an obvious step taken" to mean that the teen tried to use contraception. Carter thinks in this special case of a "mistake" being made, a teen parent isn't "a bad person" like he implicitly considers other teen parents to be.

By taking the right steps to redeem themselves after making a mistake, teen parents in Annika's "it's wrong, but" community could even experience some positive sanctions:

> *So do you think on some level there were people who were proud when somebody was pregnant and it was clear that they decided not to abort?*
>
> Oh, yeah, it was moral. You know, kind of the sentiment that, "I made a mistake, but now I'm going to stand up and be a, you know, take responsibility and take care of it." And so it was kind of like, "Oh, good for you, you're growing up," kind of thing.

"Growing up" in Annika's community, unlike many others, entails "standing up" for your mistake by "taking responsibility"—not having an abortion.

But the redemption that can come from calling one's behavior a mistake and taking responsibility for it is not available to everyone. Logan's peer group in an "it's wrong" community took for granted that teen sex and pregnancy are mistakes, but that didn't excuse anyone. He said that premarital sex "was always kind of held in derision in our group . . . Not that you were a lesser person for doing it, but it was kind of a stupid mistake to make." The interviewer asked, "And so when people talked about it, they just talked about it as a mistake?" Logan replied, "Yeah. Especially the pregnancy part." Like others, Patton explicitly ruled out the likelihood of an "innocent" mistake when talking about the kinds of girls who got pregnant in his "be careful" community: "That was looked on to be the girls that would sleep around. I mean, you didn't usually hear about girls that had sex one time and accidentally got pregnant. I think the viewpoint of a lot of people was if they got pregnant, they were probably sleeping around a lot, and this wasn't their first time, and it was bound to happen because they were the ones that were sleeping around a lot." As Abby said earlier, teens don't often inquire about the facts—rather, rumors about the promiscuity of pregnant girls are accepted as truth.[46]

Although many interviewees unquestioningly accepted the rumors that prevented pregnant girls from claiming a valid "mistake," they would often excuse their own friends in similar situations. Bethany disapproved of teen parents in her "it's wrong" community and laughed about the "skank-like behavior" that people implied a pregnant teen in her school exhibited. But she had a different story to tell about her own friend's pregnancy scare: "I remember that I went to buy a pregnancy test with one of my friends, and that still happens to this day. I think people try to be responsible, but now and in high school, maybe for different reasons, people would make mistakes and scares would happen. In high school, maybe just because they don't really know what they are doing." In contrast to teen parents whom she thinks should be judged and laughed at, Bethany's friends are "trying to be responsible," but they can be excused because they "make mistakes." The mistake justification is thus a flexible narrative that teens can try to claim, but the success of that claim for reducing negative sanctions is conditional on who you are and what evidence there is of what you did.

A second strategy young people who violate sexuality norms sometimes use in trying to minimize negative sanctions is to disassociate themselves from other norm violators by explaining why they are better.[47] The justification of making a mistake is part of this distancing—if you didn't violate a norm on purpose, then you're better than other people who did. But there are other ways teens can try to demonstrate that the perceived negative consequences of norm violation don't apply to them. Teen father Fabian—who earlier used a particularly convincing version of the "mistake" justification—also used the distancing justification in his interview by disassociating himself from the "problem teens" associated with young parenthood:

> Every person that I know growing up, minus probably about three people, myself being one of those three, all of my friends—either they fell off into gangs and ended up being deceased, or they fell off into drug sales and then drug use, and they became squatters or whatever, you know, homeless people and things of that nature. And so I think to a great extent, my children saved me. I could have possibly—you know, there's always the possibility there that I could have been involved in some of those same things that was there, you know, because when you see these guys over here making $100,000, they got these big, brand-new cars with the gold rims and everything that's alluring to the eye, it's easy to fall into that. "Hey, I'm willing to take a little risk, I'm not doing anything wrong."

Fabian is sympathetic about the young men all around him who end up "falling into" major problems, but he says that "my children saved me." This strategy distances him from the negative stereotype of the kind of guy who becomes a teen dad, and it also rejects the idea that teen parenthood is such a bad thing.

Besides abstaining from criminal behavior, being mature and succeeding in school are two other common ways teen parents distance themselves from negative stereotypes. Layla told us in retrospect that becoming a mother "really matured me a lot. It made me think about what I need to do in changing my life, so I can give them [her children] a better life.... I don't feel like it ruined my life. I feel like it pushed me to do more in my life." Like Fabian, Layla combines an argument that her maturity has helped her build a good life with a rejection of the idea that teen parenthood is negative. Education is another important tool some teen parents use to talk about why they are better than a stereotypical teen mom or dad. Adriana talked about how she responds to the many people who sanction her throughout her everyday life: "I'm like, 'I still go to school.' I can throw that in their face, because I still do what a lot of girls who don't have babies do. And I have a baby, and that makes me stronger than they are, because I have something that would possibly hold me back, and I still do it." Adriana not only distances herself from negative stereotypes of teen mothers, but she compares herself favorably to girls who don't have children. Flaunting their actual or aspirational success in education, work, or parenting "in the face" of people who have negatively sanctioned them is a common theme in the interviews with teen parents.

But like the mistake justification, the distancing justification only succeeds at reducing negative sanctions if the people around a teen *accept its validity*. This does not seem to be the case for many teen parents. Young mothers who engage in typical "good" parenting activities like taking their children for a stroller ride, to the park, or to the doctor face a multitude of negative sanctions for those behaviors from the strangers they encounter. Rochelle's, Bryce's, and other interviewees' negative reactions to the mere presence of teen mothers in public do not suggest any acceptance of the idea that they might be good parents for bringing their children to parks, social events, or doctors' offices. And the justification that succeeding in school makes a teen parent less worthy of negative sanctions also seems to backfire in my interviewees' reactions. For example, the award given to a teen mother at Bethany's high school graduation aroused anger in the other students. Bethany said, "I remember we thought that it was stupid, because why did she get an award above everyone else for making what we considered a mistake? . . . None of us got awards for *not* getting pregnant and finishing high school." Adriana thinks succeeding in school as a teen mom makes her more deserving of praise than girls who did not have a baby, while Bethany and her friends think the opposite. It's clear from Adriana's account that her distancing justification hasn't gotten her very far in avoiding negative interpersonal sanctions, so Bethany's view may be more widespread.

Finally, and often in combination with other justifications as was shown above, teens who violate sexuality norms can refuse to internalize the norm and work to distance themselves from reference groups that hold the norm. In its strongest form, this means being proud of your norm violation. Nicole uses this strategy:

> Just of course walking down the street, people would look at you. I think maybe because I'm really short, people think I'm, like, twelve, and they're like, "Oh, my God!" I used to always—my mom would always point it out to me

that I always walked with my head down. She was like, "Put your head up. It's okay." And sometimes I still kind of do that, put my head down. But a lot of times it's like, "I'm proud to be a mom. That's what I am, and I'm going to be proud of it."

For Nicole, this process strengthens her identity as not deserving of sanctions, yet people still sanction her. This internal process can still be powerful and can also spur changes in teen parents' relationships with other people. Christian said that during his girlfriend's pregnancy, her family members "were treating me pretty bad, like, what am I gonna do? I didn't have a job at the time. But I ended up getting a job and everything was better. I was misjudged by a lot of people. . . . It felt good to put some salt in their wounds. . . . Everybody I know knows that I'm a good father, as well as I know that I'm a good father."

Adriana, whose negative experiences with strangers and whose attempts to distance herself from negative stereotypes of teen mothers were described earlier, also refuses to internalize the norm sanctioning her behavior. But she has gone farther by working actively to surround herself with people who do not think she is deserving of negative sanctions. One such reference group is her family—even though some family members reacted badly at first, with the exception of one person who cut off ties, they now support her. Adriana said, "I'm always with my family. I'm a family person." The other supportive reference group is the adults and teens in her school for young mothers: "The main reason that I've stuck here [stayed in this school] is because, when I was pregnant, they really treated me like I was normal. [laughs] Not like, 'Oh, she's pregnant.' They understood me." Many other teen mothers talked about the supportive normative climate at the school as a major positive influence in their lives. Yet especially if like Adriana they don't have access to a car, students must face regular humiliation on public buses to and from school and are thus unable to isolate themselves from negative sanctions.

CONCLUSION

With little unmonitored time and a lot of parental interest in their activities, many college student interviewees felt that as teens there was considerable adult control over their lives.[48] Teen sexuality is a particularly strong focus of this control, even though the particular norms being enforced vary from one place to the next. Yet by the end of high school, most teens have had sex despite attempts at social and physical control. To accomplish this while holding onto their "sexual respectability,"[49] teens need to overcome difficult practical barriers, internally reconcile their violation of adults' norms, and conceal their behavior from the people who would sanction them. They do some of this work themselves, but many enlist the help of friends. Peers are complicated because they can either reinforce adults' attempts at controlling teens' behaviors or help teens avoid adult control. But overcoming all these obstacles can be challenging to accomplish without support.

In all the ways teens negotiate their normative climates, they strategize to behave the way they want while avoiding negative sanctions from people around them. But these efforts are constrained by the power adults, peers, and institutions hold over them. On one hand, teens hold a lot of power by making the ultimate decisions over their sexual behaviors. On the other hand, sexual behaviors come with a risk of negative sanctions, and those sanctions can often be severe. Teens can try to justify their norm violations to themselves and others as not being problematic, but if the people around them don't accept their arguments, they will face negative sanctions anyway. Those negative sanctions are often more harmful than the sexual behaviors themselves, a fact that in many ways gives adults and institutions the upper hand in the struggle over teenagers' sexuality.

But at the same time, most teens have sex before finishing high school. So do they have the upper hand in this struggle after all? From the stories the interviewees told, it seems like many teens do successfully navigate these hurdles and have sex without experiencing severe negative consequences. But others run into trouble—and who ends up in which situation isn't randomly determined. Teens from higher-status social categories can get away with "mistakes" in which they violate norms but face fewer sanctions for it, especially because so many of them are encouraged to quietly abort any accidental pregnancies. Less advantaged teens are more likely to carry a pregnancy to term, but they can sometimes even have their reputations tarnished without any factual basis.

Beyond reputational concerns, the current normative situation entails other problems for teens. Compared to other countries with similar rates of teen sex, U.S. teenagers use contraception less often, use less effective methods, and have much higher rates of pregnancy and STIs. They're also less likely to report satisfaction with their sexual experiences, and rates of intimate partner violence and forced sex are high. It certainly seems that teens aren't paranoid for being afraid of the social and practical consequences of their sexual behaviors. This stalemate between concerned adults and scared teens is a focus of the next chapter.

8

CONCLUSION

TEENS IN THE United States hear mixed messages about sexuality from the people and institutions around them. These norms focus on different sexual behaviors, like sex, contraception, abortion, or pregnancy. But sexuality norms coming from the same people are often internally conflicting, too. People communicating a practical rationale may say, "Don't have sex, but use contraception." The moral rationale is equally contradictory, saying, "Don't have an abortion, but don't become a teen parent." Metanorms about how to treat teen parents are also inconsistent, often encouraging teens both to shun and to support them.

Even though sexuality norm sets are internally contradictory, they are still social norms, which means that people who violate them experience social sanctions. It's clear from interviewees that families, peers, schools, and communities all strategize to control teens' behaviors and bring them in line with their particular norm sets. Their norm enforcer strategies are different depending on the power they have over teens, but young people feel this control keenly and work to achieve their own goals while avoiding sanctions.

Who is winning this struggle between teens and the people who want to control their behavior? I argue that nobody is. Most teens are waiting throughout much of high school before they have sex, thus conforming to community norms. But most of them do end up having sex before finishing high school, many don't use contraception consistently, and many end up inadvertently pregnant. The norm enforcers around them aren't achieving their goals. This social control does have lots of unintended consequences, though, many of them negative. Teens don't communicate much about sex with their parents—and often not even with their peers—so they miss concrete information that could be crucial for them to avoid health risks. They hide their sexual activity from their parents, which means that it's hard to use long-acting contraception and that sex is often happening in situations that can be unsafe and conducive to sexual violence. People and institutions around teens are often preoccupied with sanctioning them if they get into sexual trouble, which conflicts with the goal of supporting them and ensuring a bright future.

Nobody is winning. But what can we do about this state of affairs? This chapter concludes the book by addressing norms and social control around teen sexuality, the changing context of teen sexuality, and some potential ways forward in the future.

THE IMPLICATIONS OF NORMS AND SOCIAL CONTROL

Analyzing teen sexuality in the United States today yields a complicated picture of norms and social control with many new ideas. Rather than identifying a single norm controlling a single behavior, I have shown that teen sexuality norms come in sets that regulate a variety of related behaviors, portrayals of behaviors, emotions, and sanctions against norm violators. The normative prescriptions in the set seem internally contradictory until their underlying rationale for *why* they are appropriate is taken into account. Two rationales, the moral and the practical, dominate U.S. society, provide consistent logics undergirding sets of norms in different communities, and lead to divergent normative prescriptions for regulating teen sexuality.

Many different norm enforcers strategize to bring teens' sexuality (their behaviors, emotions, portrayals, and sanctions) in line with the norms they espouse. Teens, in turn, have their own strategies—which are often shaped by norms they have internalized from the people around them—and may comply with or resist this social control. Well-known processes of conformity, norm violation, and sanctioning are part of these strategies. But in articulating norm enforcers' and norm targets' strategies, I also introduce new ideas about how norms and metanorms are communicated and how enforcers and targets maneuver teens' social relationships and resource dependencies to control normative processes. Learning about a teenager's available reference groups, his level of surveillance by different norm enforcers, his opportunities for norm violation, and his resource dependence on norm enforcers provides a sense of what the teen's norm outcomes may look like in a specific social setting. This helps us understand how most teenagers go from not having heterosexual intercourse early in high school to having sex but not portraying that activity publicly by the end of high school, despite their normative climates remaining similar.

My perspective on the struggle between adults' and peers' social control and teens' negotiation strategies is inherently conflict-focused, bringing with it new ideas about social norms that are less static. This conflict is not just intragroup among the people surrounding a teen. It is also intergroup, between those who espouse a practical rationale for regulating teen sexuality and those who champion a moral rationale. Political conflicts and those within and between religious and nonreligious organizations reflect this struggle for power over norm communication and social control at the state and societal level. The outcomes of those conflicts can lead to change in norms, as some messages to teens are strengthened and others silenced. But the rationales underlying norm sets can themselves change in response to shifts in material circumstances, such as an economic recession; legal circumstances, such as the legalization of abortion; or cultural circumstances, such as a strengthening anti-abortion movement. All of this means that norms and social control can both reflect and reinforce social inequalities. As tools of power, normative messages and social control tend to be wielded by the powerful and give less voice to others. A teen's place in a social hierarchy shapes how she behaves and portrays her behavior publicly, what norms are communicated to her, and how people interpret and sanction her behavior.

This book can help us understand the circumstances under which norms are likely to be effective versus ineffective. Sometimes teenagers comply to sexuality norms, and sometimes they violate them. But the book also complicates what the effectiveness of a norm means. Teens who have heterogeneous social contexts can choose which reference group's norm to comply to, or because norm sets are internally inconsistent they can decide which norm in the set to follow. Young people may comply to norms in their public portrayals of behavior and their sanctioning of norm violators, but not in the private behavior itself. Norms may also be effective if they serve the purposes of powerful people and institutions by keeping teens silent about their private behaviors and making norm violations less visible.

The approach outlined in this book contributes to the life course perspective.[1] This multidisciplinary theoretical framework conceptualizes human lives as a series of life phases and transitions, with institutions, other people, and age norms shaping people's lives across time and space. The life course perspective is important for understanding teen sexual behaviors, many of which are accepted or even welcomed when a person is older but stigmatized in adolescence.[2] Situating individual biographies in their historical and cultural context, as I do here, is a key principle of the life course perspective. I argue that age norms against teen sexuality are encoded in formal institutions such as schools, religious organizations, and healthcare providers, and they also permeate informal institutions like families and communities. All of these norm enforcers exert social control over teens in an attempt to regulate their behaviors and portrayals. But as the life course perspective's focus on agency might suggest, teens agentically use alternative ideas about what's "normal" at a given age to push back against that control and create a space for their own sexuality. As the life course perspective would expect, these processes are dynamic, changing over time and varying in different places. This book's findings address critiques of age norms in the life course perspective that were made in the 1980s, updating ideas about age norms to strengthen them as a theoretical tool for understanding human lives.[3]

What is likely to happen to norms and social control around U.S. teen sexuality in the future? Our country is in a time of rising socioeconomic inequalities and social segregation based on SES. At the same time, religious, racial, and political divides are increasingly separating our social interactions and the normative messages we hear. I argue this is likely to lead to increased segregation among the four community types described in this book. Community-level SES and religious influence shape communities' norm sets, and these two characteristics are separating communities from one another more than ever. With the increasing consensus around norm sets that these changes may create within communities, teens may end up conforming to their particular community's norm set more and more. This could lead to a strengthening of the divergent patterns of sexual behaviors along geographic lines that journalist Margaret Talbot calls "red sex" and "blue sex."[4] Diverging legal contexts around reproductive health, which are largely following political lines, may strengthen this dynamic. All of this suggests that differences in U.S. teenagers' sexual behaviors may grow. As norm sets in communities become less contested and strengthen, sanctions against the many teens who violate those norms may increasingly disrupt their futures. And because sanctions are more likely when teens are more disadvantaged, sanctioning based on teen sexuality may continue to play a key role in the intergenerational transmission of social advantage and disadvantage in the United States.

THE CHANGING CONTEXT OF TEEN SEXUALITY

To better understand our normative future and how we might change it, it is first important to consider recent trends. The United States is a unique place in terms of teen sexual behavior, and it has undergone a lot of change in recent decades. U.S. teenagers tend to have sex at similar ages as their peers in other developed countries, but they are much less likely to use contraception, especially more effective long-acting methods. Only a quarter of sexually active teens used the more effective hormonal/long-acting pregnancy-prevention methods like birth control pills and intrauterine devices when they last had sex, and 40 percent of sexually active high school students didn't use a condom—the only commonly used contraceptive that offers protection from STIs—the last time they had sex.[5] Largely because of these differences in contraceptive use, the United States has much higher rates of teen pregnancy and childbirth than other developed nations. The teen abortion rate is also high compared to other countries.[6]

Although these patterns persist, since my interviews were conducted, there have been some changes in U.S. teens' sexual behaviors. The percentage of high schoolers who have ever had sex has held steady,[7] but the teen birth rate has fallen by more than a third since 2009.[8] The decrease in the teen birth rate over the early 2000s has been attributed primarily to improvements in teens' longer-acting contraceptive use.[9] What has changed in the past several years that might have spurred this new trend? The first major change is the severe recession starting in 2008 that disproportionately affected younger, less educated Americans.[10] Women of all ages, and not just teenagers, reduced their childbearing sharply during this time.[11] Researchers know that people often respond to economic hardship by postponing their fertility,[12] and teenagers seem to be no exception.

The second major change during the past few years is national sex education policy. The George W. Bush administration of 2001–2009 funded "abstinence-only" sex education programs that did not include concrete information about contraceptive use. In contrast, the Obama administration has funded more "abstinence-plus" or comprehensive sex education programs that teach teenagers about contraceptive use, while continuing to fund some abstinence-only programs.[13] My interviews with young people who were high school students during the Bush administration found that their sex education curricula were split between the two types and generally reflected community norms. Policy changes toward more comprehensive sex education programs may be partly responsible for the changes in teens' sexual behaviors since then, and these changes may also have led to a decoupling of school-based sex education curricula from communities' norm sets.[14] The decrease in the teen birth rate seems to be due in part to improvements in U.S. teens' contraceptive use.[15]

Some policies to make effective contraception more available and affordable have shown success. Colorado implemented a widespread experimental program to supply free long-acting contraceptives to teenagers, and it has experienced among the largest drops in the teen birth rate of any state.[16] The teen abortion rate also fell sharply in Colorado, while teens were no more likely to start having sex than they had been before the program. During the past few years when the Colorado program was so successful, teens may have been more motivated to avoid pregnancy because of the faltering economy at the same time that free and particularly effective contraception was made available to them—and this combination of factors may have contributed to the program's success.

There is strong evidence that teens' behaviors change in response to socioeconomic opportunities and contraceptive policies, but these factors are shaped by political context. The successful Colorado contraceptive program (which was privately funded) was severely threatened because of political battles around contraception. Although a bill to fund the program had bipartisan sponsorship in the state legislature, Republican opposition in committee prevented the bill from being brought to the floor in 2015, but in 2016 the program was funded with a lower budget.[17] The conflicting views of the program from politicians mirror normative divisions in U.S. society. In addressing teen sexual behavior, people with a moral rationale want to focus on premarital sex (and now also abortion) being morally wrong, so they aren't necessarily inclined to spend money on programs that reduce the negative consequences of morally wrong sex for teens.[18] In contrast, those with a practical rationale mostly want to reduce the negative consequences of risky sex, so they focus on contraceptive behaviors and tend to support programs that reduce teen pregnancy and abortion. The mixed societal message that results from these two perspectives—don't you dare have sex, but be really careful if you do—is confusing to teens and apparently somewhat ineffective at controlling their behaviors. And as was the case with the Colorado program for a while, it can lead to political deadlock. Like the sponsors of the Colorado contraceptive bill, the Obama administration has tried to bridge these two cultural perspectives by focusing on an apparent point of agreement: reducing teen pregnancies and abortions through proven policy interventions.[19] But programs that address these goals are still facing political opposition because of larger normative conflicts around teen sex and contraception.

National media attention to the Colorado contraceptive program and the political battles surrounding it has opened a larger, ongoing debate about policies that target teens' sexual behaviors.[20] But that debate may only be resolved after new policies are put in place—as we know from the implementation of equal opportunity laws and other policies, new norms often follow policy changes rather than causing them.[21] Changing normative messages may also be a way forward for influencing teens' behaviors. Recent research suggests that popular reality shows like *16 and Pregnant*, which highlight the struggles of young parents, played a part in the recent reductions in the teen birth rate.[22] These shows were associated with increases in Internet searches and tweets about contraception and abortion, suggesting that teens sought out information about avoiding pregnancy and parenthood after viewing the show. What's most interesting about this research is that the television show is communicating cultural messages that discourage teen pregnancy, but there are no sanctions attached to these messages. Simply changing the message, with no associated change in sanctions, may be enough to change teens' behaviors. It's unclear whether changes in *norms*, which have sanctions attached, would result in more change in teens' behaviors or would somehow backfire. Both because they affect teens' sexual behaviors and because they can change norms, I argue that solutions for improving teenagers' sexual health should focus on economic, educational, and policy factors as well as on norms.

Norm-focused solutions face considerable challenges. Among interviewees, teen sexuality norms and related sanctions don't seem to affect young people's actual sexual behaviors as much as they do their public portrayals of those behaviors. But norms do play an important role in understanding what happens to teens in terms of the stigma those who violate norms experience. This book's findings suggest that although social norms aren't particularly successful at regulating teens' sexual behaviors, they are often very effective at silencing teen sexuality and negatively sanctioning teens who violate the rules, thereby worsening their lives. Because these sanctions are applied unequally to teens from different demographic groups and because of their negative effects, I argue that it's worth rethinking whether our current normative contexts are taking the best approach. Strengthening norms against teen sexual behaviors may lead to little behavioral change but a lot of damaging sanctions against young people who violate them, which may be counterproductive as teen parents are already marginalized.

BARRIERS AND SOLUTIONS TO IMPROVING TEEN SEXUAL HEALTH

Although most Americans would agree that our teenagers' sexual behaviors are problematic, figuring out how to change them is challenging because we think they are problematic for different (moral versus practical) reasons. I have argued that strengthening norms against teen sexual behaviors isn't likely to solve the problem alone. Policies and socioeconomic improvements can be more effective, but normative conflicts often make it hard to implement change. Recognizing these difficulties, I suggest four strategies for improving U.S. teens' sexual health across cultural divides. Echoing the recent changes that have helped drive the rapidly falling teen birth rate, these strategies seek both to increase attractive alternatives that motivate teens to avoid pregnancy and to give teens practical tools to turn these motivations into reality.

First, we should implement policies that give all teens, and not just those from privileged families and communities, attractive life alternatives to early parenthood. Most young people from all walks of life do not want to become parents as teens, but research has shown that those who have attractive alternatives to parenthood are most able to translate that motivation into action and avoid pregnancy.[23] This is also true in my interviewees' communities—community socioeconomic opportunities, rather than norms, religion, or other factors, were associated with lower levels of teen parenthood in the community. Researchers recognize that some of the best programs for reducing teen pregnancy are broad-based educational initiatives that seek to reduce school dropout and improve educational opportunities for all teens.[24] Improving teens' involvement in school and motivation to get a good education leads to less risky sexual behavior.[25] Raising the quality of our schools, especially those in less privileged communities, has a wide range of benefits and should also reduce teen pregnancy. And improving educational access and affordability beyond high school, as some new governmental initiatives are seeking to do, may well reduce pregnancy among older teens who have finished high school.

Second, alongside efforts to improve teens' educational experiences and options, I suggest that we shift our policy focus away from teen pregnancy, abortion, and parenthood and toward teen sex and contraception. Although it may seem that different ideological viewpoints could agree on the importance of reducing teen pregnancy, abortion, and parenthood, examples like the Colorado contraceptive program suggest that it's not so easy. But as statistics from many other countries show, implementing effective policies around teen sex and contraception can result in there being little need to address these other issues. If rates of teen sex are low or rates of effective teen contraception are high, then pregnancy, abortion, and parenthood will be rare. In 2014, for example, just 6 per 1,000 teen girls in Sweden, 3 in Switzerland, and 10 in Canada had a baby, compared to 24 in the United States.[26] Contraception rates and use of more effective types of contraception are responsible for much of this difference, and higher education in places like Sweden is free and readily available. Focusing on the earlier links in the chain of teen sexual behaviors may be controversial, but judging from other countries' experiences, it can yield strong results.

Third, as part of the focus on sex and contraception, I suggest that policies focus on sex education and free access with the goal of getting sexually active teens consistently using a long-acting contraceptive plus a condom.[27] This policy goal is an amended version of the main focus of the practical rationale, which encourages consistent contraception but tends to treat different contraceptive methods as if they're equal. In fact, statistics collected based on typical use show large differences in the effectiveness of different methods for preventing pregnancy.[28] For example, with typical use 15 percent of women who use male condoms alone for contraception will have an unintended pregnancy within a year, compared to 8 percent for birth control pills and less than 1 percent for IUDs. In terms of pregnancy prevention, long-acting contraceptives are much more effective and less prone to user error, making them an attractive option for many teens. And condoms are the only common contraceptive method that helps stop the spread of STIs. STIs are a very widespread problem for today's teens, yet interviewees were not focused on STI risk.[29] Their two major concerns were the risk of pregnancy and the risk of their parents finding out that they were having sex. Educating teens about the importance of STI prevention and contraceptive effectiveness, while making effective contraceptive tools available, is an important goal for improving their sexual health.

To make sex as low risk as possible in terms of both pregnancy and STIs, the combination of a long-acting contraceptive (such as an IUD; birth control pills; or hormone injections, rings, implants, or patches) and condoms is the safest strategy. But especially for the most popular option of birth control pills, it isn't realistic for a girl to be using contraception without her parents finding out. A primary reason for this is cost, which is a major barrier because of the upfront expenses associated with many of these methods.[30] These difficulties are reflected in teenagers' actual contraceptive use. Just 5 percent of currently sexually active high school students in the United States use long-active methods (Depo-Provera, NuvaRing, Implanon, or an IUD), and another 18 percent use birth control pills. Even more problematically, less than 1 in 10 sexually active students uses one of these methods together with a condom (the best strategy for preventing both pregnancy and STIs).[31] The combination of long-acting contraceptives with condoms is also beneficial because in heterosexual relationships, it tends to put the responsibility for contraception on both girls (for the long-acting method) and boys (for condoms). When interviewees were asked how they preferred to have responsibility for contraception divided, most wanted it to be shared.

The final, perhaps most challenging policy strategy is to open up a national and community-level conversation about what norms we want to communicate to teens about sexuality, what sanctions are appropriate, and what effects we think those norms and sanctions will have. Evidence suggests that many parents are eager for guidance.[32] Although strengthening norms against teen sex, pregnancy, abortion, and parenthood is not likely to be particularly effective and exacerbates stigma and marginalization, other norm changes might be more productive. Although their perspectives on teen sexuality differ, U.S. parents and communities are working hard to communicate with teens and ensure the best futures for them. Making this communication more effective, in part through communicating norms that can help teens improve their sexual outcomes, is an important goal. Echoing normative changes that have happened in other countries over fairly short periods of time, I suggest that we communicate a message to teens that they should wait to have sex until they personally feel completely ready.[33] This normative focus reinforces the ways many teens already think about their sexual decision making,[34] and it bridges the moral and practical rationales. Being ready for sex is something that depends on teens' personal values about when they believe a person is ready to be sexually active. If teens believe that shouldn't happen until marriage, as the moral rationale teaches, then they won't feel ready until marriage. If they instead believe that being ready means being able to avoid risky sex, as the practical rationale teaches, then they may feel ready earlier. This message leaves room for variation in different communities' norms while leaving the ultimate decision to the teen.

The message of "wait to have sex until you're ready" should be paired with, "and when you're ready, use effective contraception." As other countries have experienced, if a blanket proscription against teen sex is replaced with a strong norm to wait until you feel completely ready, parents and community members can be more helpful with getting teens the contraceptive protections they need once they do become sexually active. This is because the teen won't then have violated a strong norm, so lines of communication are likely to be more open.[35] This normative focus is also helpful because it teaches young people to take responsibility for their own behavior and make reasoned, agentic decisions about sexuality.[36] Current norms against sex are often so strong that teens may find it a safer strategy to make spur-of-the-moment decisions to have casual sex that they can later disavow as one-time "mistakes." This strategy allows them to better conform to a moral or practical rationale, but it can lead to riskier behaviors than a more deliberate approach would. In their seminal work on the effects of virginity pledges, Peter Bearman and Hannah Brückner found that some groups of teens who took a pledge delayed first sex substantially compared to peers, but when they eventually had sex, they were less likely to use contraception.[37] This makes sense because a teen who has publicly pledged to remain a virgin is being deeply deviant if she plans ahead of time to have sex and obtains contraception, while a one-time "mistake" may seem more forgivable. But unplanned sex can put teens at risk for STIs, sexual violence, and negative emotional repercussions.

Replacing a strong norm against all teen sex with a strong norm that you should wait until you're completely ready would motivate teenagers to plan their sexual behaviors. With this kind of norm, a teen who spontaneously engages in casual sex (which is often riskier in terms of STIs and sexual violence) would anticipate negative sanctions, while a teen who engages in a long planning and decision-making process before having sex and who uses effective contraception would not. This norm might also make it easier for teens and parents to communicate about sex. Shifting normative messages from the internally contradictory "don't have sex, but if you do . . ." message that stems from both the practical and moral rationales, to a consistent "don't have sex until . . ., and when you do . . ." message, should improve effective communication with teens. Polls show that teenagers prefer to get information about sex and contraception from their parents,[38] so ending "conspiracies of silence" and opening up this line of communication are important.

This four-pronged proposal—improving educational opportunities, focusing policies on teen sex and contraception, encouraging teens not to have sex until they're completely ready, and making it feasible for them to use long-acting contraceptives plus condoms if they are—presents different challenges and opportunities for different community types. Improving education systems would yield the most positive results among lower-SES "it could be you" and "it's wrong, but" communities. Replacing an abstinence norm with a norm that teens should wait to have sex until they're personally ready would be a greater challenge in the more religious "it's wrong" and "it's wrong, but" communities. Gaining clinical access to long-acting contraceptives would make the biggest difference in rural communities and places where teens have less access to independent transportation, while offering these contraceptives for free would likely create the most positive change for teens from lower-income families and those whose parents disapprove of sex or contraception. Across all communities, shifting to a norm that teens should wait to have sex until they feel completely ready should increase sexual agency for teens and improve communication with adults.

These policy strategies do not suggest that every teen should feel it's appropriate to be having sex. Teens' own values, formed in conversation with their families, peers, schools, and communities, determine readiness. And the focus on reducing pregnancy and STIs among teens who do have sex may be something most people can support. Some people with conservative religious beliefs that discourage contraception will not be in favor of encouraging long-acting contraceptives. The recent *Burwell v. Hobby Lobby* decision by the U.S. Supreme Court revolved around the highly religious owners of two corporations' objections to certain long-acting contraceptives that they consider a form of abortion—IUDs and emergency contraceptives, sometimes known as "Plan B."[39] After the Supreme Court decision, "closely held" private companies can choose to refuse to cover these methods for their employees. But the owners did not object to covering other types of contraception, some of them effective hormonal methods such as birth control pills. Indeed, both Catholic and Evangelical Protestant women in the United States overwhelmingly use contraception—for example, just 3 percent of married Catholic women who do not want to get pregnant use natural family planning methods.[40] This suggests that even though some people may disapprove of particular types of contraceptives, few are likely to object to contraceptive use across the board.

But can communities change their norms just by having conversations and making decisions about what to communicate? I argue that past evidence says they can. Finn said his community actively changed its norms about teen abortion and parenthood after an extensive discussion process. Sociologist Amy Schalet details how the Dutch shifted from a normative context that was similar to "it's wrong" communities to a radically different norm set and enforcement strategies over the course of a single generation.[41] And over a relatively short period of time, workplaces responded to new federal laws prohibiting sexual harassment by starting discussions and formal training mechanisms that rapidly changed workers' norms and attitudes about sexual harassment.[42] Because changing norms can be difficult, especially in an ideologically diverse society like the United States, only one of the four strategies relies on norm change. The others echo what previous research says can be effective, by working to set policies and assume that norm change will follow.

These four strategies need to be backed up by other policy supports. Non-heterosexual teens need communication rather than silence, so normative messages need to be inclusive of diverse sexualities and different gender identities. If teens are being asked to wait to have sex until they are completely ready, then we need to ensure that sexual violence doesn't rob children and youth of the opportunity to make their own decisions about when to have sex.[43] And if we want sexually active teens to use long-acting contraceptives plus condoms, we need to make sure they know how to use these methods. Past evidence suggests that making contraception available to teens and teaching them how to use it doesn't lead teens to have more sex; instead, it tends to help those who are having sex anyway have safer sex.[44] Beyond improving educational experiences and options, we need to make sure that all teens believe there are other promising opportunities for their future lives so that risky sex in fact feels like a risk to their future. Ensuring the socioeconomic prospects of all teens, including those from less privileged backgrounds, is important for making this strategy work.

MAKING A CHANGE

Policy changes can be high impact, but they are also hard to implement. People who interact with teens, and teens themselves, can also work to make changes. First, what kinds of steps can *parents* take to change the norms and enforcement teens are experiencing and improve their sexual health? I argue that the two most important ones are ending conspiracies of silence and climates of fear. Teens want to learn from their parents about sex and contraception, so opening lines of communication can be a good strategy.[45] In many families, for this to happen, the climate of fear needs to be removed. When parents threaten severe sanctions if teens have sex, both parents and teens are boxed into a corner: Teens have to try to keep their sexual activity secret from parents or they may end up sanctioned, and parents have to follow through with the threats if they find out about it or they lose their credibility. According to interviewees, these threats also don't seem to be very effective at preventing teenagers' sexual activity. Removing these threats makes it possible for teens to risk disclosing their activities and for parents to react in a constructive way. But at the same time, silence isn't enough. If parents don't threaten teens but rather say nothing, teens may assume parents will have a strong negative reaction by looking at the families around them. So communicating a clear expectation that teens should be honest with parents about their sexual health may be useful.

What can *schools* do to support more productive norms and enforcement and better sexual health? One of my suggestions has to do with schools' role as instructional institutions, and the other has to do with their role as settings for teenagers' peer interactions. First, schools can ensure that students have a thorough information base to support the normative messages being communicated. This means learning about different contraceptive methods. It also means learning about human psychological development, negotiation skills, and strategies for engaging in "planful competence," all of which are necessary for understanding when a person is ready to engage in intimate relationships and new and potentially risky behaviors. Second, schools can work to reduce bullying, stigmatization, and social exclusion in their halls. By turning a blind eye to the sanctioning of teens who violate sexuality norms, many of whom are wrongly assumed to have done so, schools help perpetuate the unequal and unproductive social exclusion of teens on the basis of gender, class, race, and sexual orientation. Most of all, schools should stop practicing this social exclusion themselves by encouraging pregnant and parenting girls to leave or shifting them to special programs that keep them out of the public life of the school.

What can *communities* and community organizations such as government and churches do to help? I focus on their opportunities for opening up conversations to rethink normative messages and for filling gaps in teens' support. Whether from the pulpit or by showing a free movie with thought-provoking discussion afterwards, community organizations can ask their members to come together and talk through the norms and sanctions they are communicating to teens and what their intended and unintended consequences are. Community-level movements to improve those processes may result. As Finn and Logan showed, many religious organizations are already leading the way. Communities can also work to identify gaps in the support teens need to be sexually healthy and try to provide that support. Reproductive health clinics that work to provide effective contraception to teens are a good example that is already in place, and teen births have declined rapidly as a result of some programs.[46] Another gap teens experience is in not having a reliable adult to go to with questions about sex and contraception. Teens in that situation turn to peers, who may not give them accurate advice. In Boulder, Colorado, a coalition of sexual health organizations together with Boulder County Public Health has started a program to train "askable adults."[47] Askable adults are meant to be beacons of accurate information for teenagers who aren't able to get it from other sources, perhaps because negative norms preclude communication.

Finally, what can *teenagers* themselves do? I make two seemingly contradictory suggestions: asking for help, and working to become more sexually autonomous. Sexual activity is a decision that should not be taken lightly, and engaging in it in less risky ways requires a lot of information and support. Teens need to realize this and seek out the information they need to behave responsibly. Teenage friends are often not a reliable source of information about sex and contraception, but adults may not feel safe to ask. Indeed, in the current U.S. normative climate, teens may face serious consequences for going to the wrong adult for support. But there are safe adults to be found everywhere, and teens should find them and ask them for help. At the same time, though, only a teen himself knows if he is completely ready to have sex. Teenagers need to ask themselves a lot of questions and make a careful, well-considered decision before they engage in sexual activity. Discussing readiness with safe adults is a very good idea, but this decision is something teenagers need to devote time and energy to. Finally, research suggests that if even a few teens change their public behaviors to go against existing norms, the norms themselves may begin to change. If teens feel safe being more open about their sexual behaviors, they may have the power to change their local culture.[48]

Teenagers' sexual health is improving in some ways, but we still lag far behind other developed countries. Although the United States is becoming more politically polarized,[49] there is also increasing agreement that it's becoming harder and harder for young people to achieve a successful life.[50] The institution of new educational standards and healthcare laws suggests that Americans may be ready to try changes that improve everyone's chances of success.[51] Improving the conditions for sexual health—not having sex until you're ready and using dual contraceptives when you are—is an ideal many communities may now be willing to discuss. Norms and policies happen at the group level, and group-level solutions may be the most effective for the future.

Research Methods

COLLEGE STUDENT INTERVIEWS

This book is primarily based on 57 in-depth qualitative interviews with college students at a large public university in the western United States. Students discussed norms and attitudes about and experiences with sex, contraception, and pregnancy during high school. This retrospective approach had the advantage of recruiting interviewees when they were no longer in their high school settings, allowing them to see the norms and social control they had been immersed in more easily than if our research team had tried to talk to them while they were still immersed. Interviewers asked participants for accounts of the norms in their social contexts and stories about teens they knew, as well as information about their own experiences. The interviews, which received institutional review board approval from the University of Colorado Boulder, were conducted in two phases. The first phase consisted of 43 peer interviews conducted during 2008–2009. Undergraduate students in two senior-level sociology classes received training in qualitative interviewing techniques and were given specific instructions for collecting data for this research project. They then conducted a semi-structured in-depth interview with a college student acquaintance of their choice.[1] A minority of students chose a friend from their high school community, and most selected an interviewee with whom they already had rapport. A detailed interview guide specified the main interview questions, as well as suggested probe and follow-up questions. I also encouraged interviewers to ask their own follow-up questions when interesting information or comments arose in the interviews. This resulted in peer interviews that were fairly standardized but also customized to each interviewee's unique situation. Peer interviewers recorded post-interview field notes describing the interviewee's appearance and reactions during the interview, the setting, their thoughts on anything of note that happened, and their take on what was interesting about the interview. The student interviewers then transcribed the interviews according to specific templates, as well as submitting an audio file of the interview.[2]

There were many advantages to the peer interviews. The interviewer-based sampling resulted in a group of interviewees that came from all over the United States and had a wide variety of backgrounds, rather than coming from shared social networks as a snowball sampling strategy would have yielded. The interaction between peer interviewer and interviewee also provided different information than did the second-phase interviews in which the interviewers were adult strangers. Peer interviewing techniques have been used successfully for sensitive topics, such as sexual behavior, that may result in a less managed presentation of self and more open disclosure with a familiar peer interviewer than with an older stranger.[3] This project certainly seemed to benefit from including peer interviews. For example, two interviewees disclosed previous pregnancies and abortions to the peer interviewers, but none did so to adult interviewers. Interviewees also used more openly negative language when talking about teen parents with peer interviewers than with adult strangers. The minority of interviews that were conducted with a peer who had gone to the same high school yielded interesting data, as the shared experiences of interviewer and interviewee seemed to result in greater detail and richer description.

Alongside their many benefits, the peer interviews had two main drawbacks that prompted my decision to collect additional interview data: A small minority of peer interviewers had done a perfunctory job (asking far fewer probe and follow-up questions than I would have done), and the set interview guide didn't allow me to change the questions as themes emerged from the data. Thus, to supplement the peer interviews, I conducted a second phase of 14 in-depth, less structured interviews that employed a purposive sampling strategy. I led a female research team that included a graduate student and a senior undergraduate student who had participated earlier as a high-quality peer interviewer. My research team conducted interviews with 14 undergraduates, who were paid $10 each. We worked alone or in pairs, and I conducted more than half of the interviews.

Phase two students were recruited through a campus-wide student email list, which generated a pool of 89 potential respondents. Recruitment emphasized the project's particular interest in first-generation college students and students who came from a rural or poor community. This focus was intended to balance out the sample because these groups were underrepresented in the university's student population, but other students were also included.[4] The 20 students selected to be interviewed were split evenly between the targeted lower-SES or rural population and the overall sample, and 70 percent of those contacted completed an interview. Although the interviewees and interviewers were strangers, which may have hampered the disclosure of sensitive information, this phase of data collection permitted more detailed probing about important themes that arose inductively in the first round of interviews. This strategy of "abduction" is useful for developing and testing theoretical ideas as they evolve.[5] I used an interview guide that went into greater depth and allowed for more customized follow-up than did the interview guide for the first phase. If interviewees addressed a theme that had been identified as emerging from the first round of interviews, the interviewer sometimes articulated that theme and asked them for feedback about whether that made sense to them. This often yielded detailed information to expand on a theme.[6] Interviews continued until saturation was reached.[7]

Both phases of interviews focused on teens' experiences during high school. The topics covered included interviewees' perceptions of norms about teenage sex, contraception, and childbearing in their peer groups, families, schools, and communities during high school; how these norms were communicated; how they influenced their own and their peers' sexual behaviors; and what sanctions violators of these norms faced. My research team asked about communication with parents and peers about these issues, as well as for stories about peers' experiences. I replaced a section from the first phase's interview guide that had asked interviewees about their current support from family members with a new section asking them to compare their high school's normative climate around sexuality with the normative climate at their current university. This yielded interesting data that highlighted the consistently negative messages about sex communicated to teenagers in all communities, but not to college students. Questions about norms started out open-ended so teens could identify normative messages and targeted behaviors on their own, and the interviewer followed the open-ended questions with extensive probe questions. Although the bulk of the interview concerned events and attitudes from the past and was therefore probably subject to some degree of recall bias, interviewees' high school experiences were still fairly recent, and they seemed to have little trouble recalling them.[8] About a third of interviewees came from the same city as at least one other interviewee, and sometimes they had even attended the same high schools. Their hometowns fit into the same community type in a clear majority of cases, bolstering my confidence in the reliability of interviewees' accounts of community norms.

Peer interviewers in phase one, and three graduate students and one undergraduate student in phase two, transcribed all interviews. The research team imported the transcripts into QSR NVivo qualitative analysis software. Transcripts were then coded using three techniques. First, the research team coded responses by interview question, including simple distinctions between answers (e.g., positive versus negative attitudes toward teen sex among the interviewee's close friends). Second, I read all of the transcripts and identified important themes that emerged from the data. These themes were then coded in other transcripts. Third, I identified key characteristics of interviewees and their communities and compared findings across categories. Community-level SES and religion and teens' sexual experience emerged through this process as important for understanding the findings. The four predominant community types described in Chapter 6 arose in the second stage of coding and were connected with demographic variables during the third stage. A graduate student member of the research team and I coded cases into these community types independently, arriving at 88 percent initial agreement. We then discussed discrepant cases to arrive at a final coding decision. Fourth, I read all the transcripts one at a time to conduct whole-case analyses that linked themes together. Finally, I searched the body of electronic transcript files for key terms to make sure particular quotes hadn't been missed in earlier coding. Some of these steps were conducted multiple times at different points in the analysis and writing process.

I compiled demographic information at both the community and individual levels. Table 1.1 in Chapter 1 shows interviewee characteristics on a variety of factors, and Table A.1 displays the age distribution of interviewees.

Ninety-two percent of interviewees identified as heterosexual or straight at the time of the interview. Of the sexual minority interviewees, half identified as gay or bisexual and half as "mostly heterosexual." This latter group receives less recognition as sexual minorities but experiences a wide range of disadvantages compared to heterosexual individuals.[9] It seemed that many or most of the sexual minority respondents had started self-identifying as such sometime after

TABLE A.1

College student interviewees' ages

Age	% of Interviewees
18	4
19	12
20	20
21	38
22	16
23	8
24	2

TABLE A.2

Interviewees' sexual experience in high school, by gender

Gender	% of Interviewees	Within Gender, % Not Sexually Experienced	Within Gender, % Always Used Contraception	Within Gender, % Didn't Always Use Contraception
Female	63	42	42	16
Male	37	37	37	26

finishing high school. For this reason, unfortunately, the interviews didn't include enough data on the high school experiences of sexual minority students to permit analysis. This is an important topic for future research.

None of the interviewees had become parents, though two told us they had aborted a pregnancy. These proportions are lower than in the general population of young people, likely because the interviewees were all college students—few teen parents end up in four-year colleges.[10] A similar proportion of interviewees had heterosexual intercourse in high school compared to national estimates (Table A.2). Forty percent of interviewees (42 percent of women and 37 percent of men) reported remaining sexually abstinent throughout high school. Another 40 percent (again, 42 percent of women and 37 percent of men) were sexually active, but they or a partner always used contraception. Twenty percent of interviewees (16 percent of women and 26 percent of men), or one third of all sexually active interviewees, had sex without contraception at least once during high school.

Table A.3 shows that interviewees' sexual experience also varied by community type (described in Chapter 6). I do not include information on the sexual experiences of the very small group of interviewees with hybrid community types, although the theoretically important hybrid communities were analyzed in Chapter 6. Interviewees in the generally lower-SES "it could be you" and "it's wrong, but" communities had higher percentages of inconsistent contraception and lower percentages of sexual abstinence than those in the higher-SES community types. Thus, the starkly different norm sets in these two community types were not reflected in differences in sexual behavior. Interviewees from the generally higher-SES, highly religious "it's wrong" communities reported the highest levels of sexual abstinence (50 percent of interviewees in this group) and the lowest prevalence of inconsistent contraception (13 percent).

TABLE A.3

Interviewees' community types, by sexual experience in high school

Community Type	% of Interviewees	% Not Sexually Experienced	% Always Used Contraception	% Didn't Always Use Contraception
"It could be you"	18	30	40	30
"Be careful"	35	44	38	19
"It's wrong"	30	50	38	13
"It's wrong, but"	12	29	43	29
Hybrid	5	–	–	–

TEEN PARENT INTERVIEWS

I use interviews with teen mothers and fathers to illustrate normative processes and norm enforcer and norm target strategies among people who have violated teen sexuality norms. By having a child before age 20, these interviewees had all violated societal norms against teen sex, inconsistent contraception, and teen childbearing. My research team conducted in-depth interviews with current and former teen mothers and teen fathers (the latter is a particularly difficult group to reach), combined with limited participant observation, at a school and a clinic in the Denver metropolitan area.[11] With teen mothers accounting for 12 percent of all births, Denver is fairly typical of U.S. cities.[12] The interviews were conducted in the fall and winter of 2008–2009, with University of Colorado Boulder institutional review board approval. The researchers, who conducted interviews alone or in pairs, consisted of Professor Janet Jacobs and I, one male and one female graduate student, and one undergraduate who had been a teen mother. To be eligible, interviewees had to have had a child before turning 20. Most had babies or toddlers, but a few had older children, allowing us to observe both short- and long-term experiences of teenage childbearing. Fifty-five interviewees had been teen mothers, and 21 had been teen fathers.

When studying a population such as teen mothers and especially teen fathers that is hard to reach because teen parents make up a very small percentage of the overall population, qualitative researchers tend to rely on either samples drawn from sites serving the populations or snowball samples. Our research team chose the former strategy because we could reach a wider variety of interviewees, both mothers and fathers, who were not from the same social networks and neighborhoods. We selected the sites because they permitted access to a large pool of teen fathers and mothers from around the metropolitan area; because they served different populations in terms of race/ethnicity, age, geographic location, and educational aspirations; and because they provided quite different levels of resources to young parents. We conducted 28 interviews at a school for pregnant and parenting teen girls that offered considerable resources to its typically financially needy students, including onsite childcare, basic medical and psychological services, career counseling, and a "school store" to exchange attendance credits for diapers and other items. The school also had a satellite program for young fathers. Another 48 interviews were conducted at a hospital-based medical clinic for privately insured and Medicaid patients that provided tandem healthcare to teen mothers and their children. Despite the considerable support provided by the school, many of the school-based interviewees were younger and appeared to have fewer personal and family resources than those from the clinic. Reflecting their substantial social disadvantage, substantial minority of interviewees from both sites talked about personal backgrounds of incarceration, substance abuse, victimization, or mental health problems, and these issues were even more common in their families.

We recruited young parents by distributing flyers at the sites and giving them to interviewees to share with friends (though this latter strategy resulted in very few interviews). Staff at the sites also handed out flyers and described the study to parents they identified as eligible. Interviewees' ages ranged from 15 to 38, but only four were older than 24. Our interviewees had their first child between ages 14 and 19 with an average of 17. This is younger than the average age for teen births in the United States, tapping into a more marginalized population.[13] The average age of their oldest child was two. Two thirds of mothers and half of fathers had just one child, and most had grown up in or around Denver. Ten interviewees identified as multiracial or multiethnic, while others described themselves using a single racial or ethnic label: 36 self-identified as Latina/Hispanic/Mexican American, 21 as African American/Black, 3 as White, 2 as Native American, and 1 as Middle Eastern. Compared to Denver's 2006 teen births (of which 75 percent were to Latina mothers, 12 percent to White mothers, and 11 percent to Black mothers), our sample likely overrepresents African Americans and underrepresents Latinas and Whites, though our inclusion of multiracial identities makes comparison difficult.[14] In analyzing our data to examine the role of race/ethnicity, we found considerable similarity in Denver-area teen parents' experiences across categories. Forty interviewees were enrolled in school, and 26 were working for pay. Eighteen interviewees (24 percent) were married at the time of the interview; among all Denver teen mothers, 23 percent were married at the time of their child's birth.[15] Twenty interviewees were single, and the others identified themselves as dating, in a relationship, living with someone, or engaged. Nearly all mothers and about half of fathers were living with at least one of their children. More than one third lived with a parent or parent-in-law, about one third with a sibling or sibling-in-law, and about one third with some other adult, such as an aunt or stepparent. Many lived with people from more than one of these categories.

Our research team took an ethnographic approach to the interviews and sites, observing the sites and interactions involving interviewees during our visits to meet with staff and conduct interviews, and taking field notes. Interviews about interviewees' experiences with teen parenthood lasted about 45 minutes, and they received a $30 gift card. The interviews tended to include the same questions, but they were often asked in a different order depending on the direction the conversation went. We also asked follow-up questions to flesh out interviewees' accounts, and many of these were unique for each interview. Interviews were digitally recorded and transcribed. Topics covered during the interview included interviewees' perceptions of messages about teen pregnancy from their peers, families, communities, and broader society; their fertility decisions and behaviors; and people's reactions to the pregnancy. Their experiences before, during, and after pregnancy were discussed, as well as their ideas of what a good parent is. Interviewees described the resources available to them, who provided them, how these arrangements were negotiated, and how available resources had affected their lives.

Transcribed interviews were kept in searchable electronic format and were manually coded in the NVivo qualitative software package. First, the research team coded responses to each question, making simple distinctions between answers (e.g., a certain family member's positive versus negative reactions to the pregnancy). Second, I read whole transcripts and identified important emergent themes, which were then coded for all transcripts. Third, I searched for key words and phrases to make sure all instances of a theme had been captured by coding.

HOW THE STUDY CAME ABOUT

I have studied teen parenthood for more than 15 years, analyzing national longitudinal surveys and in-depth open-ended interviews to examine two topics: the consequences of teen parenthood for women and men and their children, and norms and stigma around teen parenthood. In my first years of research on the topic, through statistical analyses of nationally representative surveys I identified socioeconomic, racial/ethnic, and gender influences on individuals' perceived norms against teen pregnancy; linked these norms to the withholding of needed resources from teen parents; and found that a lack of resources after the birth largely explains why teen mothers' and fathers' educational attainment is compromised.

While doing this quantitative research, I felt strongly that it would be important to talk to young parents about their life experiences to flesh out the processes that had been identified using these large surveys. Qualitative interview data complement quantitative survey data. While the latter can statistically demonstrate significant relationships between two or more researcher-identified factors, such as norms against teen parenthood and the provision of resources to teens, interviews can reveal how people make sense of what is actually happening beneath the numbers, highlighting factors that may have been initially overlooked by the researcher.[16] Qualitative interview data can capture a more complete picture of the complex and intertwined factors that figure into a teenager's experiences. It can also show how young people talk about teen sexuality and parenthood.[17] Together with my colleague and mentor Janet Jacobs and a research team, I set out to conduct in-depth interviews with teen mothers, fathers, and couples. These interviews are the supplemental data used throughout the book and are described below. Hearing about the experiences of young parents yielded many important insights beyond those included here.[18]

But conducting the interviews with teen parents left me convinced that an important piece of the puzzle was still missing. I had heard about normative messages and social control of teens who were sexually active, didn't use contraception consistently, didn't get an abortion, and became parents. Both their experiences and their communities—almost all urban and of low SES—were unusual compared to the majority of teens in the United States. I needed a second set of interviews as a counterweight to these. I wanted to talk to teens who had a variety of sexual experiences, who hadn't become parents, and who came from a more diverse set of communities and social contexts.

This approach is quite different from nearly all the existing research on teen sexuality and parenthood. That research tends to fall into one of two camps: statistical analyses of large-scale survey data that examine relationships between variables that the researchers have identified, or qualitative research (observations and/or interviews) that examines a particular community—almost always one that is considered high risk—in detail. I would characterize the former approach (which I have often taken) as "an inch deep and a mile wide," providing a broad and informative national picture of a specific outcome or relationship. The latter approach is "an inch wide and a mile deep," yielding a rich understanding of one particular social context without comparison to others. In this approach, "typical" lower-risk groups of teens tend to be ignored.

STRENGTHS AND LIMITATIONS OF THE STUDY

The analytic space between these two approaches interested me for this project. I wanted to gather a moderate amount of qualitative detail about a large and diverse set of communities. The goal is not for the findings to be generalizable to a broader population, nor can they provide anywhere near the depth that single-site ethnographic studies can.[19] Yet they do provide *breadth* for understanding differences and similarities in messages about teen sexuality and social control of teens in the United States today. Because the findings represent individuals and communities from around the country, their reach is quite broad for a qualitative study. I think this strategy can help elucidate complex processes underlying social norms that regulate teen sexual behavior, and these theoretical tools may be of use to researchers working in other settings or studying other phenomena.

Especially because I purposively sampled additional people from low-SES and rural communities (who are underrepresented in the college student population), the interviews with college students better characterize the national diversity of normative climates around teen sexuality than the interviews with teen parents do. For that reason, the college student interviews are the book's primary data source. But the teen parent interviews are an important supplementary dataset because they can tell us about what happens when teens violate the strongest teen sexuality norms—those that proscribe teen parenthood—thereby illuminating sanctioning processes. I was surprised by the consistency in descriptions of normative climates and social control between the two sets of interviews, since most of the interviewees came from very different walks of life. For example, almost no adults anywhere are giving teens encouragement to be sexually active or to become pregnant in their teenage years. My data reinforce Amy Schalet's assessment that in the United States, pretty much everyone views teen sex as inherently risky and perceives teen sexual behavior as a struggle of adults against teens and boys against girls.[20] Having such a wide variety of communities in the samples allows me to identify these kinds of universal normative messages, as well as many messages that are not universal.

Although my data collection strategy has many advantages, there are also drawbacks. First, relying on people's own reports of social phenomena, as both in-depth interviews and surveys do, means that the data represent an altered version of social reality that has been "filtered" through the respondent's own perception and verbal account.[21] I make use of that perspective in this book. Using self-reported data from interviews or surveys means that the researcher has to accept people's accounts of their own and others' behaviors and motivations, seeing them as important narrative constructions that articulate culture. Interviewees' representations of their sexual behaviors could be exaggerated or untrue, a problem that also applies to surveys. But these accounts can also be an advantage for studying culture (of which norms are a part) because they capture people's justifications for their behavior.

Second, I chose to do retrospective interviews with both the college students and teen parents, which means that interviewees' accounts are probably different than they would have been at the time an event occurred. But an advantage of retrospective interviewing is that the interviewees have gained some distance from the events in question. Social norms tend to be invisible to people until they are violated or until people are put in a different normative climate. So it can be helpful to talk to people when they are in a different time and place—and hopefully thereby a different normative climate—and can perceive and articulate the earlier situation's norms more clearly. The college student interviewees often contrasted their normative climates during high school with those in college, whether prompted to do so or not. This suggests that the contrast helped shed some light on their high school experiences, making their surprisingly articulate accounts of those normative climates easier to talk about.

Third, the standpoints of both the interviewees and my research teams shaped both the data that were collected and my analysis of the data. Even if some of them came from less privileged communities, all of the interviewees in my primary dataset were still college students. This means that they either came from privileged communities or occupied at least a partial "outsider" and presumably more privileged position in their less privileged communities. Because being an outsider—who probably has access to an alternative set of norms or attitudes—can also help make norms more visible, it may have been helpful for sharpening interviewees' accounts in less privileged communities. But it also probably shaped those narratives, for example because inter- viewees' close friends were also more likely to be college-bound and not typical of less privileged communities.

My standpoint also matters. I am a White woman and was in my early thirties at the time of data collection. Like those of the sample, my experiences represent considerable breadth in norms around sexuality. I grew up in a solidly low-SES, highly religious rural community like many of the "it's wrong, but" communities in Chapter 6. Since then, I have lived in Sweden for four years, attended two private universities in different regions of the United States, and spent a decade working at a public university in a liberal, highly educated city. I have had the advantage of being exposed to radically different normative climates regarding sexuality and adolescence, and these experiences have shaped my reading of the data. I worked to triangulate standpoints in data collection and interpretation by relying on many different peer interviewers and giving the interviewers some leeway in what questions they asked. I approached coding and data analysis from a variety of different angles and worked with collaborators to improve the reliability of some key coding decisions.

CONCLUSION

The data analyzed in this book are meant to fill several gaps in previous research. I sampled inter- viewees from a wide variety of communities, included boys as well as girls, and focused primarily on fairly typical teens rather than those from particularly marginalized urban communities who had violated norms against teen parenthood. Combining interviews with college students and those with teen mothers and fathers broadens the reach of the study, engaging demographically distinct kinds of communities and including both people who did and people who did not violate teen sexuality norms. Yet the norm sets described by the college students and the teen parents sounded very similar when they came from similar communities. The goal of this book was to document U.S. normative climates around teen sexuality and their links to social control and norm enforcer and norm target strategies. This goal required a broad approach. Next steps for future research include examining particular communities in greater depth to more fully articulate these dynamics of norms, social control, and agency in specific settings, as well as applying the ideas about norms to other phenomena.

Notes

CHAPTER I

1. CBS News 2008; Pilkington 2008.

2. The perspectives of teens themselves are relatively understudied and important for understanding teen sexuality in the United States (García 2012; Thompson 1996).

3. To preserve their anonymity, all interviewees' names and some potentially identifying details have been changed.

4. García (2012) has noted the preoccupation with girls' sexuality in the literature. See Martin (1996) for an exception.

5. For example, see Thompson (1996) and Tolman (2009). In her ethnographic study of Latina girls' sexuality, Lorena García (2012) has analyzed some of these contexts.

6. Social norms (sometimes also called injunctive norms) are rules for how people ought to behave. It's important not to assume that these rules exist just by looking at people's prevalent behaviors. For example, a lot of people drink coffee, but that doesn't mean that tea drinkers are breaking a social rule. Descriptive or statistical norms, which describe how most people behave, can also influence people's behaviors, but there are no negative sanctions attached to violations of descriptive norms. See Bendor and Swistak (2001); Horne (2009); Marini (1984); Tinkler (2013); Willer, Kuwabara, and Macy (2009).

7. Merton 1968.

8. Fine 2001.

9. For example, see Hechter and Opp (2001a, 2001b); Horne (2001a, 2001b, 2001c); and Willer, Kuwabara, and Macy (2009). Horne et al. (2015) and Horne, Dodoo, and Dodoo (2013) manipulated norms using an experimental design within a survey.

10. Horne 2001c; Marini 1984.

11. Vaisey 2009. But there are exceptions, such as Fine (2001).

12. One book by Cancian (1975) has examined social norms in the field and from the point of view of individuals, based on her research in the Mayan community of Zinacantan. Sexuality norms were not the book's main focus, but it illustrates interesting processes that link norms to social identities.

13. Durkheim 1951; Marini 1984; Merton 1968; Settersten 2004.

14. Eaton et al. 2012; Foucault 1978; Perper and Manlove 2009.

15. Sennott and Mollborn 2011. But it is still common for teens who have taken a virginity pledge to end up having sex (Bearman and Brückner 2001).

16. Black (1993) identified features of groups that affect social control, including inequality of economic resources or other sources of power/prestige, group segmentation into social categories, social distance (extent of interaction), functional unity (interdependence), and immobility (geographic constraint).

17. Harding 2007, 2011. "Agency" is a complicated and heavily debated concept, and it is hard to separate individual preferences from internalized social norms; see Hitlin and Johnson (2015) for a discussion of the term.

18. Cancian 1975; Feldman 1984.

19. Bettie 2003.

20. Anderson 1989, 1990; Hechter and Opp 2001b; Mollborn and Sennott 2015. Hechter and Opp articulated the idea of systems of norms, making a strong call for people to analyze them and saying there's little work in the area. Anderson's research on codes, and other work on cultural heterogeneity, implicitly looks at systems of norms but doesn't lay it out explicitly. My research with Christie Sennott used the term "bundles of norms" to introduce a similar concept.

21. Horne 2001b.

22. The social stakes for norm enforcers are higher in more cohesive groups, so these groups have more social control (Horne 2001b).

23. Quantitative research on large national samples has found this. See Brückner, Martin, and Bearman (2004); Cherlin, Cross-Barnet, Burton, and Garrett-Peters (2008); Mollborn (2009, 2010b). Qualitative research has focused mostly on single ethnographic sites and not on norms per se, but on communities' reactions to teen childbearing and young mothers' lived experiences. See Burton (1990); Edin and Kefalas (2005); Gregson (2009); Jacobs (1994); Kaplan (1997); Ladner and Gourdine (1984).

24. Mollborn 2009, 2010b.

25. Mollborn 2009.

26. Mollborn 2010b; Mollborn, Domingue, and Boardman 2014a.

27. Mollborn, Domingue, and Boardman 2014a.

28. Bettie 2003.

29. A 2013 poll found that three quarters of Americans believe in God (Shannon-Missal 2013).

30. Mollborn, Domingue, and Boardman 2014a.

31. Mollborn, Domingue, and Boardman 2014b. These relationships predict norms and teen pregnancy prevalence differently in multivariate models, suggesting that race and SES partly explain some of the correlations with fundamentalist beliefs.

32. Strayhorn and Strayhorn 2009. Studying family formation more generally, Glass and Levchak (2014) found that individual- and county-level conservative Protestantism increased people's early family formation and divorce risk.

33. Bearman and Brückner 2001.

34. Others have articulated one or both of these differing perspectives on teen sexuality in the United States and elsewhere (Bearman and Brückner 2001; Koffman 2012; Macvarish 2010a, 2010b; Talbot 2008).

35. Furstenberg 2003; Smith and Hindus 1975.

36. Bailey 1989; Rosenfeld 2009.

37. Coontz 1992; Smith and Hindus 1975.

38. Furstenberg 2003; Mollborn 2011; Ventura, Mathews, and Hamilton 2001.

39. In 2012, the teen birth rate for ages 15 to 19 was 29.4 births per 1,000 women. The birth rate for ages 10 to 14 was 0.4 births per 1,000 women (Martin et al. 2013).

40. Arnett 2000; Rosenfeld 2009.

41. Johnson, Berg, and Sirotzki 2007; Johnson and Mollborn 2009.

42. For example, Gallup polls show that 58 percent of U.S. adults in 2015 thought same-sex marriages should be legally recognized, an increase of over 30 percentage points in 20 years (Gallup n.d.).

43. England, Shafer, and Fogarty 2007.

44. Kost et al. 2008; Ricketts, Klinger, and Schwalberg 2014.

45. Thirty-seven percent of respondents to a poll said they didn't know when asked what had happened with the U.S. teen pregnancy rate in "the last few years." Of the rest, 56 percent incorrectly thought the teen pregnancy rate was increasing and 24 percent correctly thought it was decreasing. These findings are nationally representative of U.S. adults (Sex Education in America Survey 2003).

46. Furstenberg 2003. See Wong (1997) for more discussion about the social construction of teen mothers as a relevant social category.

47. Martin et al. 2013; Mollborn 2011.

48. Science and Integrity Survey 2004.

49. Office of Adolescent Health 2014.

50. Kost and Maddow-Zimet 2016.

51. Slightly more boys (49 percent) than girls (46 percent) had had sex (Eaton et al. 2012).

52. The figure for seniors quite closely matches the 60 percent of my interviewees who had sex by the time they finished high school (Eaton et al. 2012).

53. Hoffman 2008.

54. Eaton et al. 2012. This is probably an underestimate.

55. Abma, Martinez, Mosher, and Dawson 2004; Schalet 2011.

56. Human papillomavirus (HPV), which can increase cancer risk, was the most common infection (Forhan et al. 2009).

57. Darroch, Singh, and Frost 2001; Hoffman 2008.

58. Advocates for Youth 2011.

59. Martin et al. 2013; World Bank Group 2016.

60. Advocates for Youth 2011; Martinez, Abma, and Copen 2010.

61. Roper Center 2003.

62. Roper Center 2007.

63. Ibid.

64. Sex Education in America Survey 2003.

65. Fields 2008; Irvine 2004.

66. Gallup n.d.

67. Ibid.

68. Brewster, Billy, and Grady 1993; Kirby 2002; Mollborn 2010b.

69. Everett 2015; Mojola and Everett 2012.

70. Martin et al. 2013.

71. Eaton et al. 2012.

72. Mollborn and Dennis 2012b.

73. Brewster, Billy, and Grady 1993; Mollborn 2010b.

74. Pugh 2013.

75. Ibid:64.

76. I thank the research team: Christie Sennott, Laurie James-Hawkins, Aleeza Zabriskie Tribbia, Danielle Denardo, Kathryn McCune, and undergraduate peer interviewers. Published articles from these data include Mollborn 2015; Mollborn and Sennott 2015; Sennott and Mollborn 2011.

77. I thank the research team: Janet L. Jacobs, Leith Lombas, Devon Thacker, and Nicole Moore. Published articles from these data include Jacobs and Mollborn 2012; Mollborn 2011; Mollborn and Jacobs 2012, 2015.

78. Kane, Morgan, Harris, and Guilkey 2013; Mollborn 2007.

79. For example, Elliott 2012; Fields 2008; Irvine 2004; Luker 1996, 2006; Schalet 2011.

80. Even though they may not fit within normative processes, potential media influences on sexuality are interesting and changing rapidly. See boyd (2014) and Brown, Steele, and Walsh-Childers (2001) for more information.

81. See Nack (2009) for more information about women who live with chronic STIs.

82. Fine 1988; Fine and McClelland 2006; Tolman 2009.

83. In contrast, as others have shown (e.g., Ingraham 2005), heterosexuality is normative and is taught to children from a young age.

84. Birkett, Espelage, and Koenig 2009; Kosciw, Greytak, and Diaz 2009; Pearson, Muller, and Wilkinson 2007; Rivers 2001; Russell, Seif, and Truong 2001; Wilkinson and Pearson 2009.

85. This figure, though representing inductively identified social contexts among young people, is quite similar to the ecological systems identified by Bronfenbrenner's (1986) situating of families in their social contexts.

86. Willer, Kuwabara, and Macy 2009.

87. Fields 2008; Irvine 2004.

CHAPTER 2

1. Gary Alan Fine and Brooke Harrington (Fine 2014; Fine and Harrington 2004) call small groups "tiny publics" and argue that they represent a powerful site for understanding broad sociological processes.

2. Emirbayer and Mische 1998; Hitlin and Johnson 2015; Marini 1984; Valocchi 2005. This important debate largely revolves around how much human agency is independent of versus created by structural influences.

3. Books on social norms are few and tend to be edited volumes (e.g., Hechter and Opp 2001a; Xenitidou and Edmonds 2014) or abstract or lab-focused (e.g., Bicchieri 2006; Horne 2009). An exception is Cancian (1975).

4. Bell and Cox 2015; Hechter and Opp 2001b; van Kleef et al. 2015.

5. In contrast to an older focus on norms constraining people's behavior, many sociologists, including Ann Swidler (2001) and Gary Alan Fine (2001), have started to think about culture (and norms) in a different way. In this newer view, we each possess a cultural toolkit or repertoire that we use to make sense of and explain our own and others' situations and behaviors. Cultural influences may be conscious, unconscious, or both at once. The resources people derive from social structures are necessary for many types of action and shape people's possible strategies. So although it acknowledges social structure, this perspective allows for a lot more individual agency—letting people decide their own actions and sense making within cultural and structural constraints. But as Stephen Vaisey (2009) points out, a focus on after-the-fact sense making glosses over the classic, well-documented idea that norms can shape people's motivations for their behaviors before the fact. Like Vaisey, I think it's most realistic to conceptualize of norms as working in both ways.

6. Hechter and Opp 2001b, 2001c; Marini 1984.

7. High-quality exceptions include Fine 2001, Vaisey 2010.

8. Giving a baby up for adoption is an option that many adults and media examples discuss as a good possibility, but in reality it very rarely happens. Statistics from 1995 found that less than 1 percent of teen mothers placed their children for adoption (AdoptED n.d.). Therefore I don't include it in Figure 2.1.

9. García (2012) has argued that teen pregnancy is relatively overstudied compared to some other links in the chain.

10. Jessor 1987.

11. See van Kleef et al. (2015).

12. Hechter and Opp 2001a; S. M. Lindenberg, personal communication, September 3, 2014. In documenting this phenomenon, coauthor Christie Sennott and I (2015) used the term "bundles of norms."

13. Mollborn unpublished, analyzing the National Pregnancy Norms Study (see Mollborn 2009 for study details). See Horne (2001b) for a fuller discussion of metanorms, or norms about how to sanction norm violators.

14. Pugh (2014) emphasizes that scholarship on childhood has taught us that children and teens are active agents who negotiate their behavior within social constraints.

15. Fine 2001:161–62.

16. Such inconsistencies have been used to justify a turn away from norms. Instead, I think they should be used to try to improve our understanding of social norms and how they work.

17. The idea of rationales is similar to the "motives" concept articulated by C. Wright Mills (1940). He called motives "the reasons men give for their actions. . . . Rather than fixed elements 'in' an individual, motives are the terms with which interpretation of conduct by social actors proceeds" (p. 904). He defines motives as "accepted justifications for present, future, or past programs or acts" (p. 907) and goes on to write, "Not only does the child learn what to do, what not to do, but he is given standardized motives which promote prescribed actions and dissuade those proscribed. Along with rules and norms of action for various situations, we learn vocabularies of motives appropriate to them" (p. 907). Mills's idea of "vocabularies of motive," then, states that people are not only taught norms about how to behave, but also reasons for why those behaviors are appropriate. Teens use vocabularies of motive strategically, as I discuss in Chapter 7. Others have discussed a similar idea as well. For example, Schalet (2011) writes about the "reasoning

underlying regulation" as part of a society's sexual ethics. Miller (1999) discusses a norm of self-interest as a motivation for a person's behavior. Lerner (2003) articulates a "justice motive," which underlies norms about behaviors such as reciprocity.

18. Cancian (1975) argues that people do not internalize norms (the "theory of the socialized actor") but rather make them part of their commitment to an identity. I find evidence of both internalization and identity commitment in my data.

19. Hochschild 1979.

20. Hechter and Opp 2001b.

21. Sometimes behaviors can be regulated by the same rationale but can be more distantly related. For example, theoretical ideas about health lifestyles suggest that people subscribe to overarching rationales that tell them why it's important to conform to norms regulating their health behaviors like exercise, smoking, alcohol consumption, and diet. But each of these health behaviors is also distinct, with different norms and other rationales impacting them. A cigarette smoker and a person who doesn't exercise are both viewed as having an unhealthy lifestyle, but those two behaviors are not related enough to be regulated entirely by the same norm set.

22. Heise and Calhan 1995; Hochschild 1979, 2003; Sutton 1991.

23. Simon, Eder, and Evans 1992.

24. Haidt 2003; Tangney, Price, Stuewig, and Mashek 2007.

25. Ohbuchi et al. 2004; Siddiqui 2012; van Kleef et al. 2015.

26. Keltner and Buswell 1997; Staller and Petta 2001; van Kleef et al. 2015; Vasalou, Joinson, and Pitt 2006.

27. Wooten 2006.

28. Nunner-Winkler and Sodian 1988.

29. Sociologist Erving Goffman (2009) called the management of public portrayals "information control" and the public portrayal process "passing." A person who has a stigma but engages in passing has a "discreditable identity." Others have emphasized the fragility of a public portrayal strategy because of its mismatch with underlying identity (Vinitzky-Seroussi and Zussman 1996). Elster (2009) distinguishes between "social norms," to which people conform only if they are being observed by others, and "moral norms," to which people conform even when they are alone. I instead refer to this distinction as externally conforming to a norm versus having internalized the norm. Private behaviors that can differ from people's public portrayals make this distinction salient.

30. Pugh 2013; Swidler 2001.

31. For example, researchers such as Barriger and Vélez-Blasini (2013), Cancian (1975), and Swidler (2001) have found fairly weak links between norms and behaviors.

32. Vaisey 2009.

33. Justifications are an important feature of accounts, which help reconcile normative expectations with norm-violating behaviors (Scott and Lyman 1968).

34. Goffman 2009.

35. The term "metanorm" was used in Axelrod (1986).

36. Horne 2001b.

37. This process of internalizing a norm may happen at the conscious and nonconscious levels. Yoshida, Peach, Zanna, and Spencer (2012) suggest that nonconscious "implicit normative evaluations" are different from implicit attitudes, shape behavior, and change as people are exposed to social contexts.

38. Nye 1990; Schalet 2011.

39. Schalet 2011.

40. Swidler 2001.

41. Vaisey 2009; Yoshida, Peach, Zanna, and Spencer 2012.

42. Ajzen 1991; Johnson-Hanks, Bachrach, Morgan, and Kohler 2011.

43. Reichard 2014.

44. Cook, Emerson, Gillmore, and Yamagishi 1983; Cook and Whitmeyer 1992.

45. Forward 2009; van Kleef et al. 2015.

46. Wilkins 2008.

47. Brubaker and Wright 2006; Mollborn and Jacobs 2015.

48. Cancian 1975.

49. Cancian (1975) found norms to be strongly tied to social identities. Rather than defining norms as group-level evaluations of how people ought to behave, her definition focused on the social group's responses, as "shared beliefs about what actions and attributes bring respect and approval (or disrespect and disapproval) from oneself and others" (p. 6).

50. Michel Foucault (1977, 1978) and others have made tremendous progress in understanding how power and inequality play out in cultural phenomena, and Foucault has focused on reproduction in particular as a key site for these processes.

51. Armstrong, Hamilton, Armstrong, and Seeley 2014.

52. van Kleef et al. 2015.

53. Armstrong, Hamilton, Armstrong, and Seeley 2014; Hamilton and Armstrong 2009; Kreager and Staff 2009; Pascoe 2007.

54. Bettie 2003; Schalet 2011.

55. García 2012.

56. Tuggle and Holmes 1997.

57. Bettie 2003; García 2012.

58. Bettie 2003.

59. Kreager and Staff 2009.

60. When asked what had happened with the U.S. teen pregnancy rate in "the last few years," more than twice as many people incorrectly thought the teen pregnancy rate was increasing than correctly thought it was decreasing. These findings are nationally representative of U.S. adults (Sex Education in America Survey 2003).

61. Furstenberg 2003; Hoffman 1998; Kane, Morgan, Harris, and Guilkey 2013; Levine and Painter 2003; Taylor 2009.

62. Geronimus 2003.

63. Martin et al. 2015; Perper and Manlove 2009.

64. SmithBattle 2000:29. This language of sin shows that the "practical" rationale, while not religiously motivated, is also seen as deeply moral, which I argue is increasingly true in U.S. society.

65. Researchers estimate this overall likelihood at about 3 percent (Wilcox et al. 2001).

66. For example, the teen birth rate (age 15 to 19) for Black teens in 2006 was more than twice as high as for White teens, and the Hispanic rate was more than three times as high (Martin et al. 2009; Mollborn 2011). In contrast, in 2013, 42 percent of Black teens in grades 9 to 12 reported being sexually active, compared to 35 percent of Hispanic teens and 33 percent of White teens (Child Trends 2014). See more at Child Trends (2014).

67. Jones and Kooistra 2011.

68. Kaplan 1997; Mollborn and Jacobs 2012.

69. Roscigno 2011:349.

70. For example, just 0.4 percent of teen mothers of infants in a nationally representative sample reported being in the highest quintile in terms of household SES, and less than 20 percent were in the top three fifths of the socioeconomic distribution (Mollborn and Dennis 2012a).

71. I found in a nationally representative sample that a much higher proportion of respondents with some college education reported a norm against teen nonmarital pregnancy than those with no college education. This norm predicted negative sanctions against a hypothetical teen parent in the family (Mollborn 2009).

72. Hechter and Opp 2001b; Marini 1984; Vaisey 2010.

73. Fields 2008; Irvine 2004; Luker 2006.

74. Bettie 2003; Bowles, Riley, and Gelfand 2009; Giordano 1983.

75. Cancian 1975.

76. Risman and Schwartz 2002.

77. Research by Paluck and Shepherd (2012) supports this idea. In a high school field experiment, when a subset of teens changed their public harassment behaviors, the perceived collective norm around harassment began to change. Everyday interpersonal interaction, rather than institutionally facilitated interaction, was the mechanism for this change.

78. Mollborn and Jacobs 2012.

79. A large body of research has found this to be less true than previously believed; see Hoffman (1998); Mollborn (in press).

80. Furstenberg 2007; Kane, Morgan, Harris, and Guilkey 2013; Taylor 2009.

81. For example, more and more anti-abortion laws are being passed at the state level (see Guttmacher [2011]).

82. Nathanson 1991.

83. Tyrer 1999.

84. Solinger 1992.

85. Ducker 2007.

86. Arnett 2000.

87. College Board 2014; Lorin 2014.

88. CNN Money 2015.

89. U.S. Department of Labor 2015a, 2015b.

90. American Community Survey 2010.

91. Newhart 2013.

92. Armstrong and Hamilton 2013.

93. Rosenfeld 2009.

94. Armstrong, Hamilton, Armstrong, and Seeley 2014; England, Shafer, and Fogarty 2007; Hamilton and Armstrong 2009; Wilkins 2014; Wilkins and Dalessandro 2013.

95. Bogle 2008.

CHAPTER 3

1. A national survey confirms this, finding that teens report that their parents are the greatest influence on their sexual decision making (Albert 2007).

2. Through in-depth interviews with young women, Wisnieski, Sieving, and Garwick (2015) found that mothers were the most important source of information about sex, but fathers, aunts, uncles, and grandparents sometimes played important roles. One third of interviewees had no adult with whom to discuss sexual and romantic issues as teens.

3. Research has found that parental involvement is important for teen pregnancy prevention, but that programs intended to foster it are often ineffective (see Silk and Romero [2014] for a review).

4. Elliott (2010, 2012) has found that parents talk about most teens as highly sexualized but about their own teenage child as innocent, reflecting their anxieties in a society that has conflicting discourses about teen sexuality.

5. Mollborn and Everett 2010.

6. Albert 2007.

7. Elliott 2012.

8. The idea that it is important for young people to postpone family formation to build human capital through schooling and work has been developed by others (e.g., Hamilton and Armstrong 2009; Rosenfeld 2009). Hamilton and Armstrong (2009) identify a prevailing cultural message, called the "self-development imperative," to postpone family formation until education is done.

9. Johnson and Mollborn 2009.

10. Solebello and Elliott (2011) explore this tension between wanting boys to remain sexually abstinent and teaching them to be heterosexual in their interviews with fathers of teens. Interestingly, Dylan identified as Asian American in a predominantly White community, yet his political and religious conservatism largely mirrored that of his community. The data do not allow me to fully explore whether parents who may have felt like "others" in the community communicated messages that were different from those of the community.

11. Studies have found that young adults define adulthood more through psychological maturity (particularly being responsible and making independent decisions) than through a set of behavioral transitions (such as marriage or full-time work). For a summary, see Arnett (2000).

12. Albert 2012.

13. Schalet 2011.

14. Beersma and van Kleef 2011.

15. Research on conversational silences suggests that they do communicate norms, bringing the behavior of people who are motivated to belong to a group more in line with the group's norm (Koudenburg, Postmes, and Gordijn 2013).

16. Eaton et al. 2012.

17. The "conspiracy of silence" around teen sexuality among teens and between teens and adults was first identified by Hollingshead (1949). Others have used the term "strategic ambiguity" to refer to people talking in ways that elide their actual sexual behaviors (Currier 2013), but I argue that silence can also lend strategic ambiguity.

18. Coyne and D'Onofrio 2012; Hoffman 2008.

19. Schalet 2011.

20. Bailey 1989.

21. Schalet 2011.

22. Sennott and Mollborn 2011.

23. In 2011, the national Youth Risk Behavior Surveillance System found that 47 percent of U.S. high school students had ever had sex; 63 percent of 12th-graders, 53 percent of 11th-graders,

44 percent of 10th-graders, and 33 percent of 9th-graders had ever had sexual intercourse (Eaton et al. 2012).

24. The prevalence of having ever had sexual intercourse among high school students of all ages decreased from 54 percent in 1991 to 46 percent in 2001 and has remained steady between 2001 and 2011 (Eaton et al. 2012).

25. Statistics from 1995 found that less than 1 percent of teen mothers placed their children for adoption (AdoptED n.d.).

26. See articles by Janet Jacobs and me for more discussion of these issues (Jacobs and Mollborn 2012; Mollborn and Jacobs 2012, 2015).

27. Analyzing a nationally representative survey of U.S. adults, I found that people who had stronger norms against nonmarital teen pregnancy were less likely to give several types of support to a hypothetical teen parent in their family, including money, childcare, housing, and general support (Mollborn 2009).

28. Mollborn and Jacobs 2015.

CHAPTER 4

1. See Sennott and Mollborn (2011).

2. Hayford, Guzzo, Kusunoki, and Barber 2016; Sennott and Mollborn 2011.

3. Armstrong, Hamilton, Armstrong, and Seeley 2014.

4. Risman and Schwartz 2002.

5. Being normal may have benefits, at least in some settings. Vrangalova and Savin-Williams (2011) found in a rural community that teens who became sexually experienced "on time" at the average age compared to their peers had higher well-being than those who waited longer to have sex than most peers.

6. Fine 1988.

7. This is not always the case, however. As Rees and Wallace (2014) have found for teen drinking, friendship groups can stably include people who have a mix of behaviors, such as drinkers and non-drinkers or people who are and are not sexually active.

8. Sennott and Mollborn 2011.

9. Past research has found that many boys exaggerate their sexual exploits to peers to gain social approval (Pascoe 2007).

10. Horne 2001b.

11. Willer, Kuwabara, and Macy 2009.

12. Some of this terminology may have been learned from media, illustrating that media influences can be pervasive even if unacknowledged by teens. But media messages do not have the potential for social sanctions attached, making them unlikely to be a major player in normative processes beyond communicating societal-level norms.

13. Interestingly, this suggests they expect sexual activity to be a decision made jointly by their friendship group.

14. For example, U.S. teen mothers are more than twice as likely as mothers who were at least 20 at their first birth to have lived in households that received welfare during childhood, and they were less than one quarter as likely to have a mother with a college degree (Mollborn and Dennis 2012b).

15. Geronimus (2003) points out that the condemnation of racial minority teen mothers both serves the purposes of the dominant White group and can be perpetuated by well-meaning people who are unaware that scientific findings about the consequences of teen motherhood are "equivocal."

16. In a nationally representative U.S. sample, among mothers aged 15 to 19 at their child's birth, the average age of the father was 21 (Mollborn and Dennis 2012b).

17. One potential reason for this may be that girls from families with higher SES are more likely to abort a pregnancy if it occurs (see Singh, Darroch, and Frost [2001] for a review).

18. Bearman, Moody, and Stovel 2004.

19. Armstrong and Hamilton 2013; Armstrong, Hamilton, Armstrong, and Seeley 2014; England, Shafer, and Fogarty 2007. Even during college, Barriger and Vélez-Blasini (2013) found that students overestimate the degree to which their peers are hooking up.

20. For example, Borsari and Carey 2003; Settersten 2004. Descriptive and injunctive norms are distinct and can differ in their implications for behavior (Barriger and Vélez-Blasini 2013; Mead, Rimal, Ferrence, and Cohen 2014). In the theory of normative social behavior, Rimal and Real (2005) used injunctive norms together with perceived benefits and group identities to moderate the relationship between descriptive norms and intended behaviors, succeeding in strongly predicting college students' intentions to drink alcohol.

21. Faris 2012; Schneider and Stevenson 2000.

22. Physical proximity increases conformity to norms, as does group cohesiveness (Lott and Lott 1961; Macy 1991; Milgram 1965).

23. Kreager and Staff 2009.

24. Willer, Kuwabara, and Macy 2009.

25. Goffman 2009.

26. Armstrong, Hamilton, Armstrong, and Seeley 2014; Pascoe 2007.

27. Bettie 2003.

28. Armstrong, Hamilton, Armstrong, and Seeley 2014; Pascoe 2007.

29. Armstrong, Hamilton, Armstrong, and Seeley 2014.

30. Hardy and Zabin 1991.

31. Erdmans and Black 2015.

32. Lott and Lott 1961; Milgram 1965.

33. Willer, Kuwabara, and Macy 2009.

34. Faris and Felmlee (2011) have found that social aggression is widespread among teens, with those in the middle of a status hierarchy generally more aggressive than those at the very bottom or top. Faris (2012) found that unlike some other types of aggression, aggression toward another teen's reputation can increase a young person's social status in a hierarchy. This may help explain the high levels of social exclusion my interviewees described.

CHAPTER 5

1. Legally, religious organizations are treated equally with other student organizations in their access to facilities at public secondary schools. However, the organization needs to be student-led, and non-student leaders cannot participate in group meetings at the school (Equal Access Act of 1984, see 20 U.S. Code § 4071).

2. For example, schools have been found to be more influential than neighborhoods for understanding whether teens have sex (Teitler and Weiss 2000). My coauthors and I have found that school-level norms against teen pregnancy and school-level consensus about those norms combine to influence the prevalence of student pregnancies in schools (Mollborn, Domingue, and Boardman 2014b).

3. Bearman, Moody, and Stovel 2004; Ford, Sohn, and Lepkowski 2001.

4. Bettie 2003.

5. Lareau 2011.

6. Moody 2001.

7. Most interviewees in the college sample were White and most teen parent interviewees were not, leading to perspectives in the different samples on race relations within schools that are more one-sided than would be ideal.

8. Bettie 2003; García 2012.

9. Bettie 2003; Espiritu 2001; Lamont and Molnár 2002; McCormack 2005; Myers and Williamson 2001; Thorne 1993. Link and Phelan (2014) call the use of stigma as a resource deployed by a higher-status group to retain power over a lower-status group "stigma power." Teen pregnancy stigma seems like a clear case of stigma power at work.

10. Although some social scientists would argue that the boundary work being done on either side of a social divide can strengthen norms within each of the groups (Lamont and Molnár 2002; Thorne 1993), others focus on how a lack of consensus about the social norms within the school can lead to overall cultural heterogeneity that weakens norms. The idea of anomie, or a lack of social control, comes from Emile Durkheim's (1951) work more than a century ago. Durkheim thought that as people left traditional communities and moved to heterogeneous cities, they would be less bound by social norms regulating their behavior. More recently, the concept of "cultural heterogeneity" resulting in lower levels of norm enforcement has been studied by David Harding (2007, 2011). When people have multiple cultural "scripts" or "frames" (which may include norms) to choose among, they are less bound by the rules of any one particular group. In culturally heterogeneous contexts there is less consensus about teen sexuality norms.

This is true of schools that have one or more social divides, especially if the divide is structured around a malleable characteristic such as political ideology, rather than a less flexible one like parental SES or race. In such schools, teenagers may decide to join friendship groups or subcultures based in part on their norms about sexuality. Sociologist Amy Wilkins (2008) has shown how some middle-class White youth choose to join subcultures with their own sexuality norms, such as Goths or Evangelical Christian youth groups, as a way of creating a social identity that solves identity problems for them. One of these problems for many of her interviewees is that their sexual behavior doesn't fit conventional norms in their community—such as bisexual attraction or a desire to remain abstinent in college. They choose a subculture that fits their needs and are then socialized into conforming to the group's sexuality norms. The existence of these culturally heterogeneous groups allows them to violate conventional sex norms while still having close friends who don't socially exclude them. Yet in Wilkins's book, it is much harder for White girls who want to cross an ethnic boundary and join a Puerto Rican social group; scornfully labeled as "wannabes," they are largely excluded from both Puerto Rican and White groups. In this way, cultural heterogeneity may or may not lead to a choice of groups—and thereby a choice of social norms—depending on the nature of the social divide in the school. Crossing the ethnic boundary in Rochelle's school would be very difficult, but in Finn's school a "spiteful" attitude against the conservative community was enough to give White middle-class boys access to an alternative friendship group with more lenient norms about sex.

11. Although more research is needed, Beltz, Sacks, Moore, and Terzian (2015) have found that some state-level policies are associated with lower teen birth rates. These include access to contraception and policies to improve or expand public education. The relationship of state-level policies around public assistance, sex education, and abortion access with teen birth rates is inconclusive.

12. These newer bills legislate a comprehensive sex education approach rather than abstinence-only instruction. See Bartels (2013) and House Bill 07-1292 (2007).

13. I don't have enough data to address whether community members see schools as the most appropriate reinforcers of the future narrative, but Fields's (2008) work suggests that they do.

14. Liam identified the school's normative messages (at least in retrospect) as "propaganda," whereas others did not have a similar perspective and reinforced messages from high school (e.g., contrasting "good" and "bad" kids as Alana did) when being interviewed as college students. I don't have the data available to explore why these two groups differed, but it's possible that the former group no longer internalized the norms of their high school community while the latter group still did.

15. As of 2016, 23 states required sex education in public schools, and 33 states required HIV/AIDS education (National Conference of State Legislatures 2016).

16. In 2015, 35 states allowed parents to opt out of sex education (National Conference of State Legislatures 2015).

17. Fields 2005, 2008; Irvine 2004.

18. It is interesting to note that even though a moral rationale is being communicated, the practical language of safety is being used.

19. Researchers have called for hidden and explicit agendas for education about sex to be studied together (Fields, Gilbert, and Miller 2015).

20. García 2009.

21. For more information about the racialization of sex education in the United States, see García (2012).

22. Title IX of the Education Amendments of 1972 prohibits gender discrimination in public education. In particular, pregnant and parenting students are protected from discrimination and may not be excluded from school activities. They may not be expelled from public schools, and if they voluntarily decide to transfer to another school, it should provide comparable programming (ED.gov n.d.).

23. Wooten 2006.

24. For example, after pressure from the National Women's Law Center in 2011, the state of Michigan amended its educational policy on educational instruction for homebound or hospitalized students. This policy had previously explicitly excluded pregnant students and new mothers (National Women's Law Center 2011).

25. All school names have been changed to avoid identifying interviewees.

26. While schools' use of alternative programs in their district as a way of pushing pregnant girls out of mainstream schools is problematic in many ways, I'm not arguing that these alternative programs themselves are a problem. On the contrary, the interviews with teen mothers suggest that alternative programs offer young mothers an opportunity to learn in a normative climate that

does not treat them as deviant and that provides material support tailored to their needs, often resulting in their greater academic success (Mollborn 2011).

27. BBC News 2008; Kingsbury 2008.

28. In 2011, the number of births per 1,000 women aged 18 and 19 was 54, compared to 15 at ages 15 to 17 (Martin et al. 2015).

29. As Horowitz (1995) shows, this depends in part on the relationships between the young mothers and the program staff. An accepting and supportive relationship, rather than one based around negative sanctioning, can help create a positive environment for teen mothers in segregated programs.

30. Under Title IX law, pregnancy is a medical condition that must be treated like any other condition, with the same opportunities for excused absences and tutoring offered if the student cannot attend school (ED.gov n.d.).

31. Studying the U.S. class of 1992, I found that 75 percent of people who became teen parents at high school age had completed a high school degree or GED certificate by about age 26 (even though only one third were enrolled in school in 1992). This compares to 95 percent of all others (Mollborn 2010a).

32. Christine Horne's (2001b, 2009) program of experimental research has shown the importance of metanorms for understanding interaction in groups.

CHAPTER 6

1. This chapter focuses on "real-world" communities because they were the interviewees' focus, but online communities may be important normative contexts for some people and should be a highlight of future research.

2. Studying norm enforcement in South Africa, Kocher, Martinsson, and Visser (2012) found that different school communities, even within the same city, had strong differences in norm enforcement, which could be explained by factors like social capital in the community.

3. National statistics back up Isaac's observation about teen pregnancies disproportionately occurring in the context of committed relationships (Hardy and Zabin 1991).

4. Talbot 2008.

5. Strayhorn and Strayhorn 2009.

6. Letting people define their communities themselves is helpful for three reasons. First, research on neighborhoods has shown that objective definitions of neighborhoods—such as census tracts—often do not match individuals' own definitions of their communities (Sampson 1997; Sampson, Morenoff, and Gannon-Rowley 2002). These definitions are often less useful outside of cities, in rural and suburban areas. Second, people researching health and SES have often found subjective definitions to be powerful over and above objective ones (Idler and Benyamini 1997; Ostrove, Adler, Kuppermann, and Washington 2000; Singh-Manoux, Marmot, and Adler 2005). Third, interviewees' own definitions of their communities differed widely, sometimes centered around a school or a religious organization, sometimes a neighborhood or a network of families within a geographic area, and sometimes a whole town.

7. See Christie Sennott's and my work (2011) for a comparison of adults', peers', and close friends' norms in some of these communities.

8. Because teens' own sexual behaviors were a taboo topic in many schools and friendship groups, estimates like Isaac's are bound to be imprecise, but teens' general perceptions of each other's behaviors are still an important piece of information for understanding normative contexts.

9. I didn't approach these interviews expecting to find sets of norms regulating teens' sexual behaviors, nor did I think communities would fall into groups based on their norms and prevalent teen sexual behaviors. But that is what Christie Sennott and I (2015) found after analyzing young people's accounts.

10. A few interviewees' communities didn't fit neatly into any of the community types, and sometimes specific features of the community's norms and behaviors fell outside the ideal types described here. But almost all interviewees' descriptions of their communities fit into one of the four categories. For each community type, I include two examples to illustrate sets of norms and metanorms and the prevalent behaviors perceived by interviewees. It's possible that communities with stronger norms against teen pregnancy might have worked harder to hide teen pregnancies through abortion or through girls leaving their school, resulting in the prevalence of teen pregnancy seeming lower than it actually was.

11. Gold et al. (2001) found higher county-level income predicted lower teen birth rates. For girls ages 15 to 17 but not 18 and 19, income inequality was also associated with higher teen birth rates.

12. The ethnographic literature has been divided on the issue of whether some U.S. communities view teen parenthood as a positive life event. Some scholars assert that the communities they studied view teen pregnancy as positive. For discussions, see Burton (1990); Contreras et al. (1999); and Henly (1997). Others maintain that similar communities do not view teen pregnancy positively. See Kaplan (1997) and Mollborn and Jacobs (2012).

13. Because the interviewees were mostly White college students, even though they came from a fairly diverse set of communities, the percentage of interviewees in each community type doesn't likely reflect the actual distribution of these communities in the United States. More privileged communities are overrepresented.

14. David Harding (2007) has documented cultural heterogeneity in disadvantaged neighborhoods like these that leads to diverse frames and scripts, which control teens' sexual behavior more weakly than in more homogeneous neighborhoods.

15. García 2009, 2012.

16. Mollborn 2011; see Penman-Aguilar, Carter, Snead, and Kourtis (2013) for a discussion.

17. For example, Mann (2013) found that reproductive healthcare providers highlighted the importance of teen pregnancy as a social problem for the low-income Latina teens they served, and they sought to prevent teen pregnancy among this population.

18. In fact, a large body of research has found that the actual consequences of teen childbearing are only slightly negative on average compared to similar teens who do not have children. For a review, see Hoffman (1998).

19. It's important to note that these efforts often didn't work, as teen sex and parenthood are more prevalent in places with the demographic characteristics of "it could be you" communities than in many other places.

20. Regnerus (2007) detailed the moral objections that many Christian groups have to premarital teen sex, and he also distinguished between "religious" and "secular" motivations for sexual decision making among teens that mirror the moral and practical rationales common in my study.

21. Denial of "moral responsibility" for one's actions is associated with a weakened link between internalized norms and behavior (Schwartz and Howard 1980).

22. Confirming this dynamic in a region of the United States that had limited representation in my sample, Smith et al. (2016) found that low-income women in Birmingham, Alabama, perceived community norms that discouraged unintended pregnancy but that more strongly discouraged abortion if such a pregnancy occurred.

23. AdoptED n.d.

24. Although it may sound like Annika is describing a community in which at least some older people encourage teen pregnancy, in her interview it was clear that people were not prescribing pregnancy for teens. Rather, once a teen had violated pro-abstinence norms and gotten pregnant, some people were "excited" that she had chosen to give birth rather than get an abortion.

25. Wilson 1987.

26. Uecker and Stokes 2008.

27. Jones, Zolna, Henshaw, and Finer 2008.

28. As Chapter 3 showed, the willingness to discuss teen pregnancy among families and friends that Isaac described was unusual.

29. Benard (2012) has found that when multiple groups in a social setting are in conflict, norm enforcement within groups also increases.

30. Lamont and Molnár 2002.

31. Bash 2008. Jamie Lynn Spears was another celebrity who carried a teen pregnancy to term in 2008, and Breese (2010) has argued that these media events opened up space for public debate around teen pregnancy that may have led to changes in norms.

32. A third institution, law enforcement, is also important but was brought up by fewer interviewees. They talked about the police's role in monitoring teens who were out in public, constraining available places for sexual activity, and in particular keeping an eye on gathering places among teens of color. But most interviewees didn't explicitly identify law enforcement's role in enforcing community sexuality norms.

33. Legally, this is permissible as long as the youth group is student-run. If adults run the organization's meetings, it must not be on school grounds (20 U.S. Code § 4071).

34. Bailey 1989; Solinger 1992.

35. Phillip 2013.

36. It's important to note that like many other male interviewees, Logan anticipated severe sanctions if he were to become a father—suggesting that they aren't limited to girls.

37. Goffman 2009.

38. It's also surprising that interviewees seldom mention media influences, but as they were not an explicit part of the interview guide, they are not the main focus of this discussion.

39. David Harding's (2007) work on cultural heterogeneity finds that social control is weaker when young people are acting within competing cultural frames. His work focuses on competing frames within communities and on low-income communities in particular, but I maintain the same logic can be applied to all teens at the broad societal level.

Evidence on sexual minority youth has found that these young people are likely to move to more politically liberal, urbanized environments as they transition from adolescence to young adulthood. These moves are also associated with improvements in young people's mental health (Everett 2014). I argue that these moves illustrate young people's strategy of seeking out more understanding reference groups that better support their sexuality—they know there are multiple normative contexts around sexual behavior available in U.S. society.

CHAPTER 7

1. Sociologist Lorena García (2012) has studied how Latina teen girls, in particular, navigate the reputational risks of sex to express sexual agency.

2. The very real problem of sexual abuse experienced by many young people doesn't come up much in my interviews, so I can only speak to voluntary sexual behaviors here (Hussey, Chang, and Kotch 2006).

3. Autor, Katz, and Kearney 2008; Hout 2012.

4. Cook, Emerson, Gillmore, and Yamagishi 1983; Cook and Whitmeyer 1992.

5. There are exceptions, such as Finn, who had sex as part of a revolt against the community he and his close friends engaged in—and a supportive friendship group is often important for helping young people in non-normative subcultures manage the negative sanctions others levy against them (Wilkins 2008).

6. It's important to note that other teens who did violate norms against teen parenthood would have been much less likely to make it to a four-year residential college and join my sample.

7. Finer and Zolna 2011.

8. Mollborn and Jacobs 2012.

9. Mollborn 2007, 2009; Mollborn and Jacobs 2012.

10. Eaton et al. 2012.

11. Cesario and Hughes 2007.

12. Rosenfeld 2009.

13. Carpenter 2005; Pascoe 2007.

14. Windle 2003.

15. Schneider and Stevenson 2000.

16. Mercken, Snijders, Steglich, Vartiainen, and de Vries 2010; Schneider and Stevenson 2000.

17. This is what classic conceptions of social norms would expect them to. But especially because I talked to interviewees after their sexual behavior already happened, I can't disentangle these motivations from the other way norms affect teens—by shaping their after-the-fact justifications for why they behaved the way they did. This is the newer view of social norms articulated by sociologist Ann Swidler (2001) and others (Vaisey 2009). So I can't ask how teens decided how to behave without also asking how they decided to justify the behavior they chose.

18. Swidler 2001. A reminder on the definitions of two related terms: A rationale explains why a norm is appropriate, while a justification explains why a person behaved how they did. People can draw on a rationale when they justify their behavior (e.g., it would have been morally wrong, so I didn't do it).

19. The interviews were done in a different time, place, and climate of sexuality norms than what they experienced during high school, so interviewees' motivation to pretend to adhere to norms and rationales they didn't actually agree with should have been weak in the interviews.

20. Sennott and Mollborn 2011.

21. Camryn did believe that a lack of useful information in sex education was a major problem for teens, and she critiqued her community's bias toward ignoring homosexual sex and relationships. Because Camryn had critical ideas in other areas, her silence about the norm against teen sex and the "being smart" rationale makes me more likely to conclude that she had internalized both.

22. Marini 1984; Neugarten, Moore, and Lowe 1965.

23. Sennott and Mollborn 2011.

24. Abstinent youth often drew on close friends as influences for their behavior, but not the wider peer group.

25. Marini 1984; Settersten 2004.

26. Schalet 2011.

27. Bierbrauer 1992; Conlin, Lynn, and O'Donoghue 2003.

28. "Defensive othering" is when people disassociate themselves from stereotypes about people like them (Schwalbe et al. 2000).

29. The peer interviewer's question was leading here.

30. The interviewees who inconsistently used contraception were evenly split by gender.

31. Uecker, Angotti, and Regnerus 2008.

32. However, this may be because almost all of the college students' high school relationships were now over, while some of the teen parents' relationships were not, and even if they were, the ex-partners were still their children's other biological parents.

33. Risman and Schwartz 2002.

34. Bearman and Brückner (2001) confirmed this dynamic in a nationally representative sample, finding that teens who publicly pledged to remain virgins until marriage were less likely than others to use contraception when first having sex.

35. Welti, Wildsmith, and Manlove (2011) found that teens were more likely than young adults to have used condoms, but teen women were less likely than young adult women to have used hormonal/long-acting contraceptive methods.

36. Despite stereotypes, teens tend to be similar to adults in their perceptions of vulnerability to risks (Quadrel, Fischhoff, and Davis 1993).

37. Although the efficacy of withdrawal is usually lower than for contraceptives, it does decrease the risk of pregnancy compared to no method at all (Kost et al. 2008).

38. Trussell 2004.

39. Ostrom 2014; Tarrow and Tollefson 1994.

40. The lack of unmonitored time experienced by the teens Finn is discussing is a fairly recent phenomenon and is socially classed—parenting with constant monitoring is resource intensive.

41. In some settings there are social upsides within boys' peer groups of claiming to be sexually active (e.g., Pascoe 2007), but in my interviews this was often tempered by boys' fear of adults' reactions.

42. Cromwell and Thurman 2003; Klockars 1974; Shigihara 2013; Sykes and Matza 1957.

43. Bettie 2003.

44. Because the college students didn't publicly violate sexuality norms, I rely mostly on teen parents' accounts of attempted strategies for minimizing negative sanctions and on primary interviewees' accounts for reactions to these strategies.

45. This fits with Sykes and Matza's (1957) idea of "denial of responsibility" as a technique for neutralizing deviant behavior.

46. These rumors were likely inaccurate because so many teen pregnancies occur within the context of a long-term romantic relationship (Hardy and Zabin 1991; Mollborn and Jacobs 2015).

47. This behavior has been described through the concepts of "defensive othering" and the "metaphor of the ledger" (Eliason and Dodder 1999; Klockars 1974; Schwalbe et al. 2000).

48. High levels of monitoring and intensive parenting are relatively recent and socially classed phenomena (LeMoyne and Buchanan 2011).

49. García 2012.

CHAPTER 8

1. Elder 1994, 1998; Pavalko and Caputo 2013; Settersten 2004; Shanahan 2000. Within the realm of sexualities, newer research (e.g., Carpenter and Delamater 2013; Diefendorf 2015; Montemurro 2014) is emphasizing continuity and change across phases of the life course in a way that my data cannot allow.

2. Furstenberg 2003.

3. Marini 1984.

4. Talbot 2008.

5. Hoffman 2008; CDC n.d.

6. Darroch, Singh, and Frost 2001; Hoffman 2008.

7. Boonstra 2014; CDC n.d.

8. The 2013 teen birth rate was 26.5 births per 1,000 girls aged 15 to 19, compared to 39.1 in 2009 (Martin et al. 2011, 2015).

9. Boonstra 2014.

10. U.S. Department of Labor 2015a, 2015b.

11. Martin et al. 2015.

12. Sobotka, Skirbekk, and Philipov 2011.

13. Stein 2010.

14. Boonstra 2014.

15. Ibid.

16. Hamilton et al. 2015; Ricketts, Klingler, and Schwalberg 2014.

17. Verlee 2015.

18. Bearman and Brückner 2001.

19. National Campaign to Prevent Teen and Unplanned Pregnancy 2014.

20. Tavernise 2015.

21. Taylor 1995; Tinkler 2003.

22. Kearney and Levine 2015.

23. Mollborn 2010b; Sucoff and Upchurch 1998. Cherry and Wang (2014) found that teen birth rates were negatively related to real minimum wage but were sometimes (perhaps surprisingly) positively correlated with local employment rates for young women and men.

24. Kirby 2002.

25. For a review, see Kirby (2002).

26. World Bank Group 2016. Comparative data on teen pregnancy and abortion rates are outdated, so I don't present them here.

27. Teens engaging in same-sex activity may particularly need barrier methods of contraception, but recent research has shown that sexual minority girls are at higher risk of pregnancy than heterosexual girls, so healthcare providers should tailor their efforts to the particular teen's needs (Lindley and Walsemann 2015).

28. Trussell 2004.

29. Forhan et al. 2009.

30. Although the Affordable Care Act has expanded contraceptive coverage and reduced costs, not all methods are covered, and parents can often see what medical charges are being billed to their insurance.

31. Statistics are from 2011 for contraceptive use at most recent sexual intercourse; see Eaton et al. (2012).

32. Elliott 2012. Research also suggests that programs to improve parent–teen communication around sex can be quite successful (Santa Maria, Markham, Bluethmann, and Mullen 2015).

33. This message primarily targets older teens.

34. Sennott and Mollborn 2011.

35. Schalet 2011.

36. This is the concept of sexual autonomy that Amy Schalet (2011) lays out and argues Dutch parents already teach.

37. Bearman and Brückner 2001.

38. Albert 2007.

39. Liptak 2014.

40. Jones and Dreweke 2011.

41. Schalet 2011.

42. For a discussion, see Tinkler (2012).

43. For example, 6 percent of high school students in 2013 first had sexual intercourse at age 12 or younger; see CDC (n.d.).

44. Guttmacher et al. 1997.

45. Albert 2007.

46. For an example, see the program making long-acting reversible contraception methods available to low-income young women summarized in Ricketts, Klingler, and Schwalberg (2014).

47. Boulder County Public Health 2014; Peers Building Justice n.d.

48. Paluck and Shepherd (2012) found in a field experiment with high school students that if a subset of students changed their public harassment behaviors, peers' perceived school collective norms about harassment began to change. Everyday interpersonal interaction was the driver of this change.

49. Pew Research Center 2014.

50. Milbank 2014.

51. Common Core n.d.

APPENDIX

1. This interview was part of a graded research project for the courses, one of which was taught by a colleague and the other by me. Students could choose an alternative assignment instead of conducting the interview, and they or the interviewee could choose not to release the interview data to this research project. To avoid the possibility that students would feel coerced into releasing the data, this decision was not made known to the course instructor or me until after final grades had been submitted.

2. Students were graded on the quality of their interviews and supporting materials, as well as on a paper analyzing their interview and linking it to course materials.

3. England, Shafer, and Fogarty 2007; Tinkler 2012.

4. This strategy of "sampling for range" is useful when a particular subgroup has been identified that is important for understanding the phenomenon at hand (Small 2009).

5. Reichertz 2007.

6. Here is an example of this process at work, from the interview with Finn (after he talked about his community taking a practical approach to encouraging condom use):

So often in communities where I'm hearing this really practical attitude toward condoms, it's in places where teachers and parents are fairly resigned to the fact that teens are sexually active. Was that the case here?

Yeah. They accepted it. They never made a conscious effort to stop it because they would be chastised by the teens probably. They had the power. So if the parent was like, "Don't have sex," the teen would be like, "You're so stupid, shut up." At the same time, the smarter parents would be like, "All right, boys and girls can come over and do stuff, but leave the door open in the room. We know you're going to go in the room; just leave the door open." It was like, I guess, sort of common. It was mainly like, we weren't put in very many situations where it was possible. We don't have cars. If you do have a car we're on base and freaked out about the law. Yet to go somewhere, you don't have a bed anywhere. You have to be in the perfect scenario because every girl has grown up in this romantic paradigm, . . . it has to be perfect, you know, a beautiful bed. And so all these situations have to be good.

7. Small 2009.

8. Catania, Gibson, Chitwood, and Coates 1990; Graham et al. 2003.

9. Austin, Roberts, Corliss, and Molnar 2008; Berlan et al. 2010; Mollborn and Everett 2015.

10. Mollborn 2010a.

11. One pilot interview, recruited through a personal contact, was conducted in the first author's office.

12. Child Trends 2009.

13. Ibid.

14. Ibid.

15. Ibid.

16. Becker 1996; Small 2009.

17. For perspectives on ongoing debates about measurement and methodology in cultural and qualitative sociology, see Berezin (2014); Jerolmack and Khan (2014); Lamont and Swidler (2014); and Pugh (2013).

18. Jacobs and Mollborn 2012; Mollborn 2011; Mollborn and Jacobs 2012, 2015.

19. Small 2009.

20. Schalet 2011.

21. Becker 1996.

References

20 U.S. Code § 4071 (1984)—Denial of Equal Access Prohibited. Cornell University Law School. Retrieved from: https://www.law.cornell.edu/uscode/text/20/4071.

Abma, Joyce C., Gladys M. Martinez, William D. Mosher, and Brittany S. Dawson. 2004. "Teenagers in the United States: Sexual Activity, Contraceptive Use, and Childbearing, 2002." *Vital and Health Statistics. Series 23, Data from the National Survey of Family Growth* (24):1–48.

AdoptED. "What Path Would You Make?" Retrieved from: http://adoption-education.com/library_stats.htm.

Advocates for Youth. 2011. "Adolescent Sexual Health in Europe and the U.S.: the Case for a Rights. Respect. Responsibility.® Approach." Retrieved from: http://www.advocatesforyouth.org/publications/419-adolescent-sexual-health-in-europe-and-the-us.

Ajzen, Icek. 1991. "The Theory of Planned Behavior." *Organizational Behavior and Human Decision Processes* 50(2):179–211.

Albert, Bill. 2007. "With One Voice 2007: America's Adults and Teens Sound Off About Teen Pregnancy." Washington, D.C.: National Campaign to Prevent Teen Pregnancy.

Albert, Bill. 2012. "With One Voice 2012: America's Adults and Teens Sound Off About Teen Pregnancy." Washington, D.C.: National Campaign to Prevent Teen Pregnancy.

American Community Survey. 2010. "Figure 1. Median Age at First Marriage by Sex: 1890–2010." Source: U.S. Decennial Census (1890–2000); American Community Survey (2010). Retrieved from: http://www.census.gov/hhes/socdemo/marriage/data/acs/ElliottetalPAA2012figs.pdf.

Anderson, Elijah. 1989. "Sex Codes and Family Life among Poor Inner-City Youths." *Annals of the American Academy of Political and Social Science* 501:59–78.

Anderson, Elijah. 1990. *Streetwise: Race, Class, and Change in an Urban Community.* Chicago: University of Chicago.

Armstrong, Elizabeth A., and Laura T. Hamilton. 2013. *Paying for the Party: How College Maintains Inequality*. Cambridge, MA: Harvard University.

Armstrong, Elizabeth A., Laura T. Hamilton, Elizabeth M. Armstrong, and J. Lotus Seeley. 2014. "'Good Girls': Gender, Social Class, and Slut Discourse on Campus." *Social Psychology Quarterly* 77(2):100–22.

Arnett, Jeffrey Jensen. 2000. "Emerging Adulthood: A Theory of Development from the Late Teens through the Twenties." *American Psychologist* 55(5):469.

Austin, S. Bryn, Andrea L. Roberts, Heather L. Corliss, and Beth E. Molnar. 2008. "Sexual Violence and Victimization History of Sexual Risk Indicators of a Community-Based Urban Cohort of 'Mostly Heterosexual' and Heterosexual Young Women." *American Journal of Public Health* 98(6):1015–20.

Autor, David H., Lawrence F. Katz, and Melissa S. Kearney. 2008. "Trends in US Wage Inequality: Revising the Revisionists." *The Review of Economics and Statistics* 90(2):300–23.

Axelrod, Robert. 1986. "An Evolutionary Approach to Norms." *American Political Science Review* 80(04):1095–111.

Bailey, Beth L. 1989. *From Front Porch to Back Seat: Courtship in Twentieth-Century America*. Baltimore: Johns Hopkins University.

Barriger, Megan, and Carlos J. Vélez-Blasini. 2013. "Descriptive and Injunctive Social Norm Overestimation in Hooking up and Their Role as Predictors of Hook-Up Activity in a College Student Sample." *Journal of Sex Research* 50(1):84–94.

Bartels, Lynn. 2013. "Colorado House Passes Sex Ed Bill over Republicans' Objections." *Denver Post*. Retrieved from: http://www.denverpost.com/ci_22648570/colorado-house-passes-sex-ed-bill-over-republicans.

Bash, Dana. 2008. "Palin's Teen Daughter Is Pregnant." CNN.com. Retrieved from: http://www.cnn.com/2008/POLITICS/09/01/palin.daughter/.

BBC News. 2008. "US Fears of Teen 'Pregnancy Pact.'" Retrieved from: http://news.bbc.co.uk/2/hi/americas/7464925.stm.

Bearman, Peter S., James Moody, and Katherine Stovel. 2004. "Chains of Affection: The Structure of Adolescent Romantic and Sexual Networks." *American Journal of Sociology* 110(1):44–91.

Bearman, Peter S., and Hannah Brückner. 2001. "Promising the Future: Virginity Pledges and First Intercourse." *American Journal of Sociology* 106(4):859–912.

Becker, Howard S. 1996. "The Epistemology of Qualitative Research." Pp. 53–71 in *Ethnography and Human Development: Context and Meaning in Social Inquiry*, edited by R. Jessor, A. Colby, and R. A. Shweder. Chicago: University of Chicago.

Beersma, Bianca, and Gerben A. van Kleef. 2011. "How the Grapevine Keeps You in Line: Gossip Increases Contributions to the Group." *Social Psychological and Personality Science* 2(6):642–49.

Bell, David C., and Mary L. Cox. 2015. "Social Norms: Do We Love Norms Too Much?" *Journal of Family Theory & Review* 7(1):28–46.

Beltz, Martha A., Vanessa H. Sacks, Kristin A. Moore, and Mary Terzian. 2015. "State Policy and Teen Childbearing: A Review of Research Studies." *Journal of Adolescent Health* 56(2):130–38.

Benard, Stephen. 2012. "Cohesion from Conflict: Does Intergroup Conflict Motivate Intragroup Norm Enforcement and Support for Centralized Leadership?" *Social Psychology Quarterly* 75(2):107–30.

Bendor, Jonathan, and Piotr Swistak. 2001. "The Evolution of Norms." *American Journal of Sociology* 106(6):1493–545.

Berezin, Mabel. 2014. "How Do We Know What We Mean? Epistemological Dilemmas in Cultural Sociology." *Qualitative Sociology* 37(2):141–51.

Berlan, Elise D., Heather L. Corliss, Alison E. Field, Elizabeth Goodman, and S. Bryn Austin. 2010. "Sexual Orientation and Bullying among Adolescents in the Growing Up Today Study." *Journal of Adolescent Health* 46(4):366–71.

Bettie, Julie. 2003. *Women without Class: Girls, Race, and Identity.* Berkeley: University of California.

Bicchieri, Cristina. 2006. *The Grammar of Society: The Nature and Dynamics of Social Norms.* Cambridge, UK: Cambridge University.

Bierbrauer, Günter. 1992. "Reactions to Violation of Normative Standards: A Cross-Cultural Analysis of Shame and Guilt." *International Journal of Psychology* 27(2):181–93.

Birkett, Michelle, Dorothy L. Espelage, and Brian Koenig. 2009. "LGB and Questioning Students in Schools: The Moderating Effects of Homophobic Bullying and School Climate on Negative Outcomes." *Journal of Youth and Adolescence* 38(7):989–1000.

Black, Donald J. 1993. *The Social Structure of Right and Wrong.* San Diego: Academic.

Bogle, Kathleen A. 2008. *Hooking Up: Sex, Dating, and Relationships on Campus.* New York: New York University.

Boonstra, Heather D. 2014. "What Is behind the Declines in Teen Pregnancy Rates?" Guttmacher Institute. *Guttmacher Policy Review* 17(3). Retrieved from: http://www.guttmacher.org/pubs/gpr/17/3/gpr170315.html.

Borsari, Brian, and Kate B. Carey. 2003. "Descriptive and Injunctive Norms in College Drinking: A Meta-Analytic Integration." *Journal of Studies on Alcohol* 64(3):331.

Boulder County Public Health. 2014. "2013 Boulder County Public Health (BCPH) Annual Report." Program number 460: GENESIS Program. April 30, 2014. Retrieved from: http://www.bouldercounty.org/doc/publichealth/genesisannualreport2013.pdf.

Bowles, Hannah Riley, and Michele Gelfand. 2009. "Status and the Evaluation of Workplace Deviance." *Psychological Science* 21(1):49–54.

boyd, danah. 2014. *It's Complicated: The Social Lives of Networked Teens.* New Haven, CT: Yale University.

Breese, Elizabeth Butler. 2010. "Meaning, Celebrity, and the Underage Pregnancy of Jamie Lynn Spears." *Cultural Sociology* 4(3):337–55.

Brewster, Karin L., John O. G. Billy, and William R. Grady. 1993. "Social Context and Adolescent Behavior: The Impact of Community on the Transition to Sexual Activity." *Social Forces* 71(3):713–40.

Bronfenbrenner, Urie. 1986. "Ecology of the Family as a Context for Human Development: Research Perspectives." *Developmental Psychology* 22(6):723–42.

Brown, Jane D., Jeanne R. Steele, and Kim Walsh-Childers, eds. 2001. *Sexual Teens, Sexual Media: Investigating Media's Influence on Adolescent Sexuality.* London: Routledge.

Brubaker, Sarah Jane, and Christie Wright. 2006. "Identity Transformation and Family Caregiving: Narratives of African American Teen Mothers." *Journal of Marriage and Family* 68(5):1214–28.

Brückner, Hannah, Anne Martin, and Peter S. Bearman. 2004. "Ambivalence and Pregnancy: Adolescents' Attitudes, Contraception Use and Pregnancy." *Perspectives on Sexual and Reproductive Health* 36(6):248–57.

Burton, Linda M. 1990. "Teenage Childbearing as an Alternative Life-Course Strategy in Multigeneration Black Families." *Human Nature* 1(2):123–43.

Cancian, Francesca M. 1975. *What Are Norms? A Study of Beliefs and Action in a Maya Community.* Cambridge, UK: Cambridge University.

Carpenter, Laura. 2005. *Virginity Lost: An Intimate Portrait of First Sexual Experiences.* New York: New York University.

Carpenter, Laura, and John DeLamater, eds. 2013. *Sex for Life: From Virginity to Viagra, How Sexuality Changes throughout Our Lives.* New York: New York University.

Catania, Joseph A., David R. Gibson, Dale D. Chitwood, and Thomas J. Coates. 1990. "Methodological Problems in AIDS Behavioral Research: Influences on Measurement Error and Participation Bias in Studies of Sexual Behavior." *Psychological Bulletin* 108(3):339.

CBS News. 2008. "Teens' Pregnancy Pact Shocks Mass. Town." Retrieved from: http://www.cbsnews.com/news/teens-pregnancy-pact-shocks-mass-town-19-06-2008/.

CDC. 2015. "Results from the School Health Policies and Practices Study 2014." Retrieved from: http://www.cdc.gov/healthyyouth/data/shpps/pdf/shpps-508-final_101315.pdf.

CDC. "Teen Pregnancy Prevention and United States Students: What Is the Problem?" Centers for Disease Control and Prevention. Division of Adolescent and School Health. Retrieved from: http://www.cdc.gov/healthyyouth/data/yrbs/pdf/us_pregnancy_combo.pdf.

Cesario, Sandra K., and Lisa A. Hughes. 2007. "Precocious Puberty: A Comprehensive Review of Literature." *Journal of Obstetric, Gynecologic, & Neonatal Nursing* 36(3):263–74.

Cherlin, Andrew J., Caitlin Cross-Barnet, Linda M. Burton, and Raymond Garrett-Peters. 2008. "Promises They Can Keep: Low-Income Women's Attitudes toward Motherhood, Marriage, and Divorce." *Journal of Marriage and Family* 70(4):919–33.

Cherry, Robert, and Chun Wang. 2014. "Labor Market Conditions and US Teen Birth Rates, 2001–2009." *Journal of Family and Economic Issues* 36(3):408–20.

Child Trends. 2009. "Facts at a Glance: A Fact Sheet Reporting National, State, and City Trends in Teen Childbearing." Publication #2009-25. Washington, D.C.: Child Trends. Retrieved from: http://www.childtrends.org/wp-content/uploads/2009/09/2009-25FAAG2009.pdf.

Child Trends Databank. 2014. "Sexually Active Teens." Retrieved from: http://www.childtrends.org/?indicators=sexually-active-teens.

CNN Money. 2015. "Minimum Wage since 1938." Retrieved from: http://money.cnn.com/interactive/economy/minimum-wage-since-1938/.

College Board. 2014. "Trends in College Pricing 2014." Retrieved from: http://trends.collegeboard.org/college-pricing.

Common Core. "Preparing America's Students for Success." Retrieved from: http://www.corestandards.org/.

Conlin, Michael, Michael Lynn, and Ted O'Donoghue. 2003. "The Norm of Restaurant Tipping." *Journal of Economic Behavior & Organization* 52(3):297–321.

Contreras, Josefina M., Sarah C. Mangelsdorf, Jean E. Rhodes, Marissa L. Diener, and Liesette Brunson. 1999. "Parent-Child Interaction among Latina Adolescent Mothers: The Role of Family and Social Support." *Journal of Research on Adolescence* 9(4):417–39.

Cook, Karen S., Richard M. Emerson, Mary R. Gillmore, and Toshio Yamagishi. 1983. "The Distribution of Power in Exchange Networks: Theory and Experimental Results." *American Journal of Sociology* 89(2):275–305.

Cook, Karen S., and Joseph M. Whitmeyer. 1992. "Two Approaches to Social Structure: Exchange Theory and Network Analysis." *Annual Review of Sociology* 18:109–27.

Coontz, Stephanie. 1992. *The Way We Never Were: American Families and the Nostalgia Trap.* New York: Basic Books.

Coyne, Claire A., and Brian M. D'Onofrio. 2012. "Some (but Not Much) Progress toward Understanding Teenage Childbearing: A Review of Research from the Past Decade." *Advances in Child Development and Behavior* 42:113–52.

Cromwell, Paul and Quint Thurman. 2003. "The Devil Made Me Do It: Use of Neutralizations by Shoplifters." *Deviant Behavior* 24(6):535–50.

Currier, Danielle M. 2013. "Strategic Ambiguity: Protecting Emphasized Femininity and Hegemonic Masculinity in the Hookup Culture." *Gender & Society* 27(5):704–27.

Darroch, Jacqueline E., Susheela Singh, and Jennifer J. Frost. 2001. "Differences in Teenage Pregnancy Rates among Five Developed Countries: The Roles of Sexual Activity and Contraceptive Use." *Family Planning Perspectives* 33(6):244–50, 81.

Diefendorf, Sarah. 2015. "After the Wedding Night: Sexual Abstinence and Masculinities over the Life Course." *Gender & Society* 29(5):647–69.

Ducker, Brittany. 2007. "Overcoming the Hurdles: Title IX and Equal Educational Attainment for Pregnant and Parenting Students." *Journal of Law & Education* 36(3):445–52.

Durkheim, Émile. 1951 (original work published 1897). *Suicide: A Study in Sociology.* Glencoe, IL: Free.

Eaton, Danice K., Laura Kann, Steve Kinchen, Shari Shanklin, Katherine H. Flint, Joseph Hawkins, William A. Harris, Richard Lowry, Tim McManus, David Chyen, Lisa Whittle, Connie Lim, and Howell Wechsler. 2012. "Youth Risk Behavior Surveillance—United States, 2011." *Morbidity and Mortality Weekly Report. Surveillance Summaries* 61(4):1–162. Retrieved from: http://www.cdc.gov/mmwr/pdf/ss/ss6104.pdf.

ED.gov. "Title 34 Education." U.S. Department of Education. Retrieved from: http://www2.ed.gov/policy/rights/reg/ocr/edlite-34cfr106.html-S40.

ED.gov. "106.40: Marital or Parental Status." U.S. Department of Education Subpart D—Discrimination on the Basis of Sex in Education Programs or Activities Prohibited. Retrieved from: http://www2.ed.gov/policy/rights/reg/ocr/edlite-34cfr106.html#S40.

Edin, Kathryn, and Maria Kefalas. 2005. *Promises I Can Keep: Why Poor Women Put Motherhood before Marriage.* Berkeley: University of California.

Elder, Glen H., Jr. 1994. "Time, Human Agency, and Social Change: Perspectives on the Life Course." *Social Psychology Quarterly* 57(1):4–15.

Elder, Glen H., Jr. 1998. "The Life Course as Developmental Theory." *Child Development* 69(1):1–12.

Eliason, Stephen L., and Richard A. Dodder. 1999. "Techniques of Neutralization Used by Deer Poachers in the Western United States: A Research Note." *Deviant Behavior* 20(3):233–52.

Elliott, Sinikka. 2010. "Parents' Constructions of Teen Sexuality: Sex Panics, Contradictory Discourses, and Social Inequality." *Symbolic Interaction* 33(2):191–212.

Elliott, Sinikka. 2012. *Not My Kid: What Parents Believe about the Sex Lives of Their Teenagers.* New York: New York University.

Elster, Jon. 2009. "Social Norms." Pp. 195–217 in *The Oxford Handbook of Analytical Sociology,* edited by P. Hedström and P. Bearman. New York: Oxford University.

Emirbayer, Mustafa, and Ann Mische. 1998. "What Is Agency?" *American Journal of Sociology* 103(4):962–1023.

England, Paula, Emily Fitzgibbons Shafer, and Alison C. K. Fogarty. 2007. "Hooking up and Forming Romantic Relationships on Today's College Campuses." Pp. 531–47 in *The Gendered Society Reader*, edited by M. S. Kimmel and A. Aronson. New York: Oxford University.

Erdmans, Mary Patrice, and Timothy Black. 2015. *On Becoming a Teen Mom: Life before Pregnancy*. Berkeley: University of California.

Espiritu, Yen Le. 2001. "'We Don't Sleep Around Like White Girls Do': Family, Culture, and Gender in Filipina American Lives." *Signs* 26(2):415–40.

Everett, Bethany. 2015. "Sexual Orientation Identity Change and Depressive Symptoms: A Longitudinal Analysis." *Journal of Health and Social Behavior* 56(1):37–58.

Everett, Bethany G. 2014. "Changes in Neighborhood Characteristics and Depression among Sexual Minority Young Adults." *Journal of the American Psychiatric Nurses Association* 20(1):42–52.

Faris, Robert. 2012. "Aggression, Exclusivity, and Status Attainment in Interpersonal Networks." *Social Forces* 90(4):1207–35.

Faris, Robert, and Diane Felmlee. 2011. "Status Struggles: Network Centrality and Gender Segregation in Same- and Cross-Gender Aggression." *American Sociological Review* 76(1):48–73.

Feldman, Daniel C. 1984. "The Development and Enforcement of Group Norms." *Academy of Management Review* 9(1):47–53.

Fields, Jessica. 2005. "'Children Having Children': Race, Innocence, and Sexuality Education." *Social Problems* 52(4):549–71.

Fields, Jessica. 2008. *Risky Lessons: Sex Education and Social Inequality*. New Brunswick, NJ: Rutgers University.

Fields, Jessica, Jen Gilbert, and Michelle Miller. 2015. "Sexuality and Education: Toward the Promise of Ambiguity." Pp. 371–87 in *Handbook of the Sociology of Sexualities*, edited by J. DeLamater and R. F. Plante. New York: Springer.

Fine, Gary Alan. 2001. "Enacting Norms: Mushrooming and the Culture of Expectations and Explanations." Pp. 139–64 in *Social Norms*, edited by M. Hechter and K.-D. Opp. New York: Russell Sage Foundation.

Fine, Gary Alan. 2014. "The Hinge: Civil Society, Group Culture, and the Interaction Order." *Social Psychology Quarterly* 77(1):5–26.

Fine, Gary Alan, and Brooke Harrington. 2004. "Tiny Publics: Small Groups and Civil Society." *Sociological Theory* 22(3):341–56.

Fine, Michelle. 1988. "Sexuality, Schooling, and Adolescent Females: The Missing Discourse of Desire." *Harvard Educational Review* 58(1):29–54.

Fine, Michelle, and Sara McClelland. 2006. "Sexuality Education and Desire: Still Missing after All These Years." *Harvard Educational Review* 76(3):297–338.

Finer, Lawrence B., and Mia R. Zolna. 2011. "Unintended Pregnancy in the United States: Incidence and Disparities, 2006." *Contraception* 84(5):478–85.

Ford, Kathleen, Woosung Sohn, and James Lepkowski. 2001. "Characteristics of Adolescents' Sexual Partners and Their Association with Use of Condoms and Other Contraceptive Methods." *Family Planning Perspectives* 33(3):100–105, 132.

Forhan, Sara E., Sami L. Gottlieb, Maya R. Sternberg, Fujie Xu, S. Deblina Datta, Geraldine M. McQuillan, Stuart M. Berman, and Lauri E. Markowitz. 2009. "Prevalence of Sexually Transmitted Infections among Female Adolescents Aged 14 to 19 in the United States." *Pediatrics* 124(6):1505–12.

Forward, Sonja E. 2009. "The Theory of Planned Behaviour: The Role of Descriptive Norms and Past Behaviour in the Prediction of Drivers' Intentions to Violate." *Transportation Research Part F: Traffic Psychology and Behaviour* 12(3):198–207.

Foucault, Michel. 1977. *Discipline and Punish: The Birth of the Prison*. New York: Vintage Books.

Foucault, Michel, translated from the French by Robert Hurley. 1978, 1990. *The History of Sexuality. Volume 1: An Introduction*. New York: Vintage Books.

Furstenberg, Frank F., Jr. 2003. "Teenage Childbearing as a Public Issue and Private Concern." *Annual Review of Sociology* 29:23–39.

Furstenberg, Frank F, Jr. 2007. *Destinies of the Disadvantaged: The Politics of Teenage Childbearing*. New York: Russell Sage Foundation.

Gallup. "Gay and Lesbian Rights." Retrieved from: http://www.gallup.com/poll/1651/gay-lesbian-rights.aspx.

García, Lorena. 2009. "'Now Why Do You Want to Know about That?' Heteronormativity, Sexism, and Racism in the Sexual (Mis)Education of Latina Youth." *Gender & Society* 23(4):520–41.

García, Lorena. 2012. *Respect Yourself, Protect Yourself: Latina Girls and Sexual Identity*. New York: New York University.

Geronimus, Arline T. 2003. "Damned If You Do: Culture, Identity, Privilege, and Teenage Childbearing in the United States." *Social Science & Medicine* 57(5):881–93.

Giordano, Peggy C. 1983. "Sanctioning the High-Status Deviant: An Attributional Analysis." *Social Psychology Quarterly* 46(4):329–42.

Glass, Jennifer, and Philip Levchak. 2014. "Red States, Blue States, and Divorce: Understanding the Impact of Conservative Protestantism on Regional Variation in Divorce Rates." *American Journal of Sociology* 119(4):1002–46.

Goffman, Erving. 2009. *Stigma: Notes on the Management of Spoiled Identity*. New York: Simon and Schuster.

Gold, Rachel, Ichiro Kawachi, Bruce P. Kennedy, John W. Lynch, and Frederick A. Connell. 2001. "Ecological Analysis of Teen Birth Rates: Association with Community Income and Income Inequality." *Maternal and Child Health Journal* 5(3):161–67.

Graham, Cynthia A., Joseph A. Catania, Richard Brand, Tu Duong, and Jesse A. Canchola. 2003. "Recalling Sexual Behavior: A Methodological Analysis of Memory Recall Bias Via Interview Using the Diary as the Gold Standard." *Journal of Sex Research* 40(4):325–32.

Gregson, Joanna. 2009. *The Culture of Teenage Mothers*. Albany: SUNY.

Guttmacher Institute. 2011. "States Enact Record Number of Abortion Restrictions in First Half of 2011." Retrieved from: http://www.guttmacher.org/media/inthenews/2011/07/13/index.html.

Guttmacher, Sally, Lisa Lieberman, David Ward, Nick Freudenberg, Alice Radosh, and Don Des Jarlais. 1997. "Condom Availability in New York City Public High Schools: Relationships to Condom Use and Sexual Behavior." *American Journal of Public Health* 87(9):1427–33.

Haidt, Jonathan. 2003. "The Moral Emotions." *Handbook of Affective Sciences* 11:852–70.

Hamilton, Brady E., Joyce A. Martin, Michelle J. K. Osterman, Sally C. Curtin, and T. J. Mathews. 2015. "Births: Final Data for 2014." *National Vital Statistics Reports* 64(12). Retrieved from: http://www.cdc.gov/nchs/data/nvsr/nvsr64/nvsr64_12.pdf.

Hamilton, Laura, and Elizabeth A. Armstrong. 2009. "Gendered Sexuality in Young Adulthood: Double Binds and Flawed Options." *Gender & Society* 23(5):589–616.

Harding, David J. 2007. "Cultural Context, Sexual Behavior, and Romantic Relationships in Disadvantaged Neighborhoods." *American Sociological Review* 72(3):341–64.

Harding, David J. 2011. "Rethinking the Cultural Context of Schooling Decisions in Disadvantaged Neighborhoods: From Deviant Subculture to Cultural Heterogeneity." *Sociology of Education* 84(4):322–39.

Hardy, Janet B., and Laurie Schwab Zabin. 1991. *Adolescent Pregnancy in an Urban Environment: Issues, Programs, and Evaluation*. Baltimore: Urban & Schwartzenberg.

Hayford, Sarah R., Karen Benjamin Guzzo, Yasamin Kusunoki, and Jennifer S. Barber. 2016. "Perceived Costs and Benefits of Early Childbearing: New Dimensions and Predictive Power." *Perspectives on Sexual and Reproductive Health* 48(2):83–91.

Hechter, Michael, and Karl-Dieter Opp, eds. 2001a. *Social Norms*. New York: Russell Sage Foundation.

Hechter, Michael, and Karl-Dieter Opp. 2001b. "What Have We Learned about the Emergence of Social Norms?" Pp. 394–415 in *Social Norms*, edited by M. Hechter and K.-D. Opp. New York: Russell Sage Foundation.

Hechter, Michael, and Karl-Dieter Opp. 2001c. "Introduction." Pp. xi–xx in *Social Norms*, edited by M. Hechter and K.-D. Opp. New York: Russell Sage Foundation.

Heise, David R., and Cassandra Calhan. 1995. "Emotion Norms in Interpersonal Events." *Social Psychology Quarterly* 58(4):223–40.

Henly, Julia R. 1997. "The Complexity of Support: The Impact of Family Structure and Provisional Support on African American and White Adolescent Mothers' Well-Being." *American Journal of Community Psychology* 25(5):629–55.

Hitlin, Steven, and Monica Kirkpatrick Johnson. 2015. "Reconceptualizing Agency within the Life Course: The Power of Looking Ahead." *American Journal of Sociology* 120(5):1429–72.

Hochschild, Arlie Russell. 1979. "Emotion Work, Feeling Rules, and Social Structure." *American Journal of Sociology* 85(3):551–75.

Hochschild, Arlie Russell. 2003. *The Managed Heart: Commercialization of Human Feeling, with a New Afterword*. Oakland: University of California.

Hoffman, Saul D. 1998. "Teenage Childbearing Is Not So Bad after All. Or Is It? A Review of the New Literature." *Family Planning Perspectives* 30(5):236–39, 43.

Hoffman, Saul D. 2008. "Trends in Fertility and Sexual Activity among U.S. Teenagers." Pp. 25–49 in *Kids Having Kids: Economic Costs & Social Consequences of Teen Pregnancy*, edited by S. D. Hoffman and R. A. Maynard. Washington, D.C.: Urban Institute.

Hollingshead, August B. 1949. *Elmstown's Youth: The Impact of Social Classes on Adolescents*. New York: Wiley & Sons.

Horne, Christine. 2001a. "Sex and Sanctioning: Evaluating Two Theories of Norm Emergence." Pp. 305–24 in *Social Norms*, edited by M. Hechter and K.-D. Opp. New York: Russell Sage Foundation.

Horne, Christine. 2001b. "The Enforcement of Norms: Group Cohesion and Meta-Norms." *Social Psychology Quarterly* 64(3):253–66.

Horne, Christine. 2001c. "Sociological Perspectives on the Emergence of Social Norms." Pp. 3–34 in *Social Norms*, edited by M. Hechter and K.-D. Opp. New York: Russell Sage Foundation.

Horne, Christine. 2009. *The Rewards of Punishment: A Relational Theory of Norm Enforcement.* Stanford, CA: Stanford University.

Horne, Christine, Brice Darras, Elyse Bean, Anurag Srivastava, and Scott Frickel. 2015. "Privacy, Technology, and Norms: The Case of Smart Meters." *Social Science Research* 51:64–76.

Horne, Christine, F. Nii-Amoo Dodoo, and Naa Dodua Dodoo. 2013. "The Shadow of Indebtedness: Bridewealth and Norms Constraining Female Reproductive Autonomy." *American Sociological Review* 78(3):503–20.

Horowitz, Ruth. 1995. *Teen Mothers: Citizens or Dependents?* Chicago: University of Chicago.

House Bill 07-1292. State of Colorado. "A Bill for an Act Concerning the Adoption of Science-Based Content Standards for Instruction Regarding Human Sexuality." Retrieved from: http://www.leg.state.co.us/clics/clics2007a/csl.nsf/fsbillcont/8BE351914A5391DD8725726400804B00?Open&file=1292_ren.pdf.

Hout, Michael. 2012. "Social and Economic Returns to College Education in the United States." *Annual Review of Sociology* 38:379–400.

Hussey, Jon M., Jen Jen Chang, and Jonathan B. Kotch. 2006. "Child Maltreatment in the United States: Prevalence, Risk Factors, and Adolescent Health Consequences." *Pediatrics* 118(3):933–42.

Idler, Ellen L., and Yael Benyamini. 1997. "Self-Rated Health and Mortality: A Review of Twenty-Seven Community Studies." *Journal of Health and Social Behavior* 38(1):21–37.

Ingraham, Chrys, ed. 2005. *Thinking Straight: The Power, the Promise, and the Paradox of Heterosexuality*. New York and London: Psychology.

Irvine, Janice M. 2004. *Talk about Sex: The Battles over Sex Education in the United States.* Oakland: University of California.

Jacobs, Janet L. 1994. "Gender, Race, Class, and the Trend toward Early Motherhood: A Feminist Analysis of Teen Mothers in Contemporary Society." *Journal of Contemporary Ethnography* 22(4):442–62.

Jacobs, Janet, and Stefanie Mollborn. 2012. "Early Motherhood and the Disruption in Significant Attachments: Autonomy and Reconnection as a Response to Separation and Loss among African American and Latina Teen Mothers." *Gender & Society* 26(6):922–44.

Jerolmack, Colin and Shamus Khan. 2014. "Talk Is Cheap: Ethnography and the Attitudinal Fallacy." *Sociological Methods & Research* 43(2):178–209.

Jessor, Richard. 1987. "Problem-Behavior Theory, Psychosocial Development, and Adolescent Problem Drinking." *British Journal of Addiction* 82(4):331–42.

Johnson, Monica Kirkpatrick, Justin Allen Berg, and Toni Sirotzki. 2007. "Differentiation in Self-Perceived Adulthood: Extending the Confluence Model of Subjective Age Identity." *Social Psychology Quarterly* 70(3):243–61.

Johnson, Monica Kirkpatrick, and Stefanie Mollborn. 2009. "Growing up Faster, Feeling Older: Hardship in Childhood and Adolescence." *Social Psychology Quarterly* 72(1):39–60.

Johnson-Hanks, Jennifer A., Christine A. Bachrach, S. Philip Morgan, and Hans-Peter Kohler. 2011. *Understanding Family Change and Variation: Toward a Theory of Conjunctural Action.* Dordrecht: Springer.

Jones, Rachel K., and Joerg Dreweke. 2011. "Countering Conventional Wisdom: New Evidence on Religion and Contraceptive Use." New York: Guttmacher Institute. Retrieved from: http://www.guttmacher.org/pubs/Religion-and-Contraceptive-Use.pdf.

Jones, Rachel K., and Kathryn Kooistra. 2011. "Abortion Incidence and Access to Services in the United States, 2008." *Perspectives on Sexual and Reproductive Health* 43(1):41–50.

Jones, Rachel K., Mia R. S. Zolna, Stanley K. Henshaw, and Lawrence B. Finer. 2008. "Abortion in the United States: Incidence and Access to Services, 2005." *Perspectives on Sexual and Reproductive Health* 40(1):6–16.

Kane, Jennifer B., S. Philip Morgan, Kathleen Mullan Harris, and David K. Guilkey. 2013. "The Educational Consequences of Teen Childbearing." *Demography* 50(6):2129–50.

Kaplan, Elaine Bell. 1997. *Not Our Kind of Girl: Unraveling the Myths of Black Teenage Motherhood.* Berkeley: University of California.

Kearney, Melissa S., and Phillip B. Levine. 2015. "Media Influences on Social Outcomes: The Impact of MTV's *16 and Pregnant* on Teen Childbearing." *American Economic Review* 105(12): 3597–632.

Keltner, Dacher, and Brenda N. Buswell. 1997. "Embarrassment: Its Distinct Form and Appeasement Functions." *Psychological Bulletin* 122(3):250–70.

Kingsbury, Kathleen. 2008. "Pregnancy Boom at Gloucester High." *Time.* Retrieved from: http://content.time.com/time/magazine/article/0,9171,1816486,00.html.

Kirby, Douglas. 2002. "The Impact of Schools and School Programs upon Adolescent Sexual Behavior." *Journal of Sex Research* 39(1):27–33.

Klockars, Carl B. 1974. *The Professional Fence.* New York: Free.

Kocher, Martin, Peter Martinsson, and Martine Visser. 2012. "Social Background, Cooperative Behavior, and Norm Enforcement." *Journal of Economic Behavior & Organization* 81(2):341–54.

Koffman, Ofra. 2012. "Children Having Children? Religion, Psychology and the Birth of the Teenage Pregnancy Problem." *History of the Human Sciences* 25(1):119–34.

Kosciw, Joseph G., Emily A. Greytak, and Elizabeth M. Diaz. 2009. "Who, What, Where, When, and Why: Demographic and Ecological Factors Contributing to Hostile School Climate for Lesbian, Gay, Bisexual, and Transgender Youth." *Journal of Youth and Adolescence* 38(7):976–88.

Kost, Kathryn, and Isaac Maddow-Zimet. 2016. "US Teenage Pregnancies, Births and Abortions, 2011: National and State Trends by Age, Race and Ethnicity." Retrieved from: https://www.guttmacher.org/sites/default/files/report_pdf/us-teen-pregnancy-trends-2011_0.pdf.

Kost, Kathryn, Susheela Singh, Barbara Vaughan, James Trussell, and Akinrinola Bankole. 2008. "Estimates of Contraceptive Failure from the 2002 National Survey of Family Growth." *Contraception* 77(1):10–21.

Koudenburg, Namkje, Tom Postmes, and Ernestine H. Gordijn. 2013. "Resounding Silences: Subtle Norm Regulation in Everyday Interactions." *Social Psychology Quarterly* 76(3):224–41.

Kreager, Derek A., and Jeremy Staff. 2009. "The Sexual Double Standard and Adolescent Peer Acceptance." *Social Psychology Quarterly* 72(2):143–64.

Ladner, Joyce A., and Ruby Morton Gourdine. 1984. "Intergenerational Teenage Motherhood: Some Preliminary Findings." *SAGE: A Scholarly Journal on Black Women* 1(2):22–24.

Lamont, Michèle, and Virág Molnár. 2002. "The Study of Boundaries in the Social Sciences." *Annual Review of Sociology* 28:167–95.

Lamont, Michèle, and Ann Swidler. 2014. "Methodological Pluralism and the Possibilities and Limits of Interviewing." *Qualitative Sociology* 37(2):153–71.

Lareau, Annette. 2011. *Unequal Childhoods: Class, Race, and Family Life*. Oakland: University of California.

LeMoyne, Terri, and Tom Buchanan. 2011. "Does "Hovering" Matter? Helicopter Parenting and Its Effect on Well-Being." *Sociological Spectrum* 31(4):399–418.

Lerner, Melvin J. 2003. "The Justice Motive: Where Social Psychologists Found It, How They Lost It, and Why They May Not Find It Again." *Personality and Social Psychology Review* 7(4):388–99.

Levine, David I., and Gary Painter. 2003. "The Schooling Costs of Teenage Out-of-Wedlock Childbearing: Analysis with a Within-School Propensity-Score-Matching Estimator." *Review of Economics and Statistics* 85(4):884–900.

Lindley, Lisa L., and Katrina M. Walsemann. 2015. "Sexual Orientation and Risk of Pregnancy among New York City High-School Students." *American Journal of Public Health* 105(7):1379–86.

Link, Bruce G., and Jo Phelan. 2014. "Stigma Power." *Social Science & Medicine* 103:24–32.

Liptak, Adam. 2014. "Supreme Court Rejects Contraceptives Mandate for Some Corporations." *New York Times*. Retrieved from: http://www.nytimes.com/2014/07/01/us/hobby-lobby-case-supreme-court-contraception.html?_r=1.

Lorin, Janet. 2014. "College Tuition in the U.S. Again Rises Faster Than Inflation." BloombergBusiness. Retrieved from: http://www.bloomberg.com/news/articles/2014-11-13/college-tuition-in-the-u-s-again-rises-faster-than-inflation.

Lott, Albert J., and Bernice E. Lott. 1961. "Group Cohesiveness, Communication Level, and Conformity." *Journal of Abnormal and Social Psychology* 62(2):408–12.

Luker, Kristin. 1996. *Dubious Conceptions: The Politics of Teenage Pregnancy*. Cambridge, MA: Harvard University.

Luker, Kristin. 2006. *When Sex Goes to School: Warring Views on Sex—and Sex Education—since the Sixties*. New York: W. W. Norton & Co.

Macvarish, Jan. 2010a. "The Effect of 'Risk-Thinking' on the Contemporary Construction of Teenage Motherhood." *Health Risk & Society* 12(4):313–22.

Macvarish, Jan. 2010b. "Understanding the Significance of the Teenage Mother in Contemporary Parenting Culture." *Sociological Research Online* 15(4):1–7.

Macy, Michael W. 1991. "Chains of Cooperation: Threshold Effects in Collective Action." *American Sociological Review* 56(6):730–47.

Mann, Emily S. 2013. "Regulating Latina Youth Sexualities through Community Health Centers: Discourses and Practices of Sexual Citizenship." *Gender & Society* 27(5):681–703.

Marini, Margaret Mooney. 1984. "Age and Sequencing Norms in the Transition to Adulthood." *Social Forces* 63(1):229–44.

Martin, Joyce A., Brady E. Hamilton, Michelle J. K. Osterman, Sally C. Curtin, and T. J. Mathews. 2013. "Births: Final Data for 2012." *National Vital Statistics Reports* 62(9). Retrieved from http://www.cdc.gov/nchs/data/nvsr/nvsr62/nvsr62_09.pdf.

Martin, Joyce A., Brady E. Hamilton, Michelle J. K. Osterman, Sally C. Curtin, and T. J. Matthews. 2015. "Births: Final Data for 2013." *National Vital Statistics Reports* 64(1). Hyattsville, MD: National Center for Health Statistics. Retrieved from: http://www.cdc.gov/nchs/data/nvsr/nvsr64/nvsr64_01.pdf.

Martin, Joyce A., Brady E. Hamilton, Paul D. Sutton, Stephanie J. Ventura, Fay Menacker, S. Kimeyer, and M. S. Mathews. 2009. "Births: Final Data for 2006." *National Vital Statistics Reports* 57(7). Retrieved from: http://www.cdc.gov/nchs/data/nvsr/nvsr57/nvsr57_07.pdf.

Martin, Joyce A., Brady E. Hamilton, Stephanie J. Ventura, Michelle J. K. Osterman, Sharon Kirmeyer, T. J. Mathews, and Elizabeth C. Wilson. 2011. "Births: Final Data for 2009." *National Vital Statistics Reports* 60(1). Retrieved from: http://www.cdc.gov/nchs/data/nvsr/nvsr60/nvsr60_01.pdf.

Martin, Karin A. 1996. *Puberty, Sexuality, and the Self: Boys and Girls at Adolescence*. New York and London: Psychology.

Martinez, Gladys, Joyce Abma, and Casey Copen. 2010. "Educating Teenagers about Sex in the United States." National Center for Health Statistics Data Brief 44. Retrieved from: https://www.cdc.gov/nchs/data/databriefs/db44.pdf.

McCormack, Karen. 2005. "Stratified Reproduction and Poor Women's Resistance." *Gender & Society* 19(5):660–79.

Mead, Erin L., Rajiv N. Rimal, Roberta Ferrence, and Joanna E. Cohen. 2014. "Understanding the Sources of Normative Influence on Behavior: The Example of Tobacco." *Social Science & Medicine* 115:139–43.

Mercken, Liesbeth, Tom A.B. Snijders, Christian Steglich, Erkki Vartiainen, and Hein De Vries. 2010. "Dynamics of Adolescent Friendship Networks and Smoking Behavior." *Social Networks* 32(1):72–81.

Merton, Robert King. 1968. *Social Theory and Social Structure*. New York: Free.

Milbank, Dana. 2014. "Americans' Optimism Is Dying." *Washington Post*. Retrieved from: http://www.washingtonpost.com/opinions/dana-milbank-americans-optimism-is-dying/2014/08/12/f81808d8-224c-11e4-8593-da634b334390_story.html.

Milgram, Stanley. 1965. "Some Conditions of Obedience and Disobedience to Authority." *Human Relations* 18(1):57–76.

Miller, Dale T. 1999. "The Norm of Self-Interest." *American Psychologist* 54(12):1053.

Mills, C. Wright. 1940. "Situated Actions and Vocabularies of Motive." *American Sociological Review* 5(6):904–13.

Mojola, Sanyu A., and Bethany G. Everett. 2012. "STD and HIV Risk Factors among U.S. Young Adults: Variations by Gender, Race, Ethnicity and Sexual Orientation." *Perspectives on Sexual and Reproductive Health* 44(2):125–33.

Mollborn, Stefanie. 2007. "Making the Best of a Bad Situation: Material Resources and Teenage Parenthood." *Journal of Marriage and Family* 69(1):92–104.

Mollborn, Stefanie. 2009. "Norms about Nonmarital Pregnancy and Willingness to Provide Resources to Unwed Parents." *Journal of Marriage and Family* 71(1):122–34.

Mollborn, Stefanie. 2010a. "Exploring Variation in Teenage Mothers' and Fathers' Educational Attainment." *Perspectives on Sexual and Reproductive Health* 42(3):152–59.

Mollborn, Stefanie. 2010b. "Predictors and Consequences of Adolescents' Norms against Teenage Pregnancy." *Sociological Quarterly* 51(2):303–28.

Mollborn, Stefanie. 2011. "'Children' Having Children." *Contexts* 10(1):32–7.

Mollborn, Stefanie. 2015. "Mixed Messages about Teen Sex." *Contexts* 14(1):44–9.

Mollborn, Stefanie. In press. "Teenage Mothers Today: What We Know and How It Matters." *Child Development Perspectives*.

Mollborn, Stefanie, and Jeff A. Dennis. 2012a. "Investigating the Life Situations and Development of Teenage Mothers' Children: Evidence from the ECLS-B." *Population Research and Policy Review* 31(1):31–66.

Mollborn, Stefanie, and Jeff A. Dennis. 2012b. "Explaining the Early Development and Health of Teen Mothers' Children." *Sociological Forum* 27(4):1010–36.

Mollborn, Stefanie, Benjamin W. Domingue, and Jason D. Boardman. 2014a. "Understanding Multiple Levels of Norms about Teen Pregnancy and Their Relationships to Teens' Sexual Behaviors." *Advances in Life Course Research* 20:1–15.

Mollborn, Stefanie, Benjamin W. Domingue, and Jason D. Boardman. 2014b. "Norms as Group-Level Constructs: Investigating School-Level Teen Pregnancy Norms and Behaviors." *Social Forces* 93(1):241–67.

Mollborn, Stefanie, and Bethany Everett. 2010. "Correlates and Consequences of Parent-Teen Incongruence in Reports of Teens' Sexual Experience." *Journal of Sex Research* 47(4):314–29.

Mollborn, Stefanie, and Bethany Everett. 2015. "Understanding the Educational Attainment of Sexual Minority Women and Men." *Research in Social Stratification and Mobility* 41:50–5.

Mollborn, Stefanie, and Janet Jacobs. 2012. "'We'll Figure a Way': Teenage Mothers' Experiences in Shifting Social and Economic Contexts." *Qualitative Sociology* 35(1):23–46.

Mollborn, Stefanie, and Janet Jacobs. 2015. "'I'll Be There for You': Teen Parents' Coparenting Relationships." *Journal of Marriage and Family* 77(2):373–87.

Mollborn, Stefanie, and Christie Sennott. 2015. "Bundles of Norms about Teen Sex and Pregnancy." *Qualitative Health Research* 25(9):1283–99.

Montemurro, Beth. 2014. *Deserving Desire: Women's Stories of Sexual Evolution.* New Brunswick, NJ: Rutgers University.

Moody, James. 2001. "Race, School Integration, and Friendship Segregation in America." *American Journal of Sociology* 107(3):679–716.

Myers, Kristen A., and Passion Williamson. 2001. "Race Talk: The Perpetuation of Racism through Private Discourse." *Race and Society* 4(1):3–26.

Nack, Adina. 2009. *Damaged Goods? Women Living with Incurable Sexually Transmitted Diseases.* Philadelphia: Temple University.

Nathanson, Constance A. 1991. *Dangerous Passage: The Social Control of Sexuality in Women's Adolescence.* Philadelphia: Temple University.

National Campaign to Prevent Teen and Unplanned Pregnancy. 2014. "President Obama Releases Fiscal Year 2015 Budget Request: A Statement from the National Campaign to Prevent Teen and Unplanned Pregnancy." March 5, 2014. Retrieved from: https://thenationalcampaign.org/press-release/president-obama-releases-fiscal-year-2015-budget-request.

National Conference of State Legislatures. 2016. "State Policies on Sex Education in Schools." Retrieved from: http://www.ncsl.org/research/health/state-policies-on-sex-education-in-schools.aspx.

National Women's Law Center. 2011. "Justice for Pregnant and Parenting Students in Michigan." Retrieved from: http://www.nwlc.org/our-blog/justice-pregnant-and-parenting-students-michigan.

Neugarten, Bernice L., Joan W. Moore, and John C. Lowe. 1965. "Age Norms, Age Constraints, and Adult Socialization." *American Journal of Sociology* 70(6):710–17.

Newhart, Michelle Renee. 2013. "From 'Getting High" to "Getting Well': Medical Cannabis Use among Midlife Patients in Colorado." Ph.D. dissertation, Department of Sociology, University of Colorado at Boulder, Boulder, CO.

Nunner-Winkler, Gertrud, and Beate Sodian. 1988. "Children's Understanding of Moral Emotions." *Child Development* 59(5):1323–38.

Nye, Joseph S. 1990. "Soft Power." *Foreign Policy* 80:153–71.

Office of Adolescent Health. 2014. "U.S. Adolescent Reproductive Health Facts." Retrieved from: http://www.hhs.gov/ash/oah/adolescent-health-topics/reproductive-health/states/pdfs/us.pdf.

Ohbuchi, Ken-Ichi, Toru Tamura, Brian M. Quigley, James T. Tedeschi, Nawaf Madi, Michael H. Bond, and Amelie Mummendey. 2004. "Anger, Blame, and Dimensions of Perceived Norm Violations: Culture, Gender, and Relationships." *Journal of Applied Social Psychology* 34(8):1587–603.

Ostrom, Elinor. 2014. "Collective Action and the Evolution of Social Norms." *Journal of Natural Resources Policy Research* 6(4):235–52.

Ostrove, Joan M., Nancy E. Adler, Miriam Kuppermann, and A. Eugene Washington. 2000. "Objective and Subjective Assessments of Socioeconomic Status and Their Relationship to Self-Rated Health in an Ethnically Diverse Sample of Pregnant Women." *Health Psychology* 19(6):613–18.

Paluck, Elizabeth Levy, and Hana Shepherd. 2012. "The Salience of Social Referents: A Field Experiment on Collective Norms and Harassment Behavior in a School Social Network." *Journal of Personality and Social Psychology* 103(6):899–915.

Pascoe, C. J. 2007. *Dude, You're a Fag: Masculinity and Sexuality in High School.* Berkeley: University of California.

Pavalko, Eliza K., and Jennifer Caputo. 2013. "Social Inequality and Health across the Life Course." *American Behavioral Scientist* 57(8):1040–56.

Pearson, Jennifer, Chandra Muller, and Lindsey Wilkinson. 2007. "Adolescent Same-Sex Attraction and Academic Outcomes: The Role of School Attachment and Engagement." *Social Problems* 54(4):523–42.

Peers Building Justice. "Askable Adult Workshop." Retrieved from: http://www.peersbuildingjustice.com/askable-adult-workshop/.

Penman-Aguilar, Ana, Marion Carter, M. Christine Snead, and Athena P. Kourtis. 2013. "Socioeconomic Disadvantage as a Social Determinant of Teen Childbearing in the US." *Public Health Reports* 128(Suppl 1):5.

Perper, Kate, and Jennifer Manlove. 2009. *Estimated Percentage of Females Who Will Become Teen Mothers: Differences across States*, Vol. 2009. Washington, D.C.: Child Trends. Retrieved from: http://www.childtrends.org/?publications=estimated-percentage-of-females-who-will-become-teen-mothers.

Pew Research Center. 2014. "Political Polarization in the American Public: How Increasing Ideological Uniformity and Partisan Antipathy Affect Politics, Compromise and Everyday Life." Pew Research Center. Retrieved from: http://www.people-press.org/2014/06/12/political-polarization-in-the-american-public/.

Phillip, Abby. 2013. "Obama Backs 'Plan B' Pill for Teen Girls." ABC News. Retrieved from: http://abcnews.go.com/blogs/politics/2013/05/obama-backs-plan-b-pill-for-teen-girls/.

Pilkington, Ed. 2008. "17 Pregnancies at US School after Girls Make Baby Pact." *Guardian*. Retrieved from: http://www.theguardian.com/world/2008/jun/21/usa.

Pugh, Allison J. 2013. "What Good Are Interviews for Thinking about Culture? Demystifying Interpretive Analysis." *American Journal of Cultural Sociology* 1(1):42–68.

Pugh, Allison J. 2014. "The Theoretical Costs of Ignoring Childhood: Rethinking Independence, Insecurity, and Inequality." *Theory and Society* 43(1):71–89.

Quadrel, Marilyn J., Baruch Fischhoff, and Wendy Davis. 1993. "Adolescent (In)Vulnerability." *American Psychologist* 48(2):102.

Rees, Carter, and Danielle Wallace. 2014. "The Myth of Conformity: Adolescents and Abstention from Unhealthy Drinking Behaviors." *Social Science & Medicine* 108:34–45.

Regnerus, Mark D. 2007. *Forbidden Fruit: Sex & Religion in the Lives of American Teenagers.* Oxford: Oxford University.

Reichard, Raquel. 2014. "8 Lies We Need to Stop Spreading about Teenage Motherhood." Retrieved from: http://everydayfeminism.com/2014/07/8-lies-about-teenage-motherhood/.

Reichertz, Jo. 2007. *Abduction: The Logic of Discovery of Grounded Theory.* Thousand Oaks, CA: Sage.

Ricketts, Sue, Greta Klingler, and Renee Schwalberg. 2014. "Game Change in Colorado: Widespread Use of Long-Acting Reversible Contraceptives and Rapid Decline in Births among Young, Low-Income Women." *Perspectives on Sexual and Reproductive Health* 46(3):125–32.

Rimal, Rajiv N., and Kevin Real. 2005. "How Behaviors Are Influenced by Perceived Norms: A Test of the Theory of Normative Social Behavior." *Communication Research* 32(3):389–414.

Risman, Barbara, and Pepper Schwartz. 2002. "After the Sexual Revolution: Gender Politics in Teen Dating." *Contexts* 1(1):16–24.

Rivers, Ian. 2001. "The Bullying of Sexual Minorities at School: Its Nature and Long-Term Correlates." *Educational and Child Psychology* 18(1):32–46.

Roper Center. 2003. "Focus on the Family Sex Education Survey, Dec. 2003." Retrieved Aug. 28, 2014, from the iPOLL Databank, The Roper Center for Public Opinion Research, University of Connecticut. Retrieved from: http://o-www.ropercenter.uconn.edu.libraries.colorado.edu/data_access/ipoll/ipoll.html.

Roper Center. 2007. "Associated Press/IPSOS-Public Affairs Poll, Oct. 2007." Retrieved Aug. 28, 2014, from the iPOLL Databank, The Roper Center for Public Opinion Research, University of Connecticut. Retrieved from: http://o-www.ropercenter.uconn.edu.libraries.colorado.edu/data_access/ipoll/ipoll.html.

Roscigno, Vincent J. 2011. "Power, Revisited." *Social Forces* 90(2):349–74.

Rosenfeld, Michael J. 2009, 2007. *The Age of Independence: Interracial Unions, Same-Sex Unions, and the Changing American Family.* Cambridge, MA: Harvard University.

Russell, Stephen T., Hinda Seif, and Nhan L. Truong. 2001. "School Outcomes of Sexual Minority Youth in the United States: Evidence from a National Study." *Journal of Adolescence* 24(1):111–27.

Sampson, Robert J. 1997. "Collective Regulation of Adolescent Misbehavior: Validation Results from Eighty Chicago Neighborhoods." *Journal of Adolescent Research* 12(2):227–44.

Sampson, Robert J., Jeffrey D. Morenoff, and Thomas Gannon-Rowley. 2002. "Assessing 'Neighborhood Effects': Social Processes and New Directions in Research." *Annual Review of Sociology* 28:443–78.

Santa Maria, Diane, Christine Markham, Shirley Bluethmann, and Patricia Dolan Mullen. 2015. "Parent-Based Adolescent Sexual Health Interventions and Effect on Communication Outcomes: A Systematic Review and Meta-Analyses." *Perspectives on Sexual and Reproductive Health* 47(1):37–50.

Schalet, Amy T. 2011. *Not under My Roof: Parents, Teens, and the Culture of Sex.* Chicago: University of Chicago.

Schneider, Barbara, and David Stevenson. 2000. *The Ambitious Generation: America's Teenagers, Motivated but Directionless.* New Haven, CT: Yale University.

Schwalbe, Michael, Sandra Godwin, Daphe Holden, Douglas Schrock, Shealy Thompson, and Michele Wolkomir. 2000. "Generic Processes in the Reproduction of Inequality: An Interactionist Analysis." *Social Forces* 79(2):419–52.

Schwartz, Shalom H., and Judith A. Howard. 1980. "Explanations of the Moderating Effect of Responsibility Denial on the Personal Norm-Behavior Relationship." *Social Psychology Quarterly* 43(4):441–46.

Science and Integrity Survey. 2004. iPOLL Databank, The Roper Center for Public Opinion Research, University of Connecticut.

Scott, Marvin B., and Stanford M. Lyman. 1968. "Accounts." *American Sociological Review* 33(1):46–62.

Sennott, Christie, and Stefanie Mollborn. 2011. "College-Bound Teens' Decisions about the Transition to Sex: Negotiating Competing Norms." *Advances in Life Course Research* 16(2):83–97.

Settersten, Richard A., Jr. 2004. "Age Structuring and the Rhythm of the Life Course." Pp. 81–98 in *Handbook of the Life Course*, edited by J. T. Mortimer and M. J. Shanahan. New York: Kluwer Academic/Plenum.

Sex Education in America Survey. 2003. iPOLL Databank, The Roper Center for Public Opinion Research, University of Connecticut.

Shanahan, Michael J. 2000. "Pathways to Adulthood in Changing Societies: Variability and Mechanisms in Life Course Perspective." *Annual Review of Sociology* 26:667–92.

Shannon-Missal, Larry. 2013. "Americans' Belief in God, Miracles and Heaven Declines: Belief in Darwin's Theory of Evolution Rises." New York: The Harris Poll® #97, December 16, 2013. Retrieved from: http://www.theharrispoll.com/health-and-life/Americans__Belief_in_God__Miracles_and_Heaven_Declines.html.

Shigihara, Amanda M. 2013. "It's Only Stealing a Little a Lot: Techniques of Neutralization for Theft among Restaurant Workers." *Deviant Behavior* 34(6):494–512.

Siddiqui, Roomana. 2012. "Antecedent of Reactions to Norm Violation: Intergroup Emotions or Contextual Factors." *International Journal of Psychology* 47:711–12.

Silk, Jessica, and Diana Romero. 2014. "The Role of Parents and Families in Teen Pregnancy Prevention: An Analysis of Programs and Policies." *Journal of Family Issues* 35(10):1339–62.

Simon, Robin W., Donna Eder, and Cathy Evans. 1992. "The Development of Feeling Norms Underlying Romantic Love among Adolescent Females." *Social Psychology Quarterly* 55(1):29–46.

Singh, Susheela, Jacqueline E. Darroch, and Jennifer J. Frost. 2001. "Socioeconomic Disadvantage and Adolescent Women's Sexual and Reproductive Behavior: The Case of Five Developed Countries." *Family Planning Perspectives* 33(6):251–58, 89.

Singh-Manoux, Archana, Michael G. Marmot, and Nancy E. Adler. 2005. "Does Subjective Social Status Predict Health and Change in Health Status Better than Objective Status?" *Psychosomatic Medicine* 67(6):855–61.

Small, Mario Luis. 2009. "'How Many Cases Do I Need?': On Science and the Logic of Case Selection in Field-Based Research." *Ethnography* 10(1):5–38.

Smith, Daniel Scott, and Michael S. Hindus. 1975. "Premarital Pregnancy in America 1640–971: An Overview and Interpretation." *Journal of Interdisciplinary History* 5(4):537–70.

Smith, Whitney, Janet M. Turan, Kari White, Kristi L. Stringer, Anna Helova, Tina Simpson, and Kate Cockrill. 2016. "Social Norms and Stigma Regarding Unintended Pregnancy and Pregnancy Decisions: A Qualitative Study of Young Women in Alabama." *Perspectives on Sexual and Reproductive Health* 48(2):73–81.

SmithBattle, Lee. 2000. "The Vulnerabilities of Teenage Mothers: Challenging Prevailing Assumptions." *Advances in Nursing Science* 23(1):29–40.

Sobotka, Tomáš, Vegard Skirbekk, and Dimiter Philipov. 2011. "Economic Recession and Fertility in the Developed World." *Population and Development Review* 37(2):267–306.

Solebello, Nicholas, and Sinikka Elliott. 2011. "'We Want Them to Be as Heterosexual as Possible': Fathers Talk about Their Teen Children's Sexuality." *Gender & Society* 25(3):293–315.

Solinger, Rickie. 1992. *Wake up Little Susie: Single Pregnancy and Race before Roe v. Wade.* New York: Routledge.

Staller, Alexander, and Paolo Petta. 2001. "Introducing Emotions into the Computational Study of Social Norms: A First Evaluation." *Journal of Artificial Societies and Social Simulation* 4(1). Retrieved from: http://jasss.soc.surrey.ac.uk/4/1/2.html.

Stein, Rob. 2010. "Obama Administration Launches a Sex-Ed Program." *Washington Post.* Retrieved from: http://www.washingtonpost.com/wp-dyn/content/article/2010/10/27/AR2010102707471.html.

Strayhorn, Joseph M., and Jillian C. Strayhorn. 2009. "Religiosity and Teen Birth Rate in the United States." *Reproductive Health* 6:1–7.

Sucoff, Clea A., and Dawn M. Upchurch. 1998. "Neighborhood Context and the Risk of Childbearing among Metropolitan-Area Black Adolescents." *American Sociological Review* 63(4):571–85.

Sutton, Robert I. 1991. "Maintaining Norms about Expressed Emotions: The Case of Bill Collectors." *Administrative Science Quarterly* 36(2):245–68.

Swidler, Ann. 2001. *Talk of Love: How Culture Matters.* Chicago: University of Chicago.

Sykes, Gresham M., and David Matza. 1957. "Techniques of Neutralization: A Theory of Delinquency." *American Sociological Review* 22(6):664–70.

Talbot, Margaret. 2008. "Red Sex, Blue Sex." *The New Yorker* (Nov. 3):64–9.

Tangney, June Price, Jeff Stuewig, and Debra J. Mashek. 2007. "Moral Emotions and Moral Behavior." *Annual Review of Psychology* 58:345–72.

Tarrow, Sidney, and J. Tollefson. 1994. *Power in Movement: Social Movements, Collective Action and Politics.* Cambridge, UK: Cambridge University.

Tavernise, Sabrina. 2015. "Colorado's Effort against Teenage Pregnancies Is a Startling Success." *New York Times.* July 5, 2015. Retrieved from: http://www.nytimes.com/2015/07/06/science/colorados-push-against-teenage-pregnancies-is-a-startling-success.html?_r=0.

Taylor, Julie Lounds. 2009. "Midlife Impacts of Adolescent Parenthood." *Journal of Family Issues* 30(4):484–510.

Taylor, Marylee C. 1995. "White Backlash to Workplace Affirmative Action: Peril or Myth?" *Social Forces* 73(4):1385–414.

Teitler, Julien O., and Christopher C. Weiss. 2000. "Effects of Neighborhood and School Environments on Transitions to First Sexual Intercourse." *Sociology of Education* 73(2):112–32.

Thompson, Sharon. 1996. *Going All the Way: Teenage Girls' Tales of Sex, Romance, and Pregnancy.* New York: Macmillan.

Thorne, Barrie. 1993. *Gender Play: Girls and Boys in School.* New Brunswick, NJ: Rutgers University.

Tinkler, Justine E. 2003. "Defining Sexual Harassment: Ambiguity, Perceived Threat, and Knowledge." *Amici* 10:1–2.

Tinkler, Justine E. 2012. "Resisting the Enforcement of Sexual Harassment Law." *Law & Social Inquiry* 37(1):1–24.

Tinkler, Justine E. 2013. "How Do Sexual Harassment Policies Shape Gender Beliefs? An Exploration of the Moderating Effects of Norm Adherence and Gender." *Social Science Research* 42(5):1269–83.

Tolman, Deborah L. 2009. *Dilemmas of Desire: Teenage Girls Talk about Sexuality*. Cambridge, MA: Harvard University.

Trussell, James. 2004. "Contraceptive Failure in the United States." *Contraception* 70(2):89–96.

Tuggle, Justin L., and Malcolm D. Holmes. 1997. "Blowing Smoke: Status Politics and the Shasta County Smoking Ban." *Deviant Behavior* 18(1):77–93.

Tyrer, Louise. 1999. "Introduction of the Pill and Its Impact." *Contraception* 59(1):11S–16S.

Uecker, Jeremy E, Nicole Angotti, and Mark D Regnerus. 2008. "Going Most of the Way: 'Technical Virginity' among American Adolescents." *Social Science Research* 37(4):1200–15.

Uecker, Jeremy E., and Charles E. Stokes. 2008. "Early Marriage in the United States." *Journal of Marriage and Family* 70(4):835–46.

U.S. Department of Labor. 2015a. "Earnings and Unemployment Rates by Educational Attainment." Washington, D.C.: U.S. Bureau of Labor Statistics, Office of Occupational Statistics and Employment Projections. Retrieved from: http://www.bls.gov/emp/ep_chart_001.htm.

U.S. Department of Labor. 2015b. "Labor Force Statistics from the Current Population Survey." Washington, D.C.: U.S. Bureau of Labor Statistics, Division of Labor Force Statistics. Retrieved from: http://www.bls.gov/web/empsit/cpseea10.htm.

Vaisey, Stephen. 2009. "Motivation and Justification: A Dual-Process Model of Culture in Action." *American Journal of Sociology* 114(6):1675–715.

Vaisey, Stephen. 2010. "What People Want: Rethinking Poverty, Culture, and Educational Attainment." *Annals of the American Academy of Political and Social Science* 629:75–101.

Valocchi, Stephen. "Not Yet Queer Enough: The Lessons of Queer Theory for the Sociology of Gender and Sexuality." *Gender & Society* 19(6):750–70.

van Kleef, Gerben A., Florian Wanders, Eftychia Stamkou, and Astrid C. Homan. 2015. "The Social Dynamics of Breaking the Rules: Antecedents and Consequences of Norm-Violating Behavior." *Current Opinion in Psychology* 6:25–31.

Vasalou, Asimina, Adam Joinson, and Jeremy Pitt. 2006. "The Role of Shame, Guilt and Embarrassment in Online Social Dilemmas." Proceedings of the British HCI Group Conference: 2. London, UK.

Ventura, Stephanie J., T. J. Mathews, and Brady E. Hamilton. 2001. "Births to Teenagers in the United States, 1940–2000." *National Vital Statistics Reports* 49(10):1–23.

Verlee, Megan. 2015. "Senate Committee Rejects Bill to Fund Colorado Contraception Program." Colorado Public Radio. Retrieved from: http://www.cpr.org/news/story/senate-committee-rejects-bill-fund-colorado-contraception-program-sthash.j7VHVeyd.dpuf.

Vinitzky-Seroussi, Vered, and Robert Zussman. 1996. "High School Reunions and the Management of Identity." *Symbolic Interaction* 19(3):225–39.

Vrangalova, Zhana, and Ritch C. Savin-Williams. 2011. "Adolescent Sexuality and Positive Well-Being: A Group-Norms Approach." *Journal of Youth and Adolescence* 40(8):931–44.

Welti, Kate, Elizabeth Wildsmith, and Jennifer Manlove. 2011. "Trends and Recent Estimates: Contraceptive Use among U.S. Teens and Young Adults." Publication #2011-23. Retrieved from: http://www.childtrends.org/Files/Child_Trends-2011_08_01_RB_ContraceptiveUse.pdf.

Wildsmith, Elizabeth, Megan Barry, Jennifer Manlove, and Brigitte Vaughn. 2013. "Adolescent Health Highlight: Teen Pregnancy and Childbearing." Publication #2013-5. Washington, D.C.: Child Trends. Retrieved from: http://www.childtrends.org/wp-content/uploads/2013/11/Pregnancy-and-Childbearing-updated-12-131.pdf.

Wilcox, Allen J., David B. Dunson, Clarice R. Weinberg, James Trussell, and Donna Day Baird. 2001. "Likelihood of Conception with a Single Act of Intercourse: Providing Benchmark Rates for Assessment of Post-Coital Contraceptives." *Contraception* 63(4):211–15.

Wilkins, Amy C. 2008. *Wannabes, Goths, and Christians: The Boundaries of Sex, Style, and Status*. Chicago: University of Chicago.

Wilkins, Amy C. 2014. "Race, Age and Identity Transformations in the Transition from High School to College for Black and First-Generation White Men." *Sociology of Education* 87(3):171–87.

Wilkins, Amy C., and Cristen Dalessandro. 2013. "Monogamy Lite: Cheating, College, and Women." *Gender & Society* 27(5):728–51.

Wilkinson, Lindsey, and Jennifer Pearson. 2009. "School Culture and the Well-Being of Same-Sex-Attracted Youth." *Gender & Society* 23(4):542–68.

Willer, Robb, Ko Kuwabara, and Michael W. Macy. 2009. "The False Enforcement of Unpopular Norms." *American Journal of Sociology* 115(2):451–90.

Wilson, William Julius. 1987. *The Truly Disadvantaged: The Inner City, the Underclass, and Public Policy*. Chicago: University of Chicago.

Windle, Michael. 2003. "Alcohol Use among Adolescents and Young Adults." *Alcohol Research & Health* 27(1):79–85.

Wisnieski, Deborah, Renee Sieving, and Ann Garwick. 2015. "Parent and Family Influences on Young Women's Romantic and Sexual Decisions." *Sex Education* 15(2):144–57.

Wong, James. 1997. "The 'Making' of Teenage Pregnancy." *International Studies in the Philosophy of Science* 11(3):273–88.

Wooten, David B. 2006. "From Labeling Possessions to Possessing Labels: Ridicule and Socialization among Adolescents." *Journal of Consumer Research* 33(2):188–98.

World Bank Group. 2016. "Adolescent Fertility Rate (Births Per 1,000 Women Ages 15–19)." United Nations Population Division, World Population Prospects. Retrieved from: http://data.worldbank.org/indicator/SP.ADO.TFRT.

Xenitidou, Maria, and Bruce Edmonds, eds. 2014. *The Complexity of Social Norms*. Heidelberg: Springer.

Yoshida, Emiko, Jennifer M. Peach, Mark P. Zanna, and Steven J. Spencer. 2012. "Not All Automatic Associations Are Created Equal: How Implicit Normative Evaluations Are Distinct from Implicit Attitudes and Uniquely Predict Meaningful Behavior." *Journal of Experimental Social Psychology* 48(3):694–706.

Index

Made in the USA
Monee, IL
27 January 2021